ASEPTIC PHARMACEUTICAL MANUFACTURING
Technology for the 1990s

Edited by
Wayne P. Olson
Hyland Therapeutics
Division of Travenol Laboratories
Los Angeles, California

Michael J. Groves
College of Pharmacy
University of Illinois at Chicago
Chicago, Illinois

Printing History:
Aseptic Pharmaceutical Manufacturing - First Edition, 1987

© Copyright, July 1987 by Interpharm Press Inc.,
P. O.Box 530,
Prairie View, IL 60069–0530, USA

ISBN: 0-935184-06-6

Aseptic Pharmaceutical Manufacturing Technology for the 1990s

Contents

Preface

The first two Pharmaceutical Technology Conference Symposia on aseptic pharmaceutical processing (1984 and 1985) were chaired by the editors. It became clear during those meetings that existing texts covering aseptic pharmaceutical manufacturing defined "state-of-the-art" as that of a decade earlier. Many technological developments have been implemented since that time, but have not been systematically and adequately described in texts currently available. Thus, form-fill-seal systems has revolutionized sterile pharmaceutical packaging; isolator technology has changed our concepts of clean room design and use; Clean-In-Place and Sterilize-In-Place technology have altered aseptic work methods and significantly improved probabilities of product sterility assurance. The objective of this present book is to provide the reader with a sound background to the theory and practical applications of these and other developments of the late 1970's and 1980's.

It may be anticipated that, in a later edition, the traditional aseptic filling line and control of the microbial and particulate environment will receive more attention. However, as advances continue in form-fill-seal and isolator technologies, problems associated with aseptic filling will diminish, and the failings of the traditional filling lines will become less significant factors in product quality and patient safety.

Another example of an anticipated development has been the use of robots in aseptic pharmaceutical manufacturing and quality control procedures. This area is anticipated to be a key development for the remainder of the present decade, but is only touched in passing in this volume.

The technology associated with aseptic processing is an expanding and developing area. To facilitate development of the subject into the next decade, we hope to have encapsulated current technology in this present text. What the future actually brings may be another matter but we have tried to anticipate new technologies. Time will tell.

Wayne P. Olson and Michael J. Groves
Los Angeles and Chicago, July 1987

Acknowledgments

This text started at the urging of Dr. Michael Faith (Bionetics Research, Chicago) and received very strong support from Steve Holst (Hyland Therapeutics). Many colleagues and friends provided helpful suggestions; among them Frank Inman (Glaxo), Al Bustos (Hyland Therapeutics), and so many others that a comprehensive list would be lengthy indeed. Thank you all.

It is axiomatic that the publication of this text could not have been achieved without the extensive efforts of the contributing authors. Their intimate knowledge of their fields and their willingness to share their experience have made the tasks of the editors easier than is usual with a text of this type. For their patience and dedication to producing a quality manuscript we extend a heartfelt thanks and our gratitude.

Without the considerable editorial efforts of Michael Anisfeld and Joanne Decker, a presentable text would not have been completed and published; again our appreciation.

Wayne P. Olson and Michael J. Groves

Contributing Authors

Dr. Neil R. Anderson
Merrell Dow Research Institute
9550 N. Zionsville Road
Indianapolis, IN 46268, USA

Dr. Henry Bondi
Process Consultant
CN 777
Princeton, NJ 08540, USA

Dr. Michael Groves
UIC – College of Pharmacy
833 South Wood Street
Chicago, IL 60612, USA

Dr. Michael S. Korczynski
Scientific Affairs [AP4A-D488]
Abbott Laboratories
Abbott Park, IL 60064, USA

Frank Leo
Automated Liquid Packaging
2200 West Lakeshore Drive
Woodstock, IL 60098, USA

Patrick Oles
la Calhene
252 Main Street
Goshen, NY 10924, USA

Wayne P. Olson
Hyland Therapeutics
4501 Colorado Blvd.
Los Angeles, CA 90039, USA

Dr. Frederick Pearson
Travenol Laboratories
Wilson Road at Route 120
Round Lake, IL 60073, USA

Gerry Prout
Parenteral Society
6 Frankton Gardens, Stratton
Swindon SN3 4LU, United Kingdom

Dale A. Seiberling
Seiberling Associates, Inc.
11415 Main Street
Roscoe, IL 61073, USA

Douglas Stockdale
American Pharmaseal
27200 N. Tourney Road
Valencia, CA 91355, USA

Dr. Ronald Tetzlaff
Food and Drug Administration
60 Eighth Street, N.E.
Atlanta, GA 30309, USA

Chapter Reviewers

The following colleagues have contributed to this book by performing the essential function of peer review of each chapter.

Of their professional competence, their countless suggestions on enhancing the text, and their freely given time; we express our deepest respect and gratitude.

Dr. James Harris
Glaxo Research
Triangle Park, NC, USA

Dr. Kal Horvath
Cutter Laboratories
Berkely, CA, USA

Dr. Ingelise Kvorning
Novo Industri A/S
Bagsvaerd, Denmark

Dr. Thomas Novitsky
Associates of Cape Cod
Woods Hole, MA, USA

Dr. Theodore Odlaug
Miles Laboratories
Elkhart, IN, USA

Dr. Kai Purohit
Stork-Amsterdam
Amsterdam, Netherlands

Dr. James Ralston
Ivex Pharmaceuticals
Antrim, Ulster, United Kingdom

Paul X. Shaughnessy (retired)
Bristol-Myers
Syracuse, NY, USA

Dr. John Wasynczuk
Pfizer Inc.
Terre Haute, IN, USA

1

Introduction

Michael J. Groves
College of Pharmacy,
University of Illinois at Chicago, IL, USA

1. Introduction

Administration of a medicinal substance or drug to the body by a route that bypasses the defense mechanisms requires that the patient who receives the product is not at any time placed at risk because of an inherent fault or failure in the product. Parenteral drugs are administered directly into the veins, muscles or under the skin, or more specialized tissues such as the spinal cord. That parenteral products must be quality products, is an essential demand. "Quality" defined somewhat loosely as a relative degree of excellence is expressed in quantitative terms, even in some situations as numbers when applied to parenteral products.

This monograph discusses one way in which some types of parenteral products are prepared. Before we advance to the technical aspects of the subject, it is essential that the reader orient him or herself to the key aspect of the subject. The bottom line is that these products bypass the defenses of the body of patients who are already unhealthy in some respect and they must never increase the hazard to which the patients are already exposed.

Attempts to infuse drug solutions into man were made in the 17th century following the discovery of the blood circulation by William Harvey. Routine administration by injections of drugs into sick patients became realistic only after Alexander Wood of Edinburgh invented a graduated glass syringe fitted with a hollow needle in 1853. Successful treatment of dehydrated cholera victims with intravenous saline solutions by Latto dates from about the same period. However, it was not until the turn of the century that injections became common and were included in pharmacopoeial monographs.

The first injections were morphine solutions, followed by vaccines, cocaine and ergot, administered mainly by the intramuscular route. Except for saline, the intravenous route was hardly ever used before the 1900's. Intravenous administration techniques improved so that by the time of the Great War (1914–1918), paraldehyde was used for intravenous anesthesia and experiments

1

were carried out with artificial blood expanders. Intravenous dextrose solutions were used routinely by the mid-1920's and intravenous heparin was introduced in 1930 for anticoagulant therapy. The parenteral therapy of today is based on only a half century of continued and continuous development.

Although "cleanliness" of the injected product was recognized to be an essential requirement from the onset of parenteral therapy, sterility was not required until the 1920's. Initially it was realized that injectable solutions should be sterilized by a heat or chemical treatment to prevent mold growth in the product. It is not certain when the argument was extended to a realization that contaminating microorganisms were hardly desirable from the point of view of the recipient. The pioneering microbiological investigations of Pasteur and Tyndall showed the way in which solutions of drugs could be prepared free from viable microorganisms.

In time, the official monographs specified tests for sterility and provided guidance about methods by which sterilization could be accomplished.

The associated technology has expanded and improved over the years, as has the recognition of the critical nature of injectable products. As we approach the end of this century of technological advancement, we are faced with increasing demands for improved quality in injectable products. Quality considerations demand that not only must solutions injected into the patient be completely free of viable microorganisms but they must also be free of pyrogenic materials and substantially free of inert particulate matter.

Concepts change and, hopefully, improve with time. The earliest "sterile" products were certainly prepared under conditions that would be described as unsatisfactory by the standards of today. In general, the producer relied upon the final heat sterilization process to destroy microorganisms initially present in the product. Samples from the batch of product were tested to see if the sterilization process had been carried out successfully. These tests were insensitive and the occasional contamination detected could often be blamed on the inadequate testing methodology of the time. It became evident that a simple testing procedure at the end of a production process was statistically inadequate to provide assurance that the batch as a whole was sterile. A number of incidents served to emphasize this point when, for various reasons, sterility processes failed and patients died from infected products.

Governmental regulatory authorities such as the Food and Drug Administration in America intervened and demanded that "quality" be built into a product throughout the production process. The net effect of this intervention over a 20 year period has been to heighten awareness of the critical nature of injected products, to improve production facilities to state-of-the-art technology and, inevitably, to cause a significant increase in the cost of these products to the patient.

We have a greater understanding of the processes used to produce sterile materials. However, it is essential that the advantages of this knowledge are not thrown away by ignorance on the part of the user (for whom the product, incidentally, is not intended). Careless manipulation by the pharmacist, technician, physician or nurse can negate a whole technology designed to protect the patient. Continual education and vigilance is required at all levels to ensure that the product given to the patient is not contaminated.

The stated purpose of this monograph is to provide information about the way a product can be produced aseptically and to provide a basis for understanding aseptic manipulative procedures in general.

2. Chemical and Energetic Sterilization of Drug Products

Although this book is not an appropriate place to provide a complete review of methods of sterilization, the "why" of Aseptic Processing is answered by considering what happens to a product or material during a sterilization process.

Most biological materials are inactivated or destroyed by interaction with certain classes of chemical. The earliest of this group was phenol which was demonstrated to sterilize or kill many pathogenic microorganisms. This observation, for example, dramatically improved the success of surgical procedures during the Victorian era but the disadvantages of phenolic materials led to a search for other chemical sterilants. Contact with antibiotics (as a class), heavy metal salts, quaternary ammonium compounds, alcohols and phenols are all used today, as are biocidal gases such as formaldehyde and ethylene oxide. Powerful oxidizing agents such as chromic or nitric acid are also effective sterilants but it is evident that these materials are often toxic to the patient as well as to the microbe. The fact that chemical sterilants are able to destroy living cells irrespective of their origin is a disadvantage when using a product parenterally. Small quantities of phenolic biocidal compounds maybe used in multiple dose products such as vaccines or eyedrops, but generally these materials are too toxic to be used for injections that would result in significant quantities being given to the patient. Some compounds are chemically reactive and interact with the drug entity itself, thereby reducing "activity," however that term is defined in the context of the drug.

Another problem associated with the use of chemical sterilants is the effect of concentration. Microorganisms are often killed outright at a particular concentration of a certain chemical entity. The microorganism is dead by any definition; it has no metabolic processes that are intact and cannot reproduce itself under any conditions. However, at lower concentration, the organism is incapable of reproducing itself but may recover when environmental conditions are improved, for example by dilution, so that the inhibiting chemical concentration is reduced to ineffective levels. This situation may also appear when considering the application of heat. The thermal inactivation may appear to stultify growth for a while, with the net effect that the numbers of microorganisms in a system will not increase under those conditions. It could be argued that this is perhaps satisfactory from the point of view of a parenteral product since inhibition of growth is really all that is required. The numbers of organisms can be reduced by some other means such as filtration. Although only a small number of microorganisms may be introduced into a patient and in principle these could be dealt with by the reticulo-endothelial system, this system is the last line of defense. If the organism were a pathogen such as anthrax, unlikely but conceivably possible, a major complication is introduced. The human body, in principal, makes an excellent growth medium for a microorganism to recover from a chemical or thermal shock. Dilution occurs, the temperature is generally right and the environmental nutrition level is optimal. A sick patient is not going to be helped by an additional microbiological complication due to administration of a few microorganisms during treatment.

Gaseous chemicals are effective in sterilizing surfaces but less effective when used for liquid products. Beta-propriolactone was suggested at one time as being a chemical entity that could be used to sterilize solutions but has since been implicated as a carcinogen. Although not necessarily carcinogenic, residues of biologically reactive substances such as formaldehyde and ethylene oxide are obviously undesirable in an injected product. For these reasons, all chemical sterilants or preservatives are basically undesirable in parenterals and should be limited in use to a small number of products such as vaccines in multidose containers.

For a container sealed to prevent ingress of external environmental microorganisms, the application of sufficient heat energy in the presence of moisture generally is sufficient to ensure complete killing of all microorganisms present in the product at the time the heat is applied. Dry heat (in excess of 160°C) is sufficient to cause complete desiccation of microbial protein and loss of vital function if applied for a sufficient length of time. In addition, dry heat will eventually result in the loss of pyrogenic or fever-producing activity associated with fragments of bacterial cell walls. However, it will be obvious that the application of dry heat will be appropriate for components or materials coming into contact with the product but is inappropriate for the product itself.

The combination of water and heat is capable of progressively denaturing protein and the process may be generalized by the familiar kinetics of a chemical reaction. If the microbial death rate is a first order reaction, dependent upon the concentration of the reactants, the Arrhenius equation provides an approximate relationship in the form

$$k = A_e^{(-E/RT)}$$

where k is the reaction rate; A is a constant, the Arrhenius coefficient; E is the activation energy level necessary to initiate the reaction; R is the gas constant; T is the absolute temperature; and $_e$ is the base of natural logarithms.

It is experimentally feasible to make measurements of both A and E for bacterial species. When considering sterilization processes, the most resistant spore-forming organism likely to be present in the system will be evaluated.

is usually taken to be *Bacillus stearothermophilus* for which values of A between 10^{38} and $10^{55.9}$ min^{-1}, and for E, of $67.7 - 100.9$ Kcal/mole have been reported. These values enable us to compare activation energies for the stability of drugs.

For example, considering the kinetics of acid-catalyzed degradation of hyoscine, representing a typical drug, the value for A is 5.37×10^{55} min^{-1} and E 288.3 Kcal/mol. (data taken from Kondritizer and Zvirblis, J. Am. Pharm. Ass, 46, 531 (1957)).

Although the rates of the two "reactions" may be different, the activation energy or the energy level that must be exceeded before the reaction proceeds are similar. In this situation, it will be evident that autoclaving a solution of hyoscine will kill the microorganisms but will also produce some degradation. This is because energy in the form of heat has been supplied to the system. The increased energy level necessary to destroy microorganisms may also result in degradation of the product components. When considering the application of energy, a balance has to be made between what is necessary to sterilize the product and what is likely to produce unacceptable degradation of the product. Sodium chloride in a sealed system can be heated indefinitely whereas a penicillin cannot be heated at all. Dextrose lies between these two extremes. Dextrose solutions are sterilized by autoclaving but will caramelize readily if the heat treatment is prolonged unduly. There is a need for a sterilization process that avoids the application of heat to a thermolabile substance but which effectively removes all microorganisms. This may be achieved by "sterile" filtration of solutions of the drugs or by aseptic assembly of the product using presterilized components—the Aseptic Processing discussed in this monograph.

3. Aseptic Processing

Assembly of a final drug delivery product potentially occurs in two stages. The first may be the preparation of a product by the manufacturer who has determined that the drug is unstable and requires special precautions to maintain its identity, purity, potency and efficacy from manufacture to delivery. The second stage often occurs at the delivery point when, for clinical reasons, it has been determined that the patient requires combinations of drugs. These drugs may not be unstable but are given to the patient through an already existing intravenous catheter in which saline or dilute dextrose are being administered.

The first type of aseptic processing is imposed upon the manufacturer by the inherent properties of the drug. As this book will demonstrate, the process is involved and complicated and, for these reasons, expensive. The need for the second type of aseptic manipulation is determined by the clinical situation and the requirements of the patient. The operation has little to do with the inherent properties of the drug or drugs that are mixed. However, like the manufacturer at one end of the distribution chain and the pharmacist (or clinician or nurse) at the other, the product is assembled from sterile components and must retain the sterile integrity of these components. The manufacturing process is described at some length. This introduction to the subject concludes with a discussion of the hospital aspects since it is not completely covered elsewhere.

4. Aseptic Practice

As noted, in the hospital or clinical situation, drugs are added to intravenous saline or dextrose solutions as determined by the needs of the patient. A wide variety of these drugs cannot be injected directly into the patient, but must be added to an intravenous solution, either prior to setting up at the patients bedside or into a pre-existing intravenous set already connected to the patient's vein.

5. Assembling an Intravenous Solution

After surgery or trauma, a patient is likely to be in a state of shock, with all of the associated metabolic disturbances and dehydration. The intravenous route is used to supply whole blood, plasma or plasma substitutes as well as physiologically normal saline, other electrolytes or dextrose. If the patient is debilitated, intravenous sources of calories such as dextrose, amino acids and triglyceride emulsions will be administered. If diuresis is required, urea or mannitol may be given or a diuretic drug injection added to the drip. A prophylactic antibiotic such as a cephalosporin, penicillin or gentamycin will be given to prevent sepsis following surgery. If the patient has cancer, an antineoplastic such as mitomycin or doxorubicin may be added to the intravenous drip. If cardiovascular dysfunction is present, the drugs are likely to include digoxin or nitroglycerin. From a chemical standpoint, there are potentially a wide variety of different entities present, providing a number of possibilities for interaction. This aspect of the subject will be returned to later, since it forms an important part of the discussion.

An intravenous administration set is comprised of a number of component parts. Individually, these components will have been sterilized by a suitable process and protected from microbial contamination by an appropriate package.

The constituent parts are:

1. The intravenous needle or catheter
2. A terminal filter (not always feasible and by no means universal)
3. The administration set, including a drip chamber and/or a peristaltic pump
4. The glass bottle or plastic bag containing the carrier fluid such as saline or dextrose
5. The plastic minibag or small vial containing the additive(s).

After removal from the protective package, each part requires connection to the next part in the above sequence. There is a defined sequence of assembly to be followed, with careful checks at each stage to ensure the patient's safety. This final stage of drug delivery, perhaps the most critical, is generally carried out by a physician or nurse who is likely to have little if any formal training in the principles of aseptic processing. Furthermore, assembly is, of necessity, carried out at the bedside of the patient, in a non-sterile environment and therefore subject to contamination once the sterile container or package has been opened and exposed. Techniques are critical here. Poor technique is the main reason a percentage of catheters and needles are associated with thrombosis, phlebitis and sepsis around the area of insertion into the vein. At the extreme end of the distribution process, sterile integrity is negated by poor technique on the part of an individual who, perhaps, does not fully appreciate the underlying technology. Hopefully this is less likely to occur higher up the line where the technical knowledge level increases progressively. Unfortunately, the potential danger to the patient is directly related to the knowledge or awareness level of the manipulator at a particular stage. The purpose of this monograph and others like it, is to increase the awareness and diminish the risk factor.

Most additions of other drugs to a large volume parenteral (i.e. greater than 100mL volume) will have occurred at the stage immediately prior to the bedside, either in the ward or in the pharmacy. In the ward, additions will be made by either a nurse or a pharmacist; in the pharmacy, by a pharmacist or a pharmacy technician. Attempts to control the external microbiological environment are made at this stage. Usually care is taken when exposing a sterile surface, a needle previously protected by a sleeve, for example, or the entry port of a sterile container. Surfaces will be swabbed with a sterilizing chemical such as an iodophore or alcohol.

Ideally, and more likely within the pharmacy itself, all manipulations will be undertaken in laminar air flow units. Air flowing under laminar flow conditions, after first being passed through a suitable filter (e.g. HEPA), will not be necessarily sterile. However, it will be unlikely to contain many airborne organisms and those that are in the airstream are even less likely to cross streamlines and contaminate an open container. Technique can significantly influence the situation; for example, solid objects downstream of the manipulation point can disturb the streamlines, possibly allowing cross-contamination.

Currently, most hospital pharmacies use horizontal laminar flow units that produce air blowing towards the operator. Manipulations occur at a point where undisturbed air flows. This is highly undesirable when handling antineoplastic drugs, themselves now considered to be potent carcinogens. For these reasons, vertical laminar flow units are being installed in some hospitals. This type of unit is also preferred in industrial aseptic operations since there is a reduced chance of disturbing the downstream flow regimen.

6. Difficulties Associated with Manipulating the Product Container

Product containers vary in volume from 1mL to 1000mL and are made either from all-glass or all-plastic or from glass or plastics with elastomeric seals. A plastic container, especially if made from polyvinyl chloride (PVC) collapses when the contents are withdrawn. A glass container does not and, if integrity is to be preserved, a filtered air-inlet is required. For the incoming air to be sterile, the air inlet through the elastomeric seal to the bottle will have to be fitted with a sterile filter, usually a hydrophobic membrane. If this filter is strong enough, the solution inside the bottle can be supported while allowing air to enter. One such filter type is the Gelman "Acropor" filter made of PVC/acronitril copolymer supported on a nylon matrix.

All-glass and all-plastic containers such as the newer rigid or semi-rigid plastics have to be opened completely to allow the contents to be withdrawn. The problem with an all-glass ampoule is that glass fragments and shards are generated in the process of ampoule opening. These may often end up in the product and, sometimes, in the patient. A more prevalent danger is that viable microbiological material on the outside of a product container may contaminate the sterile contents. Accordingly, it is essential that the outside surface of an ampoule be sterilized at the point of opening immediately prior to breaking. A hypodermic needle may be inserted directly through the wall of a plastic ampoule or bag to allow product withdrawal, making external contamination less of a problem. However, the plastic is not elastomeric and the hole is not self-sealing. The product is therefore compromised once the needle has been withdrawn and should be discarded or the remaining contents used within a few hours.

Large volume parenterals packed in glass with rubber seals are under vacuum. It has been reported that inserting an airway into a bottle upside down carries with it the risk of an explosion due to a water-hammer effect. Even if this does not occur, the sudden rush of air into the container may rupture the protective filter on the airway. Insertion of a hollow needle through a rubber seal may also result in coring in which the needle punches out a central core of rubber. This can contaminate the sterile contents if the external surface has not been sterilized immediately prior to needle insertion. Plastic containers which lack mechanical rigidity and strength require care in handling. For example, holding a PVC bag tightly may cause the contents to squirt out when the needle is inserted or non-sterile air to be drawn in, either effect being undesirable.

7. Drug Incompatibilities

As noted earlier, a wide variety of chemical compounds may be present in the final solution entering the patients vein. Even a single drug entity is likely to be formulated with preservatives, antioxidants, electrolytes or pH control agents and contain contaminants inadvertently present such as those extractables from an elastomeric closure. Addition of two drug entities, each with their own advertent and inadvertent additives potentially results in a number of interactions taking place. Interactions are two broad types, physical and chemical. Biological interactions mean that the product is biologically contaminated and physiological incompatibility suggests that two drugs may be mutually antagonistic from a physiological standpoint. Physical interactions take the form of a visible precipitation or crystallization, an increase in turbidity or a change of color. These reactions in themselves may not be detrimental to the physiological action of the drug unless, for example, the drug is precipitated out of solution and filtered out of the product. Lipid emulsions may be destabilized by inappropriate addition of electrolytes, leading to an increased risk of embolism in the patient. Changes of pH in a system, on the other hand, may affect the degradation rate of a drug or result in the precipitation of a less soluble form.

Chemical interactions may be manifest as direct, polymerizations, conjugations or effects on stability. Example of direct interaction are the tetracycline antibiotics that rapidly form insoluble salts in the presence of magnesium or calcium ions. Cephaloridine tends to polymerize at acid pH and penicillins form conjugates with proteins. These are visible interactions.

The invisible interactions are more difficult to detect but may be equally or more significant. For example, although the resultant mixture remains clear, a loss of therapeutic activity occurs when gentamycin is mixed with sodium ampicillin.

Tables are available listing reported incompatibilities, some listings being very comprehensive. There are situations where two drugs are reported to be incompatible but may be mixed under the correct conditions, for example by prior dilution. When dealing with a new or unfamiliar drug entity, these types of interactions have to be considered and looked for.

8. Microbiological Hazards Associated with Intravenous Therapy

As noted previously, the risk of contamination can be reduced by disinfecting the site of entry into the sterile contents of the container and using good aseptic manipulative technique. If contamination occurs during the final manipulative stages, it is desirable that the solution be used immediately before the contaminating organism has an opportunity to proliferate. It should be noted that a prepared admixture should not be stored under refrigerator conditions since common air-borne contaminants such as Pseudomonas sp. can multiply rapidly at low temperatures.

Patients have died when inadequately sterilized products have been administered, including products from containers that were incompletely autoclaved, inadvertently not autoclaved at all or contaminated by cooling water entering into the sterilized system. Glass containers that have cracked on storage or transport following a successful sterilization process have resulted in contaminated product being administered to patients. A major outbreak of septicemia in the early 1970's was attributed to a contaminated cap liner that allowed organisms to be transferred from the cap to the sterile fluid during manipulation processes. The contaminating species of the Klebsielia-Enterobacter group were capable of rapidly proliferating at room temperature in the dextrose solutions.

9. Pre-Administration Inspection and Terminal Filtration

Although visual inspection of an intravenous fluid system sometimes allows detection of precipitates or an increased turbidity, it is unlikely that a microbial contamination are as evident. Growth in an intravenous fluid has to be at levels of $10^5 - 10^6$ organisms/mL before a visible increase in turbidity can be seen. Mold colonies can be seen only if a large number of fungi are present.

Pre-administration inspection, visually or with the aid of a modest viewing device right up to the stage of the product going into the patient's vein is highly desirable. The chance of a fault being detected increases as the passage of time may allow for the growth of any contaminating organisms to a point that they can be detected by visual examination.

It is not a question of territory—"who does what?" but rather one of collective responsibility—"how often?".

Since all microbiological contamination and precipitates are physically particulate in nature, there has been a general move in the direction of placing a final filter on the delivery system immediately before the needle or catheter. Ernerot and Sandell in 1967 initiated this suggestion, noting the advantages as well as focusing attention to some of the disadvantages. Flow rate, for example, is slowed down although this is less likely to be an issue with the advent of IV pumps. Filters, likely to become blocked if micro particulates are present in the solution, cannot be used at all for emulsion products. The major advantage of a filter is that chance microbial contamination arising through faulty technique or the stress failure of a part of the delivery system can be prevented from entering the patient's vein. An additional advantage is that inadvertent air embolisms are avoided.

Trials have demonstrated a significant reduction in the incidence of systemic bacteremias, septicemias and local phlebitis when filters are used. Nevertheless it is axiomatic that the use of a terminal filter is no substitute for the use of truly sterile solutions and components of the delivery system as well as a faultless aseptic technique when making the various manipulations involved in assembling a delivery system and attaching it to the patient.

2

Container Cleaning and Sterilization

Neil R. Anderson
Merrell Dow Research Institute, Indianapolis, IN, USA

1. Introduction

The goal of an aseptic processing system is to produce an acceptable parenteral product. The acceptability of a parenteral product is based on how well the product measures up to certain product characteristics that people today deem as 'state-of-the-art'. The first characteristic is that of clinical effectiveness. This topic is much too extensive to cover in the context of this chapter. Therefore, we must simply state that clinical effectiveness includes those areas of concern for the product's efficacy, safety, and reliability throughout the product's intended useful life.

A parenteral product must be sterile, free from all living microorganisms. Such preparations must be sterile because their use bypasses the body's main line of defense, the skin. Consequently, the use of non-sterile preparations can very likely lead to serious problems for the patient.

A lack of particulate matter is another basic characteristic of parenteral products. Particulate matter may be defined as mobile, undissolved substances that are unintentionally present in parenteral preparations. Initially the concern with particulate matter was mainly for psychological reasons. What was the psychologic effect on the patient when they saw that they were receiving a solution with visible particulate material in it? What kind of conclusions might be drawn by the patient concerning the company marketing injectables with visible material (1)? More recently the concern has shifted from the psychological to the physiological effects of injecting solutions containing particulate matter. There is evidence in the medical literature that particulate matter in parenteral solutions may, injected intravenously, produce pulmonary microemboli, thrombi, or granulomas (2). While the evidence of harm from particulate matter is largely circumstantial, the parenteral industry and those who use parenteral products have taken measures to eliminate particulate matter. The quality control parameters have been made extremely clear: Particulate matter is undesirable, and constant efforts must be made to eliminate its sources and occurrence (1).

The final characteristic of a parenteral product is that of being free of pyrogens. By broad medical definition, a pyrogen is a hypothetical substance which when injected, produces fever. From the pharmaceutical standpoint, bacterial endotoxin is the most common pyrogen. The most active pyrogens of microbial origin are those produced by gram-negative bacteria.

For the purpose of this introduction, it is important to know that since pyrogens are generated in the cell walls of bacteria, microbial contamination of a product at any stage of a product's manufacture presents the risk of subsequent pyrogenic reactions from the product when used. Therefore, it is prudent in practice to assume two things about pyrogens; 1) similar to bacteria, pyrogens are ubiquitous in nature, and 2) pyrogens are cumulative in the manufacturing process itself.

How one prepares a parenteral product, the raw materials used, the procedures involved, and the care taken determine whether or not the final product will have the required characteristics described above. The required characteristics must be built into the product. No amount of end-product testing can assure a good product and the characteristics cannot be imparted to the product after it is made.

The aseptic process (often referred to as the sterile fill technique) is an alternative parenteral manufacturing process to the use of the heat-based process of terminal sterilization. While heat will sterilize a drug and the drug container/delivery system, the process may degrade the drug products(s) or render the container/delivery system unsuitable for use over the intended useful life of the product. Because the aseptic process sterilizes heat sensitive drug components by filtering the drug solutions through bacteria retentive filter membranes, the aseptic process requires that all components of the drug product and its container system by pre-sterilized. Once sterile, all of the components are brought together in an aseptic environment to create the finished parenteral drug product sealed in its container system.

Bearing in mind the basic required characteristics for a parenteral product, the aseptic process then becomes one of the most exacting operations practiced in the pharmaceutical industry. The final characteristics of the product rely upon each step in the aseptic process being totally under control to known levels of assurance that the characteristics are indeed being built into the product. How well the product's characteristics are developed is a cumulative function of all the process steps involved in the product's manufacture. The final quality level of any of the basic characteristics, for instance sterility, of the product cannot be greater than that of the processing step providing the lowest probability of sterility (3).

2. The Parenteral Container System

The role of the drug product container is much more involved than simply serving as a physical restraint system for a drug until it is used.

Containers facilitate the manufacture and sterilization of products and allow the inspection of the contents. Containers permit the shipping and storage of parenteral products as well as the convenient clinical use of the drug product. The basic objectives for a drug product container are stated in the Current Good Manufacturing Practices (CGMP) section 211.94(a)(b). "Container closure systems shall provide adequate protection against foreseeable external factors in storage and use that can cause deterioration or contamination of the drug product."(4) The primary container for a parenteral product should help maintain the product's sterility, freedom from particulates, and freedom from pyrogens throughout its intended useful shelf life. Not only must the primary parenteral container protect the product from external factors but the container itself must not threaten the product.

A number of the basic parenteral container systems made of glass or plastic used today are listed in Table I.

Table I—Basic Types of Glass and Plastic Container Systems Used for Parenteral Packaging

Glass	Plastic
Ampoules	Bottles
Vials	Bags
Bottles	Syringes
Syringes	

A. Ampoules

The glass ampoule is the oldest packaging system for parenterals. Stanislaus Limousin in the late 1800's developed the ampoule for hermetically sealing solutions for terminal sterilization (7). Ampoules are intended for single dose sterile solutions. Such solutions may or may not contain an antimicrobial preservative. The key advantage of the ampoule system, especially if Type I glass is used, is the relative non-reactivity of the container with the solution contents. Thus, the ampoule is the best choice for product formulations which will react with rubber or plastic surfaces and result in subsequent physical and/or clinical stability problems.

Ampoules potentially can be many different sizes. Most ampoule sizes are either 1mL, 2mL, 5mL, 10mL, or 20mL capacity. Empty ampoule shapes are basically identical, regardless of size, except for the neck areas.

The main problem in using ampoules involves the breaking of the neck to withdraw the contents. Not only is the process of breaking the ampoule somewhat difficult and, at times hazardous to the user (e.g. cut fingers), but also glass particles are emitted when the neck is broken resulting in particulate contamination of the solution contents. After opening, ampoules are somewhat inconvenient to use because the transfer process of the liquid contents from the ampoule into the syringe is somewhat tedious and a filtered needle should be used to eliminate the glass particles.

Ampoule manufacturers have attempted to reduce glass particulate contamination and the difficulty of breaking open the ampoules by pre-treating the ampoules allowing them to be broken easier and cleaner. Wheaton ampoules have prescored necks and Kimble ampoules are inscribed with a circle of ceramic paint. A new Japanese ampoule incorporates a one-point-cut at the narrowest point of the ampoule neck (5, 6). In each case the pretreatment weakens the glass and allows for easier and cleaner openings of ampoules.

B. Vials

Glass vials are by far the most popular container in use for packaging of sterile products. Primary reasons for their popularity include flexibility of dosage, ease in handling and decreased cost. Vials are stoppered with rubber closures, thus permitting repeated withdrawals of the contents.

Because of the rubber closure, vials do experience certain difficulties at times. Multiple penetrations of the closure could produce both microbiological and particulate contamination of the contents. Rubber closures have been shown to interact with the solution contents producing either leaching of the rubber components or adsorption of drug product components.

Vial sizes typically range from 1mL to 50mL. While the shape of the vial will vary according to the body dimensions chosen, the dimensions of the vial neck opening are typically standardized in the United States at 13mm or 20mm. Double chambered vials are also available to package a sterile powder with its sterile vehicle (Mix-O-Vial, Upjohn; Redi-Vial, Eli Lilly). Because of their larger neck size vials are easier to clean than ampoules. In addition, vials have thicker glass walls than ampoules, thus providing for greater durability.

C. Bottles

Glass bottles used to be the only container for large volume parenteral solutions (LVPs). However, with the advent of plastic bottles and bags, glass bottles are no longer the primary container system for LVPs. Glass bottles for LVP use require a rubber closure as do glass vials and hence can have similar problems.

D. Syringes

Glass syringes pre-filled with drug were developed during World War II in response to the need for having sterile medication immediately available for emergency use (7). The three major components of the syringe are the needle, the barrel and the plunger. Many prefilled syringe systems have the needle packaged separately with a rubber tip covering the opening of the syringe. The major attribute of prefilled syringes is their convenience and many parenteral manufacturers today package their products in prefilled disposable syringes (see Table II). A recent development allows a sterile powder to be packaged with but separated from its sterile vehicle in a prefilled syringe system (Hypak Liqui/Dry, Becton Dickinson). Convenience subsequently provides greater simplicity and reduces the probability of medication error and non-sterility. Dosage sizes available in prefilled disposable syringes range from 1mL to 10mL.

Table II—Examples of Prefilled Disposable Syringe Dosage Units

Manufacturer	Syringe System
Abbott Laboratories	Abboject
Eli Lilly and Company	Hyporet
Parke, Davis and Company	Steri-Dose
Roche Laboratories	Tel-E-Ject
Wyeth Laboratories	Tubex

E. Plastic container systems

Plastic dropper bottles were introduced for the packaging of sterile ophthalmic products in the 1950's. In 1971 Travenol Laboratories introduced the Viaflex plastic bag system for the packaging of intravenous fluids. In the late 1970's large volume plastic bottles became available both for sterile irrigation solutions using screw caps and for sterile intravenous solution using rubber closures. In the early 1980's Abbott Laboratories introduced the plastic vial for use with certain solutions. While most prefilled disposable syringe packages are glass, there are a few products available in plastic sterile syringes such as the Abboject system (Abbott Laboratories).

Protecting a parenteral product in a suitable container system begins by properly preparing the container to receive the drug product. The CGMP regulations (211.94c) require that:

> "Drug product containers. . .shall be clean and, where indicated by the nature of the drug, sterilized and processed to remove pyrogenic properties to assure that they are suitable for their intended use."(4)

Aseptically prepared parenteral products must be free of bacterial, pyrogenic, and particulate contamination. Therefore, it is essential that the parenteral product container be clean, sterile, particulate free, and pyrogen free when the drug product is filled into it.

3. Container Properties

A. Properties of glass

Glass is an excellent packaging material because it is readily available, economical, easily sterilized and depyrogenated, clear, relatively inert, and easily handled on high-speed production lines. Its high degree of chemical inertness compared to other packaging materials makes it the container-of-choice for injectable products (8-10).

Glass can be defined as an "inorganic product of fusion which has been cooled to a rigid condition without crystallization." Thus it is amorphous substance, and is sometimes referred to as an 'supercooled liquid'. Glass resembles a liquid in its structure, consisting of a random network of atoms, even though it is a very rigid material (11, 12).

The structure of glass is illustrated in Figure 1. The random network of silica tetrahedra comprise the backbone of this structure. Since Figure 1 is a two dimensional illustration, only three of the four oxygen atoms in the tetrahedron are shown.

Figure 1—Schematic illustration of the structure of sodasilicate glass

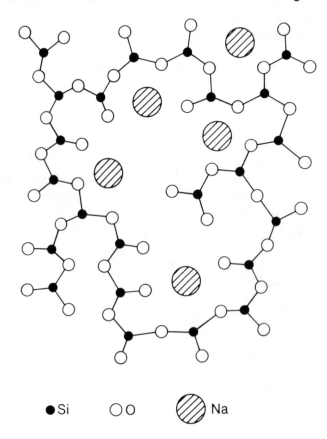

● Si   ○ O   ◍ Na

Commercial glasses are produced from inorganic oxides, chiefly silica or sand. The most chemically resistant type of glass is one that consists solely of silica tetrahedra. This glass, however, is very brittle and difficult to fabricate (12). Modifying oxides, also called fluxing agents, are added to improve the strength and workability of the glass by lowering its melting point and lowering its viscosity in the molten state. These oxides include those of sodium, aluminum, potassium, calcium, magnesium, barium and boron. Examples of formulas for glasses for pharmaceutical use are given in Table III. The type and quantity of various oxides in the glass formula affect the manufacturing process by influencing the melting temperature, ease of fabrication, and other factors. Properties of the resultant glass are also affected. Glass characteristics depend not only on the oxide content, but also on the thermal history of the glass. Two glasses with the same ratio of constituents may exhibit different densities, indices of refraction, and coefficients of thermal expansion due to differences in the rate of cooling from the molten state (9, 11, 12). The alkali oxides (chiefly of sodium) enter the spaces in the network of silica tetrahedra and decrease the bonding forces between the silicon and oxygen atoms (see Figure 1). The alkali atoms are held by weak ionic forces and can migrate through the glass matrix using relatively little energy (13). Thus, even at room temperature, sodium ions have sufficient mobility to be extracted into an aqueous solution after prolonged contact with the solution. Oxides of divalent, trivalent, or quadrivalent elements such as CaO and Al_2O_3 will produce a glass with higher chemical resistance than alkali oxides because they are more strongly held in the glass matrix. The melting and molding properties, however, will not be as greatly improved as with the alkali oxides. These oxides will improve the abil-

Table III—Compositions (%) of Some Glass Containers for Pharmaceutical Use

	Glass Type			
Ingredient	1 Borosilicate	2 Borosilicate	3 Soda-Lime	4 Soda-Lime
SiO_2	69.15	71.1	72.3	71.63
Na_2O	8.6	8.3	13.4	13.6
B_2O_3	10.8	11.5	0.3	0.54
Al_2O_3	5.9	4.6	2.7	1.95
CaO	0.8	1.36	10.3	9.25
K_2O	1.2	0.7	0.5	—
BaO	2.5	2.42	0.2	0.54
Fe_2O_3	<0.05	<0.05	0.04	0.014
MgO	0.4	—	0.3	2.42
ZnO	0.6	—	—	—

ity of the glass to retain alkali ions (14). Boric oxide is referred to as a network former because it does not enter the spaces in the glass like the other oxides, but is incorporated into the silica network itself. When it is included in the formula for borosilicate glasses, it becomes part of the glass matrix and the boron ions are not available for release when in contact with a solution. This accounts for the high degree of chemical durability observed in borosilicate glasses compared to soda-lime glasses (9, 12, 15, 16).

The United States Pharmacopoeia/National Formulary (USP/NF) categorizes glass containers into four types. Table IV presents this classification system. The glass types are defined according to the amount of titratable alkali released from the glass under the given test conditions (17). Types I, II, and III may be used for parenteral products, while type NP is for non-parenteral packaging applications. Containers of type I glass have excellent properties of heat and chemical resistance and can be used for all types of parenteral products. Type II glass is soda-lime glass that has been treated to de-alkalize the surface for improved chemical durability. This glass is generally used for buffered solutions that have a pH of 7 or less. The suitability of type II glass for unbuffered solutions should be evaluated on a case-by-case basis (9, 17, 18). The surface de-alkalization can be accomplished in a number of ways, but the most common method is to treat the surface with sulfur dioxide (13). This treatment is carried out during the annealing stage of glass production. The container surface is exposed to SO_2 gas at high temperatures (540–650°C) and controlled humidity. The reaction that takes place may be written as follows:

$$2Na^+ \text{ (glass)} + SO_2 + 1/2O_2 + H_2O \rightarrow 2H^+ \text{ (glass)} + Na_2SO_4$$

The sodium sulfate produced by this reaction appears on the surface as a highly water soluble white precipitate. The precipitate is easily removed from the glass surface by rinsing (19). Hydrogen ions with associated water molecules are exchanged with sodium ions in the de-alkalization reaction and the resulting "hydrogen glass" on the surface is more resistant to chemical attack than the underlying material (20). When the "hydrogen glass" is exposed to further heat, dehydration of the glass causes a compaction of the silica network. The surface layer now has a higher density than the bulk of the glass and is more impervious to the diffusion of sodium ions. Mochel et al. (14) have shown that the de-alkalization process also imparts a greater physical strength to the glass as well as increasing the chemical resistance. The de-alkalization reaction is only a surface effect, however, and if the surface is in contact with a solution for a long period of time, the compacted outer layer may be penetrated or removed (10, 16, 21, 22). Type I glass may also be surface treated; and although this treatment is not necessary, it is sometimes used to enhance the durability of a container that already has excellent chemical resistance. This treatment may be especially desirable for small containers where a high surface-to-volume ratio warrants the use of glass with the lowest possible alkali content (18).

Table IV—USP Glass Types and Test Limits

			Limits	
Glass Type	General Description	Test Type	Size (mL)	MLs of 0.02N H_2SO_4
I	Highly resistant borosilicate glass	Powdered Glass	all	1.0
II	Treated soda-lime glass	Water Attack	100 or less over 100	0.7 0.2
III	Soda-lime glass	Powdered Glass	all	8.5
NP	General purpose soda-lime glass	Powdered Glass	all	15.0

Type III soda-lime glass containers are seldom used for parenteral products. These containers may be used after stability tests have established that the glass is satisfactory for the parenteral product to be packaged. Type III glass containers have been found to be acceptable for some non-aqueous products or dry powders which are dissolved just prior to use (9, 17).

To aid in the evaluation of glass containers, the USP/NF describes two tests for evaluating the chemical resistance of glass (17) and the Parenteral Drug Association has published their Technical Methods Bulletin No. 3, Glass Containers for Small Volume Parenteral Products: Factors for Selection and Test Methods for Identification (18).

The interactions of aqueous solutions with glass containers are extremely complex. In recent publications, authors have admitted that only a little is yet known about the actual mechanisms involved. No single test is adequate for comparing the durability of glasses with different compositions and the data from one study cannot be easily extrapolated to another study (18, 23, 24). Some generalizations, however, can be made.

Under normal service conditions, glass is very slowly decomposed on the surface in contact with an aqueous solution. The extraction is a preferential one in which the alkali ions are extracted first. The nature of chemical attack on glass can be viewed in terms of the structure of the glass itself. Silica is very inert and practically insoluble in water except at high temperatures. Neutral and acid solutions (except hydrofluoric acid) have little effect on silica, and the solubility of silica increases with the alkalinity of the solution. A distinction, therefore, is made between acid and water attack of glass and attack by alkaline and hydrofluoric acid solutions. Corrosion by neutral and acid solutions, called leaching, is a diffusion-controlled ion-exchange process involving certain components within the surface layer of the glass. The alkali oxides are extracted first, followed by other oxides such as the alkaline earths which exchange with hydronium ions to a lesser degree. The ion-exchange process can be represented by the following equation:

$$H_3O + Na^+_{(glass)} \rightarrow H_3O_{(glass)} + Na^+_{(aqueous)}$$

The removal of hydronium ions from solution results in an increase in pH and the formation of sodium hydroxide in the solution (25). The porous layer of hydrated silica that remains then acts as a barrier through which the liquid and extracted material must diffuse. The process slows down with time as the diffusion layer increases in thickness. A linear correlation is generally found between amount extracted and square root of time, indication that a diffusion process does indeed take place (11, 20).

The attack by alkaline solutions, referred to as etching, is much faster than attack by acidic or neutral solutions. When this occurs, the surface of the glass actually undergoes dissolution as well as extraction of alkali, Since the process is dissolution controlled, the rate of attack is constant and the amount extracted follows a linear relationship with time. Alkaline attack can be illustrated by the equation:

$$2NaOH + (SiO_2)_x \rightarrow Na_2SiO_3 + H_2O$$

The alkali silicate is soluble in water and simply diffuses away from the glass surface. When the concentration of silica in solution approaches the saturation point, the rate of attack will slow down. The reaction also indicates the manner in which glass flakes can be formed (26, 27). A large section of the insoluble porous layer may peel off under suitable conditions and be seen floating in solution. Flaking may occur during acid attack as well as alkaline attack. The acid will preferentially remove the alkali from the glass, leaving a silica skeleton which may be fragile enough to slough off and form flakes in the solution. Borosilicate glasses are very resistant to flaking (12, 20, 22).

When a glass surface is attacked by water with no added substances or neutral unbuffered aqueous solutions, the process will initially involve leaching. This results in the extraction of alkali and other basic oxides which will then lead to alkaline attack of the glass. Since alkaline attack is faster than neutral or acidic attack, the rate of corrosion of the glass will speed up until reaching a steady state. A plot of the amount extracted versus time has a diffusion profile at first, but as the attack time increases the silica network begins to dissolve, and a linear relationship is obtained. A structural re-arrangement of the silica network is believed to occur during the leaching process. Complex mathematical equations have been developed to express the time dependence of constituent release for the reaction of water with glass. These expressions became considerably more difficult when the authors considered the many variables involved including various time periods (23, 25). Some factors affecting the degree and type of chemical interactions of glass containers with solutions are listed in Table V (18, 22, 23, 28).

Table V—Some Factors Affecting the Degree and Type of Chemical Interactions of Glass Container Surfaces

---

Agitation of attacking solution	Surface-to-Volume ratio
Glass composition	Temperature
Nature of the attacking medium	Thermal history of the glass
Storage time	Washing procedure/pretreatment
Surface treatment	

The chemical composition of a specific glass is the most important factor influencing its chemical durability. This is readily illustrated by the higher chemical durability of the borosilicate glasses compared to soda-lime glasses (see Table IV).

The material packaged can have a stabilizing or deleterious effect on the rate of extraction of alkali from glass containers. The extraction of alkali from glass may be retarded or enhanced by the presence of various salts in the parenteral solution. Bacon and Raggon (29) found that citrate and other anions promoted the attack of glass by neutral solutions. Other neutral salts have been shown to promote attack, but most of the investigations regarding the effects of salts have been concerned with the more commonly observed effect, namely, inhibition of attack by various cations (23, 25, 30). Some salts which cause this inhibitory effect are salts of calcium, aluminum, zinc, potassium, lithium, sodium, and barium. The amount of inhibition is highly dependent on the salt concentration. As already discussed, the corrosion of the glass is also influenced by the pH of the solution and whether it is buffered or unbuffered (10, 13, 22, 23, 29, 31, 32, 33).

If the temperature is increased while a glass surface is being attacked, the rate of attack will increase. A general rule of thumb is that the rate of attack increases two and one-half times for every 10°C increase in temperature (11, 20, 23, 34).

The surface properties of a glass will be affected by its thermal history. The chemical reactivity may change depending on whether the glass was cooled rapidly or slowly from the molten state. Annealed glasses have been found to be more durable than glasses that were not annealed (22). Other types of heat treatments can produce pronounced effects on the chemical durability of glass (11). Tubing vials have been reported to have a tendency to release slightly more alkali than molded bottles because the additional heat treatment of the remelting of the tubing to form the vials causes some of the alkali ions to move to the surface of the glass (35).

Majeski (23) has reported vast differences between different samples of Type II glass containers. The type of surface treatment used will determine the effectiveness of the treatment. The conditions under which the treatment was given will also be an important factor.

The leaching and dissolution of glass in contact with parenteral solutions can create numerous formulation problems. Boddapati et al. (32) reported on the presence of subvisible barium sulfate crystals in parenteral solutions. These studies revealed that barium ions were released from the glass and combined with sulfate moieties in the parenteral formula to produce the undesired precipitate. Glass flakes, even at the subvisible level, may cause pathological effects when injected (16). Glass particles may be in the parenteral solution from sources other than flaking, such as mechanical damage (37). The changes in alkalinity of injectable products may produce a toxic reaction (30). Other deleterious glass effects include precipitation of alkaloids such as morphine and atropine, flocculation of colloidal substances due to pH change, degradation of esters and glucosides, re-arrangement of optically active isomers, acceleration of oxidation reactions, and precipitation of hydroxides or oxides from solutions of metal salts (20).

B. Properties of plastics

A plastic can be defined as a material that contains as an essential ingredient one or more polymeric organic substances of large molecular weight, is solid in its finished state and at some stage in its manufacture or processing into a finished article can be shaped by flow (38).

The large molecular weight organic substance is called a polymer. A polymer is a large molecule built up by the repetition of small, simple chemical units. In some cases the repetition is in a linear form, in the same way that a pearl necklace is built up from individual pearls. In other cases the repetitions are branched and interconnected to form three-dimensional networks. The starting unit of a polymer is called a monomer and the repeating unit in a polymer is usually the same or nearly the same as the monomer.

The repeat unit of poly (vinyl chloride) is $-CH_2CHCl-$;
the monomer is vinyl chloride $CH_2=CHCl$.

The repeat unit of polyethylene is $-CH_2CH_2-$;
the monomer is ethylene $CH_2=CH_2$.

The repeat unit of natural rubber (polyisoprene) is
$-CH_2CH=C(CH_3)-CH_2-$;
the monomer is isoprene $CH_2=CH-C(CH_3)=CH_2$ (35).

The process of forming polymers from their monomers is called polymerization. To be able to polymerize the monomers must be capable of forming two covalent bonds or in other words the monomers must be bifunctional. The bifunctional characteristics can be achieved by the monomer containing an unsaturated double bond like ethylene, $CH_2=CH_2$, or by the monomer having two different organic groups that can react with each other such as an amino acid, $(NH_2-CHR-COOH)$. Depending on the type of bifunctionality of the monomer, polymerization can proceed by two basic processes: condensation or addition.

Addition polymerization (also referred to as chain-reaction polymerization or free radical reaction polymerization) usually makes use of monomers containing the $C=C$ bond. A chain reaction is usually initiated by the formation of a free radical from an initiator compound. The free radical is capable of reacting to open the $C=C$ bond and add to it, with an electron remaining unpaired. Very quickly then many more monomers add to the growing chain. Finally two free radicals react with each other and stop the reaction. A great variety of polymers can be prepared by this method. The general chemical structure of the starting monomer is $CH_2=C(R_1)R_2$ where R_1 and R_2 can be $-H$, $-CH_3$, phenyl, $-COOH$, $-COOR$, $-OCOCH_3$, $-CN$, $-F$, $-Cl$, $-CONH_2$, or pyrrolidone. The polymer produced can be represented then as $-[CH_2-C(R_1)R_2]_N-$ where n indicates the average number of monomer units that make up the polymer. Teflon, $(-CF_2-CF_2-)_n$ is made by this process from the monomer tetrafluoroethylene, $CF_2=CF_2$. This monomer is unique in that all four hydrogen atoms in the ethylene molecule have been substituted with a fluorine atom. Other common polymers made by this type of reaction are polyethylene (PE), polypropylene (PP), polyvinylchloride (PVC), polystyrene (PS), and polymethylmethacrylate (PMMA) (39, 40).

Condensation or step-reaction polymerization takes place between monomers that contain two different types of functional groups to produce one larger polyfunctional molecule, with the possible elimination of a small molecule such as water. This reaction can be illustrated by the reaction of two hydroxy acid molecules to form a polyester;

$$HO(CH_2)COOH + HO(CH_2)COOH \rightarrow HO(CH_2)COO(CH_2)COOH + H_2O$$

Table 6 lists some distinguishing features of the addition and condensation polymerization reactions. Some common polymers made by this type of reaction include the polyesters (Dacron and Mylar), polyamides (Nylon), polyanhydrides and polycarbonates (39.)

Table VI—Some Distinguishing Features of the Addition and Condensation Polymerization Reactions

Addition Polymerization Reaction	*Condensation Polymer Reaction*
Growth occurs by adding monomers to the growing chain.	Growth occurs with any two species present (monomer or polymer).
Monomer concentration decreases throughout the reaction.	Monomer disappears early in the reaction.
High polymer formed quickly; long reaction times affect polymer weight very little.	Polymer weight increases throughout reaction; long reaction times are necessary for high polymer weights.

Plastics fall into two general categories: thermoplastic and thermosets. The thermoplastic family consists of those polymers which at normal temperatures are rigid but can be made to soften and take on new shapes by the application of heat and pressure. The thermoset family of plastics are stable to heat and cannot be made to flow or melt.

Thermoplastics can be modified and properties enhanced by the addition of certain additives. The additives that are most routinely used in the production of thermoplastics are listed in Table VII.

Table VII—Commonly Used Additives in Thermoplastic Polymer Formulations

Additive	Use
Lubricants	Assist processing of polymers in molding and extrusion operations; lowers melt viscosity or prevents polymer sticking to equipment. (zinc stearate, paraffin and polyethylene waxes)
Stabilizers	To retard or prevent polymer degradation with heat and light; improve aging properties. (organometallics, fatty acid salts, inorganic oxides)
Plasticizers	To impart softness and flexibility to the polymer. (phthalate esters)
Antioxidants	To retard or prevent oxidative degradation of the polymer. (BHT)
Antistatics	To prevent the build up of static charges on the plastic surface. (quaternary ammonium compounds)
Slip Agents	Added primarily to polyolefin type plastics to reduce the coefficient of friction of the plastics.
Dyes and Pigments	To impart color to the plastic materials.

The application of plastic for the primary packaging of ophthalmic and parenteral products has grown very rapidly over the last twenty years. Plastic materials have obvious advantages over glass when it comes to weight and breakage. These two factors alone have done much to stimulate the change from glass to plastic. However, problems have been encountered in the glass to plastic conversion that today make up an outline of potential problem areas that must be fully considered in any future conversion study. The problems that have occurred or may occur in the future might be ascribed to a property or properties of a specific material in contact with a product.

The first potential problem area is that of permeation. Volatile components of a product, some active ingredients, or head space gases added for protection, may be able to pass through the container to the exterior environment. Such permeation could result in decreased potency and stability. Conversely, atmospheric oxygen, water vapor, or other gases may be able to pass through the container into the interior and cause stability problems via oxidative and hydrolytic degradation (40).

Sorption of active ingredients and preservative onto plastic surfaces have been reported in the literature (41-44). Such activity can lead to a loss of drug potency and efficacy of preservation (45).

The chemical make-up of a plastic can be complex and leads to the third basic problem area of leaching. The additives and constituents from plastic containers can be leached into a product (41, 42, 46). Such leaching can change the purity of the product, the physical stability of the product, the chemical stability of the product, or cause some adverse effect when the product is administered. Other leaching activity can potentially lead to the formation of particulate matter. The reader is referred to an excellent review of parenteral packaging compatibility and stability by Wang and Chien prepared for the Parenteral Drug Association (40).

All of the above problem areas make it imperative that the final product/package be thoroughly evaluated for safety and stability. The drug product and its package should not be a health liability by producing some side effect that complicates the existing illness of a patient. This consideration becomes even more exacting considering that many parenterals are administered directly into the systemic circulation. Consequently, the pharmaceutical industry requires that a very high level of safety be established for plastic containers used for parenterals just as for the product itself.

New barrier plastic containers, originally researched and developed for the food industry, exhibit a high resistance to the molecular flow of liquids or vapors through the polymer matrix. The barrier plastics are multilayer coextruded laminates. The great advantage of coextrusion is that it makes it possible to select resins in the right combination and in exactly the necessary thickness required to obtain the desired result. American Can Company's Gamma bottle is a polypropylene/ethylene vinyl alcohol/polypropylene (PP/EVOH/PP) structured coextruded high barrier plastic bottle introduced in the food industry (barbecue sauce and catsup) in mid-1983. The EVOH layer adds a superior oxygen barrier to the laminate. Continental Groups's Plastic Container Division and Owens-Illinois have barrier plastic containers available. Also available is a five-layered sterilizable bottle with flexible or rigid side walls. The bottle is being promoted in Europe for various sterilizable ophthalmic preparations by its maker Holmia A/S of Denmark (47). Although packaging systems for food products require considerations similar to those for pharmaceutical products, the food products usually have a relatively rapid rate of turnover and, hence, relatively short shelf-life requirements. On the other hand, pharmaceutical products require an extremely long shelf-life stability that leads to the most critical technical and toxicological data for regulatory approval. However, the successes in the food packaging systems lead us to believe that pharmaceutical packaging systems have a lot to look forward to in terms of plastic containers.

Recently two new plastic intravenous infusion sets (Avon Medicals Limited, Worcester, England) have been developed to combat the problems of drug sorption and photodegradation. The 'Sureset' apparatus is made from polybutadiene and, while it has the working qualities of PVC, it does not exhibit sorption of diazepam, chomethiazole, nitroglycerin, or isosorbide dinitrate. The 'Amberset' apparatus protects light sensitive infusion solutions from ultraviolet light by utilizing two layers of PVC. The outer PVC layer has a transparent, amber, light absorbing (220 to 470 nm waveband) polymer incorporated into it. The inner layer is standard PVC. Since the amber polymer is only in the outer layer it does not come into contact with the infusion solution and thereby avoids a leaching problem (44).

4. Container Washing

As noted earlier, one of the basic characteristics of a parenteral product is that of being free of particulate matter. In the manufacture of parenteral products there are at least three generic sources of particulates: the solution and its components, the process of manufacture and its variables, and the package and its components (48). The composition of unwanted particulate matter is varied. In some cases the composition of particulate matter is common to many sources. In other cases the particulate matter is characteristic to a specific source. Theoretically, particulate contamination can come from any environmental material to which the product is exposed.

Since the final container comes in contact with the parenteral preparation, the container should not be a source of particulates. Therefore, prior to filling the container must be thoroughly cleaned. The results of the cleaning procedures for containers depend to a large extent on the amount of contamination present prior to cleaning. The more initial contamination there is the more difficult it will be to clean the container thoroughly. New, unused containers become contaminated principally with dust, fibers, and chemical films associated with their manufacture, packing, shipment, storage, and handling. The breakage of a glass ampoule or vial in a box of containers will also contaminate many of the accompanying containers.

Since newly fabricated containers are essentially free from particulate contamination, protection of the empty containers as quickly as possible can reduce particulate contamination. Exercising continued protection of the containers by the manufacturer, shipper, and user will also reduce contamination.

In the past, a chief source of contamination was the dust and debris from the cardboard boxes used to ship the empty glass and plastic containers. The manipulation of the cardboard to load and empty the glass and plastic containers generated a great deal of particulate matter (49). In recent years container manufacturers have begun wrapping their containers in a plastic film before placing them in the cardboard shipping boxes. Such packaging has been shown to reduce the particulate contamination of the containers during shipment, storage, and handling (50). Pharmaceutical users take advantage of the plastic wrap by removing the plastic wrapped containers from the cardboard boxes in an area away from the processing area and then opening the plastic wrapped containers in a clean area (37, 49).

Most particulate contamination encountered in new containers is surface contamination and relatively easy to remove, often by rinsing only. To loosen and remove the surface debris, alternating hot (preferably steam) and cold treatments are used. This thermal-shock treatment is employed to cause expansion and contraction and thus aid in loosening debris that may be adhering to the container wall. Detergents are not used with new containers to avoid the risk of leaving a detergent residue. The final water rinses of the containers must be made with high purity water to prevent pyrogens and/or particulate contamination from previous treatments being transferred to the final container. A final cleaning cycle treatment is sometimes a blast of clean air to force out any remaining water from the container (51). In some instances production cleaning processes have been designed to clean containers simply by a blast of clean air (52). Plastic ophthalmic containers and plastic wrapped containers have been successfully cleaned in this manner. The argument made for air-only cleaning is that wetting certain particulate contamination causes the contamination to cling more tenaciously to the container walls.

Optional washing pre-treatments have been explored over the years and have been adopted by some users. Ultrasonic techniques in glassware cleaning utilizes the physical action of cavitation to remove dirt and debris (both inside and outside at the same time) from glassware immersed in the cleaning medium. Ultrasonic energy transmitted in a liquid creates pressure alternations tearing microscopic holes in the liquid and then forcing them to collapse. This process is called cavitation. The cleaning occurs when effective cavitation in a liquid comes in contact with "dirt" on the glass surface.

Ultrasonic cleaning requires that the containers be totally immersed open end up. Once ultrasonically cleaned the "dirty" liquid must be separated from the container surfaces by rinsing. The ultrasonic treatment thus requires a more complex and expensive equipment installation. Large scale implementation of ultrasonic pretreatment has not taken place in the pharmaceutical industry (53).

Another aid in the washing of glass containers that has been implemented by some is an ammonium bifluoride rinse. With this washing technique, the inner container surfaces are flushed with a 0.5% to 5.0% ammonium bifluoride solution for one second at room temperature. The glass surfaces are allowed to remain wet for an additional 30 seconds prior to rinsing with water. This interval allows time for the acid to attack and actually dissolve a thin surface layer of the glass. When rinsed with water the dissolved glass layer is removed carrying away the particulate matter adhering to it (54). This type of fluoride treatment was initially reported to also improve the chemical resistance of Type I glass equivalent to a good sulfur treatment (37). However, recent studies have reported that the level of particulate contamination after fluoride treatment was not significantly better than the standard water wash (55) and that sulfur treatments produced a better chemical resistance than the fluoride treatment (10).

The container washing process of a parenteral product manufacturing system has also been studied as a possible site of treatment to further enhance other properties of the container. Feldsine et al. reported that washing techniques are an acceptable alternative to dry heat depyrogenation procedures and that such techniques can be validated (56). Depyrogenation of containers during the washing stage utilizing caustic solutions (57) or hydrogen peroxide solutions (58) is also conceivable. However, the use of these agents would require extensive depyrogenation validation and lack of residuals validation. Compatibility and stability studies would also have to be investigated following such chemical treatment (57).

In some cases the washing step has been used to apply a coating of medical grade silicone to the interior surfaces of glass vials. The main purpose of such action is to make the interior surfaces water repellent and thereby allow for a more complete emptying of the contents (37, 52, 59) and for the smooth operation of pre-filled syringes (60). A few years earlier, there was some thought that siliconization of the glass surface might increase its chemical resistance. However, studies showed no improvement in long term chemical resistance. The explanation offered was that the silicone coating is not a continuous coating thus allowing water to get through the silicone coat to the glass surface. At the surface the water produces a weak alkaline solution which eventually destroys the silicone (28).

5. Washing Machines

A variety of machines are available to carry out the cleaning of final containers. The selection and use of a particular machine will be determined largely by the physical type of the container, level of contamination, and the number of containers to be processed in a given period of time. Certain characteristics are required in any cleaning machine selected.

> The liquid or air treatment must be introduced in such a manner that it will strike the bottom of the inside of the inverted container, spread in all directions, and smoothly flow down the walls and out the opening with a sweeping action.
>
> The pressure of the jet stream should be such that there is minimal splashing, and the flow should be such that it can leave the container opening without accumulating and producing turbulence inside. Splashing may fail to clean all areas and turbulence may redeposit loosened debris. Therefore, direct introduction of the jet stream within the container with control of the flow of the jet stream is required.

The container must receive a concurrent outside rinse.

The cycle of treatments should provide for a planned sequence with alteration of very hot and cool treatments. The final treatment should be an effective rinse with good quality, filtered, distilled water followed by an optional clean air blast.

All metal parts coming in contact with the containers and with the treatments should be constructed of stainless steel or some other non-corroding and noncontaminating material. (61)

Container washing machines can be divided into two categories: batch processing and continuous processing. In a batch type of operation the containers are hand loaded into the washer, machine washed, removed from the washer by hand, loaded into metal trays, and then sterilized. In a continuous washer the containers are bulk fed by hand into the washer. The washer then aligns, washes, and discharges the containers automatically and continuously. In many instances the continuous washing machine is connected directly to and continuously feeds continuous sterilizing tunnel. The tunnel in turn is connected directly to the filling line in the aseptic filling room.

The batch operation has the advantage of being flexible. Containers for batch 1 can be sterilized while containers for batch 2 are being washed. In a continuous operation only one batch of containers can be processed at a time. A batch operation usually utilizes a batch type of sterilizer that is more compact and inexpensive than the continuous tunnels. However, the batch system exposes the container to considerable risk of particulate contamination due to

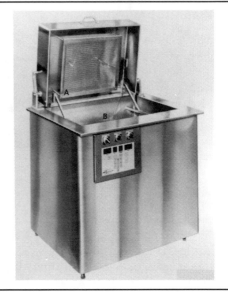

Figure 2 – A Cozzoli Ampul/Vial Washer with its cover raised to show the container hold down screen (A) and the wash nozzles (B) attached to the washing head. *(Photo courtesy of the Cozzoli Company).*

the number of handling/transfer steps involved. The continuous process, while large and expensive to install and operate, can clean large numbers of containers at a time and provide for close control of the container from start to finish, substantially reducing the particulate contamination (62).

A common batch type machine (Figure 2) for washing containers, particularly ampoules and vials, uses a stationary washing head shown in Figure 3 to which are attached an array of stainless steel, needle-like wash nozzles. Vials and ampoules are placed, inverted, into a stainless steel wash rack either by hand or by the 'dump-box' method that is illustrated in Figure 4. The wash rack is designed so that when placed in the washer each container is centered over a wash head nozzle as shown in Figure 3. For 'dump-box' loading methods washing heads are interchangeable in the machine and can be designed for various ampoule or vial sizes and to the container manufacturer's packing configuration. It is possible to wash several different sizes of containers using one wash head if the containers are loaded individually. However, this drastically reduces the overall container output rate.

Figure 3 — Metromatic Washer Wash Head. The array of wash nozzles is shown filled with vials. *(Photo courtesy of the Metromatic Company).*

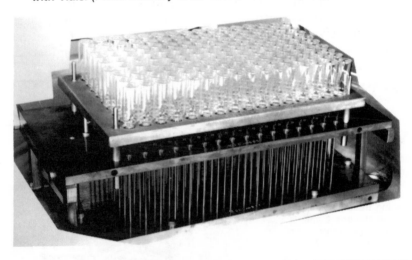

In the wash operation the alternating treatments of air, steam or water are forced under pressure through the nozzles and into the inverted containers. A stainless steel hold down screen, shown in Figure 2, adjustable to the various container sizes, prevents containers from being blown off the nozzles during the washing operation. In general, a cycle of treatments is applied to produce the

Figure 4 – Dump-box loading method.

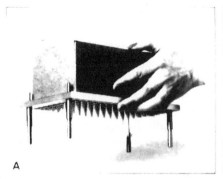 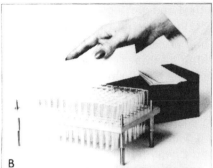

A   B

A – The loading rack and the box of ampuls are inverted. The ampuls fall into the rack, which holds the ampuls at the shoulder.
B – The ampul box and divider strips are removed, leaving the ampuls in the rack ready to be placed in to the washer.
(Photo courtesy of the Cozzoli Company).

thermal-shock that was discussed earlier. A typical wash cycle is listed in Table VIII. The actual cycle and duration of treatments will depend on the container condition and the desires of the manufacturer. Washing machines can be set up to treat containers with detergent, to deliver an application of ammonium bifluoride, to rinse plastic bottles with hydrogen peroxide, and to apply a coating of silicone. Washing machines can also be set up to use compressed air only to clean such items as plastic bottles and ophthalmic ointment tubes.

Figure 5 – The Calumatic washing machine rotating column assembly.

A – Container feed turntable
B – Containers entering the washer at station 1
C – Inverted containers at station 2
D – Cleaning treatments applied between stations 2 and 11
E – Upright containers are discharged at station 12

(Photo courtesy of the Calumatic Company).

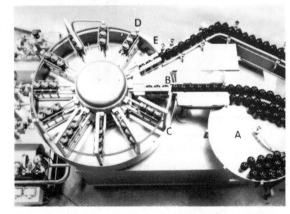

When the wash cycle is finished the washing machine lid is opened and the washed containers in their rack are placed into a covvered metal tray for sterilization.

For higher rates of output in a batch process or for incorporation into all in-line continuous washing-sterilizing-filling-sealing process, continuous washing machines are available. These machines operate in either a rotary or a conveyer belt fashion.

The operation of the Calumatic vial washer (Figure 5) is based on an intermittently rotating central column with 12 vial holders. Each vial holder can accommodate up to 9 vials depending on the diameter of the vials. Each vial holder passes intermittently through each treatment station in 12 steps.

Figure 5 shows that the vials are fed in single file from the feed turntable (A) into the vial holder at the first station (B). During the move from the first station to the second, the vial holder is rotated so that the vials are inverted (C). Between the second and 11th station (D) the cleaning treatments are applied. The vials are cleaned by rinsing inside and out with different treatment media and with blasts of air. During the move to the last station the vials are returned to their original upright position and discharged (E) from the washing machine.

Figure 6—The Strunck rotary washing machine cleaning assembly

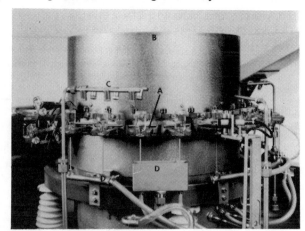

A—Container grippers
B—Central rotating column
C—External wash nozzles
D—Internal wash nozzles
(Photo courtesy of the Robert Bosch Corporation).

In the Strunck rotary washing machines containers are fed upright directly into the machine from a feed turntable or an inclined feed chute. The containers are serially indexed and each container is picked up by a gripper. As shown in Figure 6, the cam controlled grippers (A), mounted on a central rotating column (B), invert the containers and pass each container through the external (C) and the internal (D) cleaning stations. At the individual stations, spray nozzles moving in synchronism with the container enter the containers for a controlled treatment. The gripper/container alignment is maintained from the start to the finsh of a cleaning station. Cleaning tations may deliver internal and external sprays of fresh water, blasts of air, sprays of recirculated cleaner or water, and silicone treatment. After cleaning the grippers turn the containers upright and the containers are discharged.

Figure 7—The Strunck RUR Type rotary washing machine

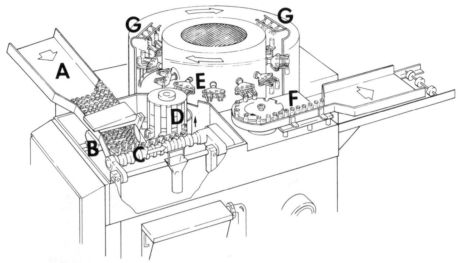

A—Feed chute
B—Ultrasonic bath
C—Indexing screw
D—Lifting device for removing the containers out of the ultrasonic bath
E—Container grippers
F—Container discharge assembly
G—Wash stations
(Drawing courtesy of the Robert Bosch Corporation).

The Strunck RUR machine (Figure 7) utilizes an ultrasonic bath to pretreat containers. Containers are fed into the machine via an inclined feed chute (A), are filled with water, submerged and treated with ultrasound (B). The containers are then serially indexed by a screw assembly (C), lifted out of the bath (D), picked up by the grippers (E), and passed on to the rinsing system as described above. After cleaning, the gripper turn the containers upright and the containers are discharged via a star-wheel device (F).

The conveyer belt type of washer handles large numbers of containers in rows. The number of containers that can be handled per row depends on the width of the conveyer and the diameter of the containers.

In operation, the machine operator places containers to be cleaned into the feed station where the containers are advanced through a guide plate via a wide conveyer (Figure 8). Some conveyer type washing machines can be adapted to give the containers an ultrasonic pre-treatment at the feed station. A schematic representation of a conveyer washing machine is shown in Figure 9. The container feed station (A) advances the containers which are then automatically picked up and inverted row-wise from the feed conveyer and placed into container transport devices attached to another wide conveyer (B). The row of containers is then advanced step-wise (C) through the various cleaning treatments. The cleaning treatments are administered through stainless steel nozzles positioned above the containers (G) or inserted into the containers at each treatment step (F). Depending on the machine, up to 12 treatment steps are available, which may be used in any way for inside/outside sprays and drip off steps. The duration of each treatment step can be adjusted within the limits of a few seconds, usually 2–10 seconds. Siliconization of the containers is usually an available option with these machines. The Cozzoli AW9 washing machine features a unique pre-cleaning system that utilizes a combination or air and vacuum. The containers are inverted and indexed through two air/vacuum cleaning stations. At these stations, noz-

Figure 8—Cozzoli Vial Washing Machine

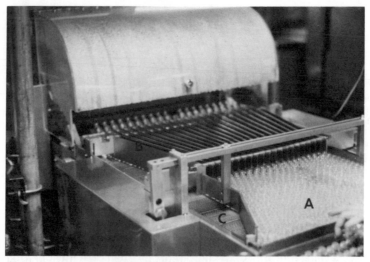

A—Hand loading of the vials into the feed conveyor
B—Vial guide plates directing the vials toward the automatic pickup site
C—Container transport conveyor

zles enter the container and blow air to loosen dirt. Simultaneously, the container is subjected to a vacuum at the container opening. The treatment is to remove paperboard matter which, when wet, clings very tenaciously to container surfaces. The container is then subjected to conventional rinsing (62).

Once the containers have been through the cleaning cycle, they are discharged row-wise from the washing machine in their original upright position. For a totally continuous process the discharge from the washing machine can be connected directly to the feed station of a tunnel sterilizer.

Figure 9—Schematic diagram of a conveyor type washing machine

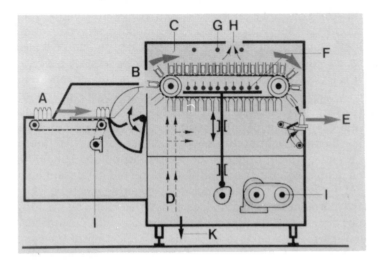

A—Container feed station
B—Automatic container transfer from the feed station to the container transport devices
C—Cleaning treatment area
D—Cleaning treatment media connections
E—Container discharge port
F—Internal wash nozzles
G—External wash nozzles
H—Air exhaust
I—Conveyor drive unit
(Drawing courtesy of Gilowy GmbH).

Once a container has been thoroughly cleaned care must be taken to keep it clean. Containers being transferred from the washer to the sterilizing tunnel must have laminar flow protection to keep the containers from being recontaminated. If the washer is used in a batch operation, then the entire discharge and sterilization staging area where the containers are placed into trays prior to sterilization must be under laminar flow protection.

The final rinse of a container must be made with a very high quality water. Water for Injection (WFI) is to be used (63, 64). Water for Injection is very expensive to produce and if only fresh WFI were used for all water input in a washing machine the consumption of water would be high and therefore expensive. To lower operating expenses, WFI is used for the final rinse only, collected at the drainage from that step and recycled through filters to be used in the initial container rinses.

When WFI is used, the United States Current Good Manufacturing Practices (CGMP) require that certain measures be taken to maintain the quality of WFI. For example, pipelines must be welded stainless steel and equipped for steam sterilization. Sanitary stainless steel fittings are required for areas in need of service disassembly. In addition WFI must be stored at a temperature of at least 80°C and be dumped to drain every 24 hours. The WFI used for final rinsing must be sampled and tested at least once every 24 hours.

With the CGMP requirements for WFI handling, a container washing machine should have certain characteristics. The washing machine should have an all stainless steel construction. The pipelines to the various treatment nozzles should not be threaded and all pipelines should be properly sloped for complete drainage during machine shutdown. Pressure gauges and flow meters are required on each treatment line and the recirculating tank should have a thermometer and heaters. Sanitary sampling ports should be present on each treatment line. Safety switches that shut down the washing machine when pressure is lost on any treatment line should also be installed (58). The washing machine should also be so designed so that the treatment nozzles, container transport devices, and other moving parts do not damage each other or the container and thereby create more particulate contamination than the washer eliminates (37).

Table VIII—A Typical Wash Cycle for the Cleaning of Glass in a Batch Type Washing Machine

Wash Step (1 minute duration)	Medium	Application
1	Hot, filtered, pyrogen-free water	Inside wash
2	Hot, filtered, pyrogen-free water	Outside wash
3	Filtered air	Inside wash
4	Hot, filtered, pyrogen-free water	Inside wash
5	Hot, filtered, pyrogen-free water	Outside wash
6	Filtered air	Inside wash
7	Hot, filtered, pyrogen-free water	Inside wash
8	Filtered air	Inside wash
9	Filtered air	Inside wash

The final rinse of the container with WFI is to prevent pyrogens and or particulate matter from previous treatments being transferred to the final product. In a recent Danish study, six vial washing machines were investigated to assess the efficiency of their final rinses. Fluorescein-sodium, monitored spectrophotometrically, was used as a tracer compound in the water of the initial container rinses of the washing machines. How well the final rinse removed the tracer compound from the vial served as a measure of rinse efficiency. A Coulter Counter was used to monitor the particulate contamination of the vial treated. Results of the study showed differences in rinsing efficiencies between washing machines and showed a correlation between the rinsing efficiency and the level of particulate contamination found (65).

The above study points out that as with any pharmaceutical process the container washing step must be under control and validated. Perhaps the hardest portion of validating a washing process is to define what "clean" and "particulate-free" means as well as to establish the detection and measurement methodology so as to develop them into acceptable and workable quality control standards. Particulate matter has been the subject of much discussion for many years but in recent years the science of particulate detection has improved dramatically (66–70) and the USP/NF has attempted to specify minimum acceptable particulate levels in large volume and small volume parenteral solutions (71). One can also have the complication of having to test for the presence of residual chemicals from such optional treatments as detergent washes, silicone treatments, and fluoride flushes. Once acceptable standards have been established the wash cycle can be validated.

The washing machine should first be checked to see that it conforms to all CGMP and WFI plumbing requirements and that the machine performs mechanically as it was designed to. The machine must be equipped to periodically monitor, check, test, and calibrate those parameters critical to its operation (72). The machine must also have those safety devices built in and working that prevent further processing should a malfunction occur in a critical processing parameter or actually prevent accidental contamination from occurring, such as opening the lid of a batch washer during the washing cycle. The machine must also be checked for appropriate design. The equipment must be designed so as to keep different treatment media separate so as not to contaminate other treatment steps. Auxiliary devices, such as water and air filter devices, must also be check to see that they are validated for the purposes that they are being used. With the washer fully inspected and qualified, the various critical operational parameters can be established and proven to provide containers that consistently meet the quality control standards for a 'clean' container. Once the validation has been performed a routine periodic inspection and testing program of the critical operating parameters will help to maintain a washing process that is under control and producing a clean container ready for sterilization and depyrogenation.

6. Sterilization

Sterilization has been defined as the process or act of inactivating or killing all forms of life, especially microorganisms (73). The state of sterility is an absolute, for there are no degrees of sterility. Determination of this state in parenteral products in the pharmaceutical industry has in the past relied on official compendial sterility tests (74). However, these are end product tests and have been shown to suffer from a great many insufficiencies (75, 76). Even if the sterility test were assured of detecting any microorganisms present, there are problems associated with the probability of detection based on the statistics of sampling.

Because of the difficulties in determining the state of sterility, the process of sterilization has become operationally defined as a probability function rather than as a method of achieving the absolute state of sterility (77). Regardless of the type of sterilization process (heat, chemical, or radiation), microorganisms, when exposed to lethal levels of such treatments, will die in an approximate logarithmic relationship between the population of the surviving cells and the treatment exposure. Using the knowledge that bacterial death occurs in an approximate logarithmic fashion, mathematical treatments have been devised which make it possible to calculate the probability of having a non-sterile unit in a given batch of product having been exposed to a given sterilization treatment (78-80). In addition, it is possible by these methods to compare the relative efficacies of various sterilization treatments.

Processing a container to render it sterile can be handled in any one of a number of methods. The choice of method employed is based, in part, on the compatibility of the sterilizing method with the container. The sterilizing methods employed are steam, dry heat, ethylene oxide gas (ETO), ultraviolet light, ionizing radiation from Cobalt-60 or electron accelerators.

A. Moist heat sterilization

Sterilization by the application of heat is recognized to be the oldest agent of bacterial destruction known (81). Sterilization by moist heat or steam sterilization is one of the most widely used methods of bacterial destruction. All living organisms can be killed by exposure to moist heat given an adequate amount of exposure. Sterilization of bacterial cells and spores by heat is generally held to be due to the denaturation of critical protein or nuclear material in the cell (82).

Steam sterilization utilizes saturated steam under pressure, usually 15 psig which results in a temperature of 121°C(250°F). The effectiveness of saturated steam is due to the instant condensation and transfer of the latent heat of vaporization when the steam contacts a cooler body. As long as the steam pressure is maintained, condensation and heat transfer will continue until temperature equilibrium is achieved throughout the load. The effective heat is retained by the condensate, maintaining the temperature, and is the lethal agent. The condensate is an accessory factor hydrating the organisms and thus making them even more susceptible to heat. Steam at 121°F kills bacteria in 15 minutes. At 134°C steam kills in 3.5 minutes.

Steam is a very dependable sterilization medium when employed properly. Steam is not suitable for moisture or heat sensitive items. Sterilizing plastic containers with steam under normal conditions may deform the containers. Glass containers can be sterilized with steam but care must be taken to eliminate air from the bottles before apply the steam. Being heavier then steam, air forms layers that resist steam penetration. While steam and air will eventually mix, the mixture does not develop the same temperature characteristics of saturated steam.

Modern designs of steam autoclaves using vacuum cycles have eliminated the inefficiencies due to entrapment of air in the chamber. Recent developments in the microcomputer field have made automation and monitoring of cycles possible for very close control of sterilization processes.

Steam sterilization is a very reliable method when properly controlled. Because it is a batch oriented method, great care must be taken to minimize possible contamination in the handling of materials upon removal from the autoclave. Although sterilization cycles are not excessively long, it must be remembered that drying and cool down cycles are necessary. Steam sterilization is an inadequate method for depyrogenation as will be discussed later.

B. Dry heat sterilization

Dry heat is a less efficient sterilization medium than saturated steam because there is no latent heat of vaporization to be released. Consequently, higher temperatures and longer times are required to achieve equivalent sterilization processes. The mode of action of dry heat depends on three major factors: water content of the bacterial spores and surrounding atmosphere, temperature, and time. Several researchers in recent years have noted the importance of moisture in sterilization by dry heat (83–86). Their research shows that there is significant variability in the death characteristics of spores depending on their water content before, during, and after treatment. Lewith (87) provided data using egg albumin showing that a temperature of 56°C caused denaturation when the protein was mixed with 50% water. When no water was present, a temperature of 160–170°C was necessary to achieve the same result. Many believe that microorganisms exposed to hot dry air may dehydrate long before their temperature reaches a point at which denaturation will take place. For this reason it is thought that dry heat sterilization is an oxidation process.

Like the steam based process, heat sensitive items such as plastic containers cannot be sterilized by dry heat. Glass containers can be sterilized with dry heat and air entrapment is not a problem in this method as it is with steam. At the end of the dry heat process the containers are dry; however, the glass containers need to be cooled down prior to placing drug products into the containers.

For a more in-depth discussion concerning thermal processing the reader is directed to Chapter 4.

C. Ethylene oxide sterilization

Sterilization by ethylene oxide gas (ETO) has been used widely in the pharmaceutical industry. Ethylene oxide has been employed primarily in the sterilization of drug products, disposable plastic items, and plastic bottles. Because of the complexities involved with this method and its practical limitations (88), sterilization by ETO is used only when other methods are not acceptable.

Ethylene oxide sterilizes by chemically reacting with (alkylating) biological compounds which are vital to normal metabolism and reproduction (89–91). Processes using ETO are more complicated than steam processes with cycles depending upon temperature, exposure time, ETO concentration, and environmental humidity. Because of its explosive nature in the pure form, ETO is used as a mixture (10–12%) with an inert gas such as Freon or carbon dioxide. In addition, ETO is a toxic substance and therefore, its use demands employee training in its proper use and handling, employee exposure monitoring, and employee medical surveillance (89–93).

Sterilization with ETO does have the advantage of being able to operate effectively at temperatures of 50–60°C. These lower temperatures make the ETO process an attractive one for sterilizing plastic containers. However, when plastic container are sterilized with ETO, they require a lengthy period of time to allow the residual ETO to desorb from the container. In addition, where chloride ions are available in the plastic material, ETO can undergo hydrolysis to form the toxic compounds ethylene chlorohydrin and ethylene glycol (94–96).

D. Ionizing radiation sterilization

Sterilization by the use of ionizing radiation has become an increasingly popular method for the sterilization of materials in the past few years (7). Recent developments in the production of safe and efficient sources have resulted in greater effectiveness and economy. Ionizing radiation is commercially produced by two major sources, those producing gamma rays and electron accelerators.

Gamma rays produce high energy electron upon striking the material to be sterilized primarily by a process known as Compton scattering (98). Compton scattering produces secondary electron, or delta rays with energies approaching 1.25 MeV. Ionization effects produced by these electrons can be severe since most chemical bonds can be altered at energies less than 10eV.

Electron acceleration produces high energy electron external to the product which lose energy primarily by ionization of molecules. In both cases, the secondary electrons produce most of the chemical changes and therefore, destruction of the molecules.

Two main theories are currently held for the bactericidal action of ionizing radiation:

1. Direct destruction of a vital molecule.
2. Indirect effects due to the action of chemical compounds formed by the radiation (99–100).

Literature reviews by Ginoza (101) and Howard-Flanders (102, 103) support the theory that DNA is the primary target for direct inactivation by ionizing radiation. The indirect effects of ionizing are thought to be the result of the hydrogen peroxide and the hydroperoxyl radical decomposition products of water (100, 104).

Gamma radiation emitted by the decay of ^{60}Co is the predominant method of ionizing radiation today (105). Most gamma radiation facilities are relatively large and provide services on a contract basis. The large size of these installations is necessitated by the intensity of radiation emitted by ^{60}Co and the need for shielding to protect personnel.

Electron accelerators are of two main types, Van de Graf generators and linear accelerators. The Van de Graf generators generate electrons by a mechanical belt or by a series of transformers and rectifiers producing very high voltages.

Linear accelerators produce electrons in a cylindrical acceleration chamber in which electrodes are fed with a voltage of very high frequency, typically by a microwave generator. The beam produced is very narrow, usually only a centimeter in width. The power of this beam is extremely concentrated and results in a dosage rate several thousand times greater than in a gamma irradiation facility (106).

While electron accelerators can process only a narrow range of small articles, it can offer several advantages over ^{60}Co sources. Lower material damage has been reported (107–109) because of the relatively short exposure time. Doses can be varied quite easily and can be carefully controlled. Electron accelerators have a very short turnaround time. Accelerators can be turned off at will without a continuous radiation danger. Gamma radiation however, remains the method of choice for heat sensitive or dense objects.

Historically, a dose of 2.5 Mrad was specified to assure product sterility (110). The rad is a measure of energy absorbed and is equal to 100 ergs absorbed per gram. This level has been reduced to a lower level for many materials depending on their relative bioburdens, uses, and physical characteristics (110).

E. Ultraviolet radiation sterilization

The ultraviolet region of the electromagnetic spectrum contains the wavelengths of interest in the sterilization of microorganisms by non-ionizing radiation. The region of wavelengths from 200 to 3100 angstroms is commonly referred to as the "abiotic region." Radiations of these wavelengths injure or kill cells easily. Because of the relatively low energies, UV radiation merely causes excitation of atoms rather than ionization by raising electrons to a higher state without removing them.

Nucleic acids are thought to be the most important absorbers of UV in cells (111, 112). All nucleic acids are aromatic and show high UV absorptivity. These compounds absorb 10 to 20 times more than an equal weight of protein. Furthermore, the alteration of a single nucleic acid, and therefore gene, may cause death or mutation in a bacteria (113). Ultraviolet induced photodimerization of thymine, a pyrimidine base found in DNA molecules, has been specifically linked to cellular inactivation (114–116).

Because of the relatively low energies involved, UV radiation does not readily penetrate most materials. Even ordinary glass in thicknesses of 1 mm or more is practically opaque to ultraviolet radiation. Due to its low penetration abilities, the use of ultraviolet light for the purpose of sterilization and disinfection has been limited to three main areas; the disinfection of air (116–119), water (112, 120, 121), and surfaces (122, 123). Because of the problems associated with assuring adequate doses of radiation for the large areas and volumes involved, most UV installations do not attempt to achieve complete sterilization, but only a reduction in the number of organisms present.

7. Sterilization and Depyrogenation of Glass

For the purposes of this chapter, we need only be concerned to know that pyrogens from bacterial sources are of primary concern to the pharmaceutical industry and that the primary source of bacterial pyrogens are gram negative bacilli. The pyrogen produced by these organisms are known as endotoxins and have been shown to originate in the cell wall of the bacteria (124). These bacterial endotoxins are very resistant to inactivation by chemical and physical means. Therefore, the production of pyrogen free parenteral products rely very heavily on preventing pyrogenic contamination. Rigid cleanliness and aseptic handling procedures are of the utmost importance. While exposure to such agents as acids, bases, and oxidizing agents have all proven to produce a pyrogen free surface, dry heat has traditionally been used to depyrogenate glassware and metal equipment. In general, the application of dry heat at not less than 250°C for not less than 30 minutes is the standard operating procedure for the pharmaceutical industry (125). Because the dry heat depyrogenation temperature is higher than that required for sterilization, the major use of dry heat in the pharmaceutical industry is for combined sterilization/depyrogenation processes. Glass containers that are to be aseptically filled are routinely treated in this manner.

The pharmaceutical industry has found that glassware received from their glassware vendors is free of detectable levels of endotoxin (120). Reports have also demonstrated that native endotoxins in the form of intact microorganisms can be removed from glassware by washing (126). Therefore, dry heat sterilization and depyrogenation is probably not necessary but used only as a precaution against some post-manufacture contamination occurring in an uncontrolled environment.

In general, the batch manufacture of a parenteral product requires that the glass containers, after washing, be packaged into stainless steel boxes and then loaded onto portable racks or carts. The loaded racks are then placed into a dry heat sterilizing oven where the entire load of glass containers are exposed to high temperatures (180° to 350°C) for a given period of time. Following a cool down period, the racks are removed from the opposite side of the oven which is in a clean room area. The loading and unloading of a batch sterilizer is manual. While the use of batch sterilizers is highly flexible, a large amount of sterile storage area is required to hold the sterile containers until used. Lengthy holding times combined with manual manipulations increased the chances of container contamination.

One type of batch sterilizer oven is referred to as a gravity convection oven. In this type of oven, air is circulated in accordance with the existing temperature differences in different portions of the oven. Heated air is less dense and rises while cooler air descends in the oven. The cooler air is then heated by the heating elements and begins to rise. This heating, cooling, and reheating of the air establishes convection air movement within the oven.

Gravity convection ovens heat the load very slowly and irregularly. A serious problem that develops is that of air stratification resulting in temperature variations in the oven and oven loads.

The other type of batch dry heat sterilizing oven is the mechanical convection or forced-air ovens. This type of oven is equipped with a motor-driven blower to mechanically circulate the air inside the oven. In such ovens the air velocity, the circulation direction, and the heat intensity can be controlled to produce a uniform temperature in the oven. The forced circulation also gives a faster heat-up and cool-down of the load in the oven resulting in shortened cycle times. Forced circulation also allows for larger and more compact loads.

Because glass containers are being sterilized and depyrogenated in these ovens, the design and construction of the ovens must be such as to seal the load from contaminants and be able to maintain cleanliness.

While forced circulation results in a more efficient oven, it also creates an area of concern in its operation. Insufficient air circulation within the oven defeats the design of the oven. Therefore, load arrangements in the oven must allow for proper circulation. The blower responsible for the forced circulation must be properly installed, operated, and maintained. In addition the air baffles that help direct and distribute the air around the oven and heaters must be properly maintained.

Ventilation fans must be properly sized, operated, and maintained. Proper ventilation aids the process cycle in several ways. Ventilation removes the humidity that builds up from wet the containers and decreases the heat-up time. The ventilation process maintains a slight positive pressure that helps prevent contamination from entering the oven. Ventilation can also aid in the elimination of air borne particulates from the interior of the oven. Of course all of the air circulation; the intake, re-circulation, and exhaust must be done through HEPA (High Efficiency Particulate Air) filters (127).

A more recent and popular means of achieving dry heat sterilization and depyrogenation of glass containers is the use of a continuous process hot air

Figure 10 – Strunck Tunnel Sterilizer *(Photo courtesy of Robert Bosch Corporation).*

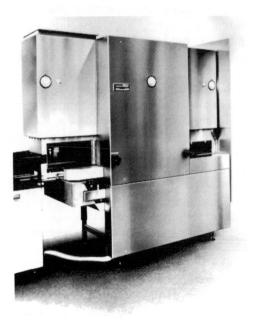

"tunnel". The containers are fed into the sterilizer directly from a washing machine. The junction between the washer and the sterilizer is protected by HEPA filtered laminar flow air. When the containers are discharged from the washer they are relatively particulate free and the laminar flow air gives protection against the containers becoming contaminated (128). As the containers travel through a tunnel on a continuously moving metal conveyer belt, they are heated to sterilizing and depyrogenation temperature (250–350°C), held at temperature for a given time, cooled down with air, and discharged into an aseptic filling area. Depending on the temperature used, the cycle time for an individual container can be as long as 45 minutes (129, 130). While the introduction of the continuous tunnel sterilizers offered a great many processing advantages, early tunnels generated particulate contamination due to bottle breakage, conveyer belt rub-off, oxidation of the heating elements, filter breakdown, gasket deterioration, and long cycle times (129, 131).

    Modern continuous tunnel sterilizers have been designed to both generate sterilization and depyrogenation temperatures and to maintain a clean en-

Figure 11—Schematic representation of the laminar air flow in a Strunck sterilizing tunnel

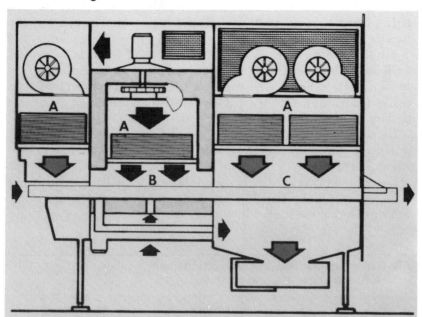

A—Laminar flow HEPA filters
B—Heating zone
C—Container cool down zone
(Drawing courtesy of the Robert Bosch Corporation).

vironment. One of the modern tunnels (Figure 10) has been designed to utilize the laminar flow (LF) technology that achieved good particulate control at normal temperatures in aseptic production areas. Figure 11 schematically illustrates the LF design. The sterilizing medium is HEPA filtered, laminar flow, high temperature air. The containers travel through the tunnel from left to right under HEPA filters (A). Air is heated and forced through the HEPA filters in a vertical downward direction (B). This hot laminar flow air stream not only helps prevent particulate contamination but also serves as a means of more efficient heat transfer. Because of the more efficient heat transfer the cycle time is reduced by being able to rapidly heat the containers to a high sterilization temperature of 350°C (which shortens the required hold time) and then to rapidly cool them to ambient temperatures (C). Another modern tunnel design has been termed a counter-flow radiant heat tunnel (132). The tunnel, shown in Figure 12 with an attached washing machine, is illustrated schematically in Figure 13. The counter-flow tunnel uses radiant heaters (C) located above and below the conveyer belt (A). These heaters are usually spiral wound nickel chrome elements enclosed in quartz envelopes to help prevent particulate shedding. Unlike the LF convection tunnels described above, the counter-flow tunnels do not have HEPA filtered air originating in the heating zone. The counter-flow tunnels use the HEPA-filtered (E) air from the cool zone (4) to generate a flow of clean air in the heating zones (2, 3). Using a system of air curtains and exhaust fans, a horizontal laminar flow of clean air moving towards the inlet of the tunnel (counter-flow) is achieved. Underberg et al. (132) found the counter-flow tunnel to be easier and more energy efficient to operate than the LF type tunnels while maintaining a Class 100 environment in the tunnel (129, 132).

The containers are cooled prior to being discharged from the tunnel. Containers exit the sterilization heating zone (2,3) into a cooling zone(4). The cooling zone uses HEPA filtered laminar flow air to maintain a Class 100 environment. The containers are gradually cooled through a combination of air velocity and mixing a percent of recirculated and fresh air. Once cooled the containers are discharged out of the tunnel into a sterile room and onto a packaging line.

Figure 12 – Gilowy tunnel sterilizer with attached vial washer.
(Photo courtesy of Gilowy GmbH).

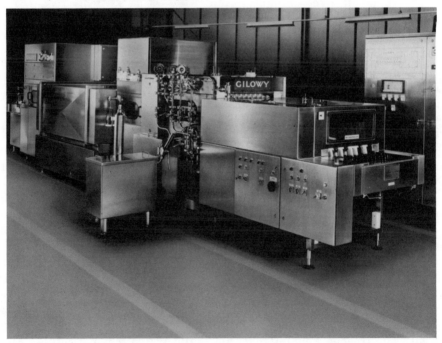

Figure 13—Schematic illustration of the Gilowy tunnel sterilizer.

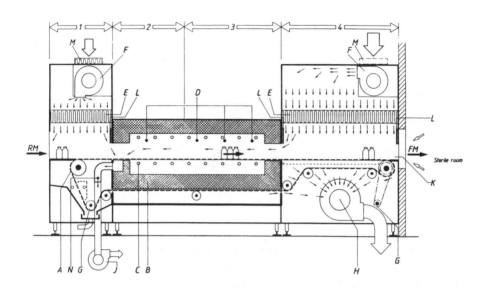

1—Feed zone
2—Heating zone
3—Sterilizing zone
4—Cooling zone
A—Conveyor belt
B—Heat insulation
C—Heating elements
D—Temperature sensors
E—HEPA filters

F—Air intake blower
G—Conveyor drive assembly
H—Exhaust fan
J—Moist air exhaust
K—Container discharge
L—Bafffles
M—Prefilters
N—Air balance sensor
RM—Preceding washing machine
FM—To filling machine

(Drawing courtesy of Gilowy GmbH).

Manufacturers of continuous depyrogenation tunnels include:

Strunck

Robert Bosch Corporation
121 Corporate Boulevard
South Plainfield, NJ 07080, USA

Cozzoli

Cozzoli Machine Company
401 East Third Street
Plainfield, NJ 07060, USA

Bausch and Strobel

PharmaSystems, Inc.
87 Midland Avenue
Montclair, NJ 07042, USA

Gilowy

Gilowy GmbH and Co.
Bussardstrasse 5
Postfach 2108
D-6078 Neu-Isenburg 2
West Germany

As mentioned earlier, both types of tunnel sterilizers are designed to supply dry heat energy in a Class 100 environment to produce parenteral glass containers that are sterile, free of pyrogens , and free of particulate contamination. In order to achieve such processing results, careful attention must to paid to numerous parameters. The Parenteral Drug Association (PDA) Technical Report No. 3 suggests that the following operational systems be checked for proper operation:

Electrical Logic–Ensure that each step is in the correct sequence
and that it is repeatable.

Cycle Set Point Adjustability–Verify limit switch sequencing.

Door Interlocks–Must work correctly, not allowing access during the
cycle.

Gasket Integrity–Check for positive/negative pressure seal of all
door gaskets.

Vibration Analysis–Check blowers for correct dynamic balancing to
minimize vibration.

Air Balance Ability–Check that baffle/linkage mechanisms can be
actuated and adjusted for balance.

Blower Rotation–Check that blowers rotate in the specified direction.

Blower RMP–Verify that the correct blower RPM is achieved.

Heater Elements–Check that all heater elements operate.

Air balance—Check that the pressure balance is positive from the sterile core to the preparation area through the tunnel.

HEPA Filters—Verify integrity of filters.

Heat Shields—Verify that all heat shields are correctly installed (radiant heat sources).

Belt Speed—Check that belt speed and belt speed recorded operate correctly (133).

Although the dry heat tunnel has become the common method of processing glass vials, dry heat sterilization and depyrogenation does pose difficulties. High temperature hot air as a sterilizing medium requires considerable time and energy for treatment cycles and it necessitates significant cool down times before the vials can be filled. It is not unusual for the processing time for an individual vial to approach 45 minutes.

Due to the relatively high speed of modern filling equipment, large numbers of containers must be washed, sterilized, and depyrogenated in advance to maintain a constant supply for the filling lines. Containers sitting open for a period of time are subject to particulate contamination. Hence, space in clean room areas is needed to store the treated containers while they are waiting to be filled.

While particulate control in the tunnels has been significantly improved the potential for particulate contamination still exists. Glass containers still rub, jostle, and bump each other, producing glass particulates. HEPA filters and electrical elements can still degrade in the hot air medium furnishing another source of particulate contamination.

Tunnels require a high capital investment and their use increases the complexity of the entire manufacturing system. The use of a tunnel system usually results in a lack of flexibility. Generally tunnels require large batch sizes. While it is possible to run small batches of containers through a tunnel, the amount of time and effort needed to initiate tunnel operation from one run to another makes it unattractive to run small batches or to use the tunnel to process a variety of different container types and sizes.

Once proper functioning of the tunnel sterilizer can be verified the validation process can continue. Validation studies conducted on dry heat sterilizers (batch and continuous) can be divided into two components. One component encompasses all of the physical processes which must be validated such as temperature control, particulate levels, and belt speeds. The second component is biological and involves studies that prove the provess destroys both microbial and pyrogenic contaminants. A number of excellent reports can be found in the literature which detail dry heat sterilization validation (129, 133-135).

8. Sterilization Processes for Plastic Containers

Plastic containers for ophthalmic use are usually washed in the same manner as glass. However, plastic containers do have some limitation that creates a difficulty in terms of sterilization. Specifically, many plastics cannot withstand the conditions imposed by the common methods of sterilization. In general plastics cannot survive the temperatures of dry heat sterilization. Many rigid plastic containers that one might choose for parenteral use cannot be steam sterilized, at least at the normal sterilization temperature of 121°C, without deforming. Therefore, plastic ophthalmic containers are usually sterilized with ethylene oxide (ETO). When ETO sterilization is used plastic containers require a long period of time for the residual ETO to desorb from the container. In addition, where chloride ions are available in the plastic ETO can undergo hydrolysis to the toxic ethylene chlorohydrin (94-96).

The ionizing radiation sterilization of plastic containers can have negative effects on the physical properties of the plastic. In some instances the radiation causes additional cross-linking of the polymer molecules and in other instances the radiation causes polymer chain scission. In either situation the physical properties such as impact strength, tear resistance, and elongation can change substantially from the non-irradiated plastic. Radiation can cause a color change in a number of different plastics. The change in color has been attributed to the capture of electrons or free radicals in the polymer crystal structure. Because polyvinylchloride (PVC) is very sensitive to radiation-induced color changes it is used as a radiation dosimeter (136-138). Because of these and other difficulties and shortcomings of current container sterilization processes, scientists continue to investigate the possibilities for increasing the speed of sterilization, decreasing the energy usage for sterilization, increasing the sterility assurance of the entire aseptic process and to find new container materials, or to eliminate problem areas such as ETO.

New technology and research is constantly being applied to stabilize many polymers that were previously sensitive to the different methods of sterilization. Additives are now available for PVC and polypropylene that enable them to be sterilized by radiation without discoloration and a recent publication reported the results of a study which investigated the hot-water and steam sterilization resistance of a series of new polymers (139).

With the exception of water and air, ultraviolet radiation is not considered to be a penetrating radiation; there, UV sterilization has only the limited application of disinfecting air, water, and contaminated surfaces. However, some polyethylene materials will transmit a percentage of UV radiation presented to it. Using this fact, researchers al Alcon Laboratories have devised a method of sterilizing natural low-density polyethylene containers. Validation of the UV sterilization process was accomplished in both a batch type sterilizer and a continuous conveyer sterilizer (140). The development of the UV process allowed

Alcon to eliminate the ETO sterilization of the bottles and the accompanying problems regarding ETO residuals, several ETO process control parameters, and higher costs associated with ETO use (141).

Researchers at Eli Lilly and Company demonstrated that an electromagnetic plasma produced inside a glass vial sterilized the vial in less the one second with little heating of the vial (143). The authors stated that the process itself was amenable to in-line processing, being fast, inexpensive, and energy efficient.

Using an improved version of the plasma system described by Tensmeyer et al. (142), Peeples and Anderson (143, 144) were able to demonstrate a larger and more lethal plasma at relatively lower power levels. The plasma system was shown to be an excellent agent for the sterilization of empty 10mL glass serum vials. Bacterial loads of 10^6 B. subtilis spores per vial were completely sterilized in less than 0.2 seconds. The mode of action appeared to be a combination of at least two mechanisms: the heating properties of the plasma resulting in microincineration and heat sterilization, and the large amounts of UV radiation emitted by the plasma. Although the exact extent of heating and incineration could not be determined, the amount of UV radiation generated in the germicidal wavelength region was measured and calculated to be sufficient to provide 47 log reductions of the the bacterial spores in 0.2 seconds. Vial heating in these short times was shown to be insignificant and the plasma did not seem to have any deleterious effects on the physical or chemical properties of the glass vials used.

Peeples and Anderson reported that although pyrogenic bacterial endotoxin was destroyed by the plasma, the levels destroyed were of little practical significance. The authors concluded that direct contact of the endotoxin by the plasma was probably necessary for destruction. Therefore, with higher power levels were probably necessary to provide for additional surface contact and hence sufficient depyrogenation for a commercial process (143, 144).

Plasma sterilization could possibly offer many advantages over currently used methods. Since the sterilization of individual vials can be accomplished in under one second with no significant heat build up, the process might be used immediately prior to filling, allowing for continuous on-line operation and would do away with the need for aseptic holding areas for containers waiting to be filled. The space required for this equipment would involve considerably less space than conventional tunnels. Due to the nature of the system, small batches of containers could be processed as easily as large ones. In addition, calculations by researchers at Eli Lilly estimated that plasma sterilization would consume less than 1/20 of the power used by conventional electric dry heat tunnels. Due to the low heat buildup of the container during plasma treatment, no cool down time for the vials would be required (as is required for vials emerging from a conventional tunnel) which would facilitate an on-line process.

Lohmann and Manique (145) investigated the feasibility of sterilizing glass vials by microwave heating. The investigators were able to show that a 10^{12}

spore reduction could be attained in three to four minutes with an end-point vial temperature of 160-170°C. A conventional dry heat sterilization process would require approximately 80 minutes to achieve the same spore log reduction at the same temperature. The investigators concluded that a selective heating of the spores takes place in a microwave field greatly reducing the processing time without raising the vial temperature to the high temperatures (350°C) as required in the tunnel sterilizers.

Some pharmaceutical companies will aseptically fill a parenteral product and then expose the product to a thermal, terminal sterilization process. The practice is to produce a product with the lowest possible probability of a non-sterile unit (PNSU). If we can assume that an aseptically produced product has but one chance in a thousand of having a non-sterile unit, or a PNSU of 10^{-3}, then subjecting the product to a steam sterilizing process that will provide a PNSU of at least 10^{-6} will result in the product having a PNSU of at least 10^{-9}. Aseptic processing in these cases presents to the terminal sterilization step a product with a very low bioburden of 10^{-3} per unit. This approach will work only for materials which can withstand the thermal treatment. However, using the aseptic filling process to lower the bioburden of a product might allow for the use of a thermal sterilization step for heat sensitive items or for plastic containers. If a suitable PNSU is considered to be 10^{-6}, then the steam sterilization process need only impart a lethality of 10^{-3}. Therefore, lower temperatures could be used to keep from deforming bottles or from degrading product.

Although the decrease in operating temperature would require an increase in exposure time, the lowered lethality requirements of the process might keep processing times reasonable for use.

Future research efforts may produce plastic containers that are more compatible with parenteral products. Advances have already been made in the area of plastic containers that can withstand ionizing radiation. Many medical devices made of and wrapped in plastic materials are routinely sterilized in this manner. Suppliers of radiation sterilization services are suggesting that the pharmaceutical industry evaluate sterilization by radiation (106, 146-149). To date, only limited work on drug stability after irradiation has been done (149) but the results are positive. With these advances it is well within the realm of feasibility to pursue the idea of aseptically filling a reconstitutable drug in dry form into a plastic container and then subjecting the container/drug product to a terminal sterilization of ionizing radiation. Such a process is a totally cool, dry operation that might easily produce a product with a PNSU of at least 10^{-6}.

9. References

1. Turco, S. and King, R.E., Sterile Dosage Forms: Their Preparation and Clinical Application, 2 ed., Lea and Febiger, Philadelphia, pages 37-54 (1979).

2. Lockhart, J.D. "The Medical Significance of Particulate Matter in Large Volume Parenterals," National Symposium Proceedings, Safety of Large Volume Parenteral Solutions, Washington, D.C., July 28-29, 1966.

3. Validation of Aseptic Filling for Solution Drug Products, Technical Monograph No. 2, Parenteral Drug Association, Inc. Philadelphia, pages 2-3 (1980).

4. Federal Register 43(190):45013, September 29, 1978.

5. Kesper, F. and Lietz, H., "Investigations into Reducing the Secondary Particle Contamination on Opening of Ampoules," Drugs Made Ger., 28:96 (1985).

6. Murakami, H. and Shimizer, H., "Present Status and Future Trends of Ampoule Manufacturing and Filling in Japan," Parenteral Drug Association Annual Meeting, Philadelphia, November 5, 1985.

7. Turco, S. and King R.E., Sterile Dosage Forms: Their Preparation and Clinical Application, 2nd Edition, Lea and Febiger, Philadelphia, pages 1-13 (1979).

8. Dean, D.A. and Corby, P.L., "The Packaging of Pharmaceuticals," in Banker, G.S. and Rhodes, C.T., eds., Modern Pharmaceutics, Marcel Dekker, Inc., New York, pages 627-647 (1979).

9. Avis, K.E., "Sterile Products," in Lachman, L., Lieberman, H.A. and Kanig, J.L., eds., The Theory and Practice of Industrial Pharmacy, Lea and Febiger, Philadelphia, pages 586-623 (1076).

10. Sanga, S.V., "Review of Glass Types Available for Packaging Parenteral Solutions," J. Paren. Drug Assoc., 33(2):61 (1979).

11. Shand, E.B., Glass Engineering Handbook, McGraw-Hill, New York, 1958.

12. Phillips, C.J., Glass: Its Industrial Application, Reinhold Publishing Corp., New York, pages 53-88 (1960).

13. Persson, H.R., "Improvement of the Chemical Durability of Soda-Lime-Silica Glass Bottles by Treating with Various Agents," Glass Technol., 3(1):17 (1962).

14. Mochel, E.L., Nordberg, M.E., and Elmer, T.H., "Strengthening of Glass Surfaces by Sulfur Trioxide Treatment, " J. Amer. Ceram. Soc., 49(11):585 (1966).

15. Holland, L., The Properties of Glass Surfaces, Chapman and Hall, London (1966).

16. Subrahmanyam, S.V. and Majeske, J.P., "The Stability of Packaged Pharmaceuticals as Related to Glass Chemical Durability," Amer. Jour. Pharm., July, page 222, (1957).

17. United States Pharmacopeia XXI/ National Formulary XVI, United States Pharmacopeial Convention, Inc., Rockville, MD., pages 1233-1235 (1985).

18. Glass Containers for Small Volume Parenteral Products: Factors for Selection and Test Methods for Identification, Technical Methods Bulletin No. 3, Parenteral Drug Association, Inc., Philadelphia, (1982).

19. Douglas, R.W. and Isard, J.O., "The Action of Water and of Sulfur Dioxide on Glass Surfaces," J. Soc. Glass Technol., 33:289 (1949).

20. Adams, P.B., "Surface Properties of Glass Containers for Parenteral Solutions," Bull. Parenter. Drug Assoc., 31 (5): 213 (1977).

21. Franz, H., "Durability and Corrosion of Silicate Glass Surfaces," J. Non-Cryst. Solids, 42:529 (1980).

22. Dimbleby, V., "Glass for Pharmaceutical Purposes," J. Pharm. Pharmacol., 5:969 (1953).

23. Scholze, H., "Chemical Durability of Glass," J. Non-Cryst. Solids, 52: 91 (1982).

24. McVay, G.L. and Buckwalter, C.O., "The Nature of Glass Leaching," Nucl. Technol., 51:123 (1980).

25. Doremus, R.H., "Time Dependence of the Reaction of Water with Glass," Nucl. Chem. Waste Mgmt., 2:119 (1981).

26. Roseman, T.J., Brown, J.A., and Scothorn, W.W., "Glass for Parenteral Products: A Surface View Using the Scanning Electron Microscope," J. Pharm. Sci., 65:22 (1976).

27. Scothorn, W.W., Roseman, T.J., and Hamlin, W.E., "Model Particulate Research Laboratory: I. Characterization of Glass for Parenteral Products," Bull. Parenter. Drug Assoc., 30(3):105 (1976).

28. Majeske, J.P., "Choice of Glass Packages for Parenteral Products," Bull. Parenter. Drug Assoc., 16(4):1 (1962).

29. Bacon, F.R. and Raggon, F.C., "Promotion of Attack on Glass and Silica by Citrate and Other Anions in Neutral Solution," J. Amer. Ceram. Soc., 42(4):199 (1959).

30. Dugger, D.L., "The Exchange of Twenty Metal Ions with the Weakly Acidic Silanol Group of Silica Gel, " J. Phys. Chem., 68(4):757 (1964).

31. Hudson, G.A. and Bacon F.R., "Inhibition of Alkaline Attack on Soda-Lime Glass," Ceramic Bull., 37(4):185 (1958).

32. Oka, Y. and Tomozawa, M., "Effect of Alkaline Earth Ion as an Inhibitor to Alkaline Attack on Silica Glass," J. Non-Cryst. Solids, 42:535 (1980).

33. Oka, Y., Ricker, K.S., and Tomozawa, M., "Calcium Deposition on Glass Surface as an Inhibitor to Alkaline Attack," J. Am. Ceram. Soc., 62(11-12):631 (1979).

34. Hinson, A.L., Smith, D.C., and Greene, J.F.,"Changes in Distilled Water Stored in Glass Ampuls," J. Am. Ceram. Soc., 30(7):211 (1947).

35. Stafficker, C.F., "A Comparison of Blown Bottles and Tubing Vials," Bull. Parenter. Drug Assoc., 17(5):31 (1963).

36. Boddapati, S., Butler, L.D., Im, S., and Deluca, P.P., "Identification of Subvisible Barium Sulfate Crystals in Parenteral Products," J. Pharm. Sci., 69(5):608 (1980).

37. Anschel, J., "General Guidelines for the Processing of Glass Containers for Parenteral Products," Bull. Parenter. Drug Assoc., 31(1):47 (1977).

38. Giles, R.L. and Pecina, R.W., "Plastic Packaging Materials," in Gennaro, A.R., ed., Remington's Pharmaceutical Sciences, 17th edition, Mack Publishing, Easton, PA, pages 1473-1477 (1980).

39. Billmeyer, F.W., Textbook of Polymer Science, 2nd edition, Wiley-Interscience, New York, pages 1-5, 280-327, 255-279 (1971).

40. Wang, Y.J. and Chien, Y.W., Sterile Pharmaceutical Packaging: Compatibility and Stability, Technical Report No. 5, Parenteral Drug Association, Inc., Philadelphia, 1984.

41. Autian, J., "Interrelationship of the Properties and Uses of Plastics for Parenterals," Bull. Parenter. Drug Assoc., 22:276 (1968).

42. Autian, J., "Plastic as a Container for Parenteral Solutions," National Symposium Proceedings, Safety of Large Volume Parenteral Solutions, Washington, D.C., July, 28-29, 1966.

43. Amidon, G.L., Taylor, J., and Sorkness, R., "A Convective Diffusion Model for Estimation Drug Loss to Tubing: Sorption of Vitamin A," J. Paren. Sci. Tech., 35(1):13 (1985).

44. "Stability of Drugs in Plastic Infusion Containers: A Solution to the Problem?," Pharm. Internat., 6(3):59 (1985).

45. Anderson, N.R. and Motzi, J.J., "Permeation of Preservative Through Rubber Membranes as a Basis of Predicting Loss of Preservative into Rubber Closures," J. Paren. Sci. Tech., 36(4):161 (1982).

46. DeLuca, P.P. and Papadimitriou, D., "The Application of Proposed Procedures for Testing for Extractables in Plastic Containers," J. Paren. Sci. Tech., 36(1):28 (1982).

47. Sacharow, S., "Developments in Barrier Plastic Bottles for Pharmaceutical Packaging," Pharm. Mfg., 2(2):12 (1985).

48. Endicott, C.J., Giles, R. and Pecina, R., "Particulate Matter: Its Significance, Source, Measurement, and Elimination," National Symposium Proceedings Safety of Large Volume Parenteral Solutions, Washington, D.C., July 28-29, 1966.

49. Portnoff, J.B., Harwood, R.J. , and Sunbery, E.W., "The Processing of Small Volume Parenterals and Related Sterile Products," in Avis, K.E., Lachman, L., and Lieberman, H.A., eds., Pharmaceutical Dosage Forms: Parenteral Medications, Vol. 1, Marcel Dekker, New York, pages 224-227 (1984).

50. Smith, J.C., "Component and Equipment Preparation Validation," Proceedings of the Second PMA Seminar Program on Validation of Sterile Manufacturing Processes: Aseptic Processing, Atlanta, March 1-2, 1979," Pharmaceutical Manufacturers Association, pages 97-125.

51. Avis, K.E., "Sterile Products," in Lachman, L., Lieberman, H.A., and Kanig, J.L., eds., The Theory and Practice of Industrial Pharmacy, 2nd edition, Lea and Febiger, Philadelphia, pages 602-612 (1976).

52. Pomeroy, C.G., "Development of a High-Speed Vial Filling Line," Bull Parenter. Drug Assoc., 18(4):21 (1964).

53. Hightower, F., "Ultrasonic Techniques in Glassware Cleaning," Bull. Parenter. Drug Assoc., 12(2):19 (1958).

54. Hinson, A.L., "Fluoride Washing of Glass Containers," Bull. Parenter. Drug Assoc., 25(6):266 (1971).

55. Nail, S.L., "Evaluation of the Effectiveness of Ammonium Bifluoride Treatment in the Cleaning of Parenteral Glassware by an Automatic Particle Counting Technique," J. Paren. Drug Assoc., 33(4):177 (1979).

56. Feldsine, P.T., Ferry, E.W., Gauthier, R.J., and Pisik, J.J., J. Paren. Drug Assoc., 33(3):125 (1979).

57. Depyrogenation, Technical Report No. 7, Parenteral Drug Association, Inc., Philadelphia, pages 78-92 (1985).

58. Koblis, R.J., "Key Considerations in Selecting Machinery for an Aseptic Packaging Line," Pharm. Manuf., 2(5):35 (1985).

59. Riffkin, C., "Siliconization: As Applied to Containers and Closures," Bull. Parenter. Drug Assoc., 22(2):66 (1968).

60. DeLuca, P.P., "Manufacturing Aspects of Prefilled Disposable Syringes," Bull. Parenter. Drug Assoc., 23 (1) (1969).

61. Avis, K.E., Parenteral Preparations," in Gennaro, A.R., ed., Remington's Pharmaceutical Sciences, 17th Edition, Mack Publishing, Easton, PA., pages 1530-1532 (1985).

62. Koblis, R.J., "Continuous In-Line Packaging Systems for Parenteral Products," Proceedings, Pharmacuetical Packaging Section, Interphex 80, September 15-17, 1980, New York.

63. United States Pharmacopeia XXI/National Formulary XVI, United States Pharmacopeial Convention, Inc., Rockville, MD., page 1123 (1985).

64. "Current Good Manufacturing Practice in the Manufacture, Processing, Packing, or Holding of Large Volume Parenterals," Federal Register, Tuesday, June 1, 1976, pages 22202-22218

65. Kvorning, I. and Manique, F., "Validation of Vial Washing Machines," Poster Session, Parenteral Drug Association, Annual Meeting, Philadelphia, PA., Nov. 7-9, 1984.

66. Knapp, J.Z. and Kushner, H.K., "Generalized Methodology for Evaluation of Parenteral Inspection Procedures," J. Paren. Drug Assoc., 34(1):14 (1980).

67. Knapp, J.Z. and Kushner, H.K., "Implementation and Automation of a Particle Detection System for Parenteral Products," J. Paren. Drug Assoc., 34(5):369 (1980).

68. Knapp, J.Z., Kushner, H.K., and Abramson, L.R., "Automated Particle Detection for Ampuls with Use of the Probabilistic Particulate Dection Model," J. Paren. Sci. Tech., 35(1):21 (1981).

69. Knapp, J.Z., Kushner, H.K., and Abramson, L.R., "Particulate Inspection of Parenteral Products: An Assessment," J. Paren. Sci. Tech., 35(4):176 (1981).

70. Knapp, J.Z. and Zeiss, J.C., Thompson, B.J., Crane, J.S., and Dunn, P., "Inventory and Measurement of Particles in Sealed Sterile Containers," J. Paren. Sci. Tech., 37 (5) (1983).

71. United States Pharmacopeia XXI/ National Formulary XVI, United States Pharmacopeial Convention, Inc., Rockville, MD., pages 1257-1258 (1985).

72. Fitzsimon, R., "Design Considerations for Parenteral Liquid Systems," Drug Dev. Comm., 2(1):1 (1976).

73. Beloian, A., "Methods of Testing for Sterility and Efficacy of Sterilizers, Sporicides and Sterilizing Processes," in Block, S.S., ed., Disinfection, Sterilization and Preservation, 2nd Edition, Lea and Febiger, Philadelphia, page 11 (1977).

74. United States Pharmacopeia XXI/National Formulary XVI, United States Pharmacopeial Convention, Inc., Rockville, MD., pages 1156-1160 (1985).

75. Brewer, J.H., "sterility Tests and Methods of Assuring Sterility," in Reddich, G.F., ed., Disinfectants, Fungicides, and Chemical and Physical Sterilization, Lea and Febiger, Philadelphia, page 158 (1957).

76. Ernst, R.R., West, K.L., and Doyle, J.E., "Problem Areas in Sterility Testing," Bull. Parenter. Drug Assoc., 23:29 (1969).

77. Bruch, C.W., "Levels of Sterility: Probabilities of Survivors vs. Biological Indicators," Bull. Parenter. Drug Assoc., 28(3):105 (1974).

78. Pflug, I.J., "Heat Sterilization," in Phillips, G.B. and Miller, W., eds., Industrial Sterilization, Duke University Press, Durham, NC., pages 239-281 (1972).

79. Pflug, I.J. and Bearman, J.E., "Treatment of Sterilization Process Microbial Survivor Data," in Pflug, I.J., ed., Microbiology of Sterilization Processes, Parenteral Drug Association, Philadelphia, pages 59-74 (1978).

80. "General Principles of Process Validation; Current Good Manufacturing Practice Draft Guideline", Federal Register, 18(81):13098 (March 29, 1983).

81. Ernst, R.R., "Sterilization by Heat," in Block, S.S., ed., Disinfection, Sterilization and Preservation, 2nd Edition, Lea and Febiger, Philadelphia, pages 481-521 (1977).

82. Fricke, H., Leone, C.A., and Landmann, W., "Role of Structural Degradation in the Loss of Serological Activity of Ovalbumin Irradiated with Gamma-Rays," Nature, 180:1423 (1957).

83. Hoffman, R.K., Gambill, V.M. and Buchanan, L.M., "Effect of Cell Moisture on the Thermal Inactivation Rate of Bacterial Spores," Appl. Microbiol. 16:1240 (1968).

84. Angelotti, R.J., Marganski, J.H., Butler, T.F., Peeler, J.T. and Campbell, J.E., "Influence of Spore Moisture Content on the Dry Heat Resistance of B. subtilis ," Appl. Microbiol., 16:735 (1968).

85. Murrell, W.G. and Scott, W.J., "The Heat Resistance of Bacterial Spores at Various Water Activities," J. Gen Microbiol., 43:411 (1966).

86. Marshall, B.J., Muarrell, W.G. and Scott, W.J., "The Effect of Water Activity, Solutes, and Temperature on the Viability and Heat Resistance of Freeze Dried Bacterial Spores," J. Gen. Microbiol., 31:451 (1963).

87. Lewith, S., "Veber die Ursache der Widerstandsfahigkeit der Sporen Gegen Hohe Temperaturen," Arch. Exp. Pathol. Pharmakol. 26:341 (1890).

88. Royce, A. and Bowler, C., "Ethylene Oxide Sterilization--Some Experiences and Some Practical Limitations," J. Pharm. Pharmacol., 13:87T (1961).

89. Ernst, R.R., "Ethylene Oxide Gaseous Sterilization for Industrial Applications," in Phillips, G.B. and Miller, W., eds., Industrial Sterilization, Duke University Press, Durham, NC., pages 78-99 (1972).

90. Kereluk, K. and Lloyd, R.S., "Ethylene Oxide Sterilization," J. Hosp. Res., 7:7, (1969).

91. Kereluk, K., Gammon, R.A., and Lloyd, R.J., "Microbial Aspects of Ethylene Oxide Sterilization II. Microbial Resistance to Ethylene Oxide," Appl. Microbiol., 19:152 (1970).

92. Kereluk, K., Gammon, R.A., and Lloyd, R.J., "Microbial Aspects of Ethylene Oxide Sterilization III. Effects of Humidity and Water Activity on the Sporicidal Activity of Ethylene Oxide," Appl. Microbiol., 19:152 (1970).

93. Phillips, C.R., "Relative Resistance of Bacterial Spores and Vegetative Bacteria to Disinfectants," Bacteriol. Rev., 16:135 (1952).

94. Cleary, D.J., "Residual Effects of Ethylene Oxide Sterilization," Bull. Parenter. Drug Assoc., 23(5):233 (1969).

95. Bruch, C.W., "Sterilization of Plastics: Toxicity of Ethylene Oxide Residues," in Phillips, G.B. and Miller, W., eds., Industrial Sterilization, Duke University Press, Durham, NC., pages 49-77 (1972).

96. Baan, E., "Ethylene Oxide Adsorption and Desorption of Elastomers and Plastics," Bull. Parenter. Drug Assoc., 30(6):299 (1976).

97. Sztanyik, L.B., "Application of Ionizing Radiation to Sterilization," in Gaughran, E.R.L. and Goudie, A.J., eds., Sterilization by Ionizing Radiation, Multiscience Publication, Montreal (1974).

98. Setlow, R.B. and Pollard, E.C., Molecular Biophysics, Addison Wesley Publishing, Reading, MA. (1962).

99. Lea, O.E., Actions of Radiations on Living Cells, Cambridge University Press, London (1956).

100. Hutchinson, F. and Pollard, E., "Physical Principles of Radiation Action," in Errera, M. and Forssberg, A., eds., Mechanisms in Radiobiology, Academic Press, New York (1961).

101. Ginoza, W., "The Effects of Ionizing Radiation on Nucleic Acids of Bacteriophages and Bacterial Cells," Annu. Rev. Microbiol., 21:325 (1967).

102. Howard-Flanders, P., "DNA Repair," Annu. Rev. Biochem., 37:175 (1968).

103. Howard-Flanders, P., "Genes That Control DNA Repair and Genetic Recombination in E. coli.," Adv. Biol. Med. Phys., 12:299 (1968).

104. Silverman, G.J. and Sinskey, A.J., "Sterilization by Ionizing Irradiation," in Block, S.S., ed., Disinfection, Sterilization and Preservation, 2nd Edition, Lea and Febiger, Philadelphia, pages 546-547 (1977).

105. Artandi, C.R., "Sources and Facilities for Radiation Sterilization of Medical Supplies," in Proceedings of the U.S.P. Conference on Radiation Sterilization, United States Pharmacopeial Convention, Rockville, MD., page 14 (1972).

106. Vroom, D.A., "Electron Beam Sterilization," Med. Device and Diag. Ind., 2 (11): (1980).

107. Chapiro, A., "Physical and Chemical Effects of Ionizing Radiations on Dolymeric Systems," in Gaughran, E.R.L. and Goudie, A.J., eds., Sterilization by Ionizing Radiations on Polymeric Systems, Multi-science Publications, Montreal, pages 367-374 (1974).

108. Bradbury, W.C., "Physical and Chemical Effects of Ionizing Radiation on Cellulosic Materials," in Gaughran, E.R.L. and Goudie, A.J., eds., Sterilization by Ionizing Radiations on Polymeric Systems, Multiscience Publications, Montreal, pages 387-402 (1974).

109. Plester, D.W., "The Effects of Radiation Sterilization on Plastics," in Phillips, G.B. and Miller, W., eds., Industrial Sterilization, Duke Univeristy Press, Durham, NC., pages 141-152 (1972).

110. Masefield, J., "Advances Made in Cobalt-60 Gamma Sterilization," in Gaughran, E.R.L. and Morrissey, R.F., eds., Sterilization of Medical Products, Vol. 2, Multiscience Publication, Montreal, pages 202-203 (1981).

111. Erreva, M., "Mechanism of Biological Action of Ultraviolet and Visible Radiations," in Butler, J.A.V. and Randall, J.T., eds., Progress in Biophysics, Vol. 3, Academic Press, New York, pages 88-130 (1953).

112. Huff, C.B., Smith, M.F., Boring, W.D. and Clarke, N.A., "Study of Ultraviolet Disinfection of Water and Factors in Treatment Efficiency," Public Health Report 80, pages 695-705 (1965).

113. Giese, A.C., "Ultraviolet Action Spectra in Perspective: With Special Reference to Mutation," Photochem. Photobiol., 8:527 (1968).

114. Setlow, R.B., Swenson, P.A., and Carrier, W.L., "Thymine Dimers and Inhibition of DNA Synthesis by Ultraviolet Irradiation of Cells," Science, 142:1464 (1963).

115. Setlow, R.B. and Carrier, W.L., "Pyrimidine Dimers in Ultraviolet Irradiated DNA's, J. Mol. Biol., 17:237 (1966).

116. Rubbo, S.D. and Gardner, J.F., Review of Sterilization and Disinfection, Lloyd-Luke, London, page 88 (1965).

117. Hart, D., "Bactericidal Ultraviolet Radiation in the Operating Room," J.A.M.A., 172:1019 (1960).

118. Wells, W.F. and Fair, G.M., "Viability of E. coli Exposed to Ultraviolet Radiation in Air," Science, 82:280 (1935).

119. Nagy, R., Mouromseff, G., and Rixton, F.H., "Disinfecting Air with Sterilizing Lamps," Heating, Piping, Air Condit., 26:82 (1954).

120. Cortelyon, J.R., McWhinnie, M.A., Riddiford, M.S., and Semrad, J.E., "The Effect of Ultraviolet Irradiation on Large Popluations of Certain Waterborne Bacteria in Motion," Appl. Microbiol., 2:269 (1954).

121. Luckiesh, M. and Holliday, L.L., "Disinfecting Water by Means of Germicidal Lamps," Gen. Elect. Rev., 47:45 (1944).

122. Widmer, W., "Three New Twists with Ray Lamps," Food Ind., 23:114 (1951).

123. Matelsky, I., "Germicidal Lamps in the Pharmaceutical Industry," Pharm. Int., 21:147 (1951).

124. Braun, V., "Molecular Organization of the Rigid Layer and the Cell Wall of E. coli.," in Kass, E.H. and Wolff, S.M., eds., Bacterial Lipopolysaccharides, U. of Chicago Press, Chicago, pages 1-7 (1973).

125. Depyrogenation, Technical Report No. 7, Parenteral Drug Association, Inc., Philadelphia (1985).

126. Feldsine, P.T., Ferry, E.W., Gauthier, R.S., and Pisik, J.S., "A New Concept in Glassware Depyrogenation Process Validation," J. Paren. Drug Assoc., 33(6):125 (1979).

127. Hauser, B., "How to Specify Equipment for Dry-Heat Sterilization and Drying of Pharmaceuticals," Pharm. Tech., 3(10):53 (1979).

128. Koblis, R.J., "Continuous In-Line Packaging Systems for Parenteral Products," in Interphex 80, Pharmaceutical Technology, Springfield, OR., pages 31-48 (1980).

129. Elias, T.F., Webb, B.H., and Taylor, F.D., "A Laminar Flow Approach to In-Line Vial Sterilization," Bull. Parenter. Drug Assoc., 33(1): 33 (1977).

130. Kruger, D.T. and Sirch, E., "Neues Wirtschaftliches zur Partikelarmen Kontinuierlichen Sterilisation von Glasbehaltnissen fur Parenterale Arzneinittel," Pharm. Ind., 39(4):372 (1977).

131. Hortig, H., "Laminar Flow in the Pharmaceutical Industry," Bull. Parenter. Drug Assoc., 27(1):38 (1973).

132. Underberg, P., Sirch, E., and Krueger, D.T., "A New Economical Process for Low Particle, In-Line Sterilization of Glass Containers," J. Paren. Drug Assoc., 32(2):84 (1978).

133. Validation of Dry Heat Processes Used for Sterilization and Depyrogenation, Technical Report No. 3, Partenteral Drug Association, Inc., Philadelphia (1981).

134. Akers, M.J. and Anderson, N.R.,"Validation of Sterile Products," in Loftus, B.T. and Nash, R.A., eds., Pharmaceutical Process Validation, Marcel Dekker, New York, pages 29-97 (1984).

135. Akers, M.J., Avis, K.E., and Thompson, B., "Validation Studies of the Fostoria Infrared Tunnel Sterilizer," J. Paren. Drug Assoc., 34(5):330 (1980).

136. Olander, J.W., "Radiation Sterilization of Plastics," Bull. Parenter. Drug Assoc., 16(4):10 (1962).

137. Foure, M. and Rakita, P., "The Stabilization of PVC Against Gamma Radiation, Part I," Med. Device Diagnos. Ind., 5(11):57 (1983).

138. Foure, M. and Rakita, P., "The Stabilization of PVC Against Gamma Radiation, Part II," Med. Device Diagnos. Ind., 5(12):33 (1983).

139. Rosato, D.V., "Polymer Resistance to Hot-Water and Steam Sterilization," Med. Device Diagnos. Ind., 7(7):48 (1985).

140. Abshire, R.L., Schlech, B.A., and Dunton, H., "The Development of a Biological Indicator for Validating Ultraviolet Radiation Sterilization of Polyethylene Bottles," J. Paren. Sci. Tech., 37(5):191 (1983).

141. Abshire, R.L., "High-Intensity Ultraviolet Radiation to Sterilize Empty Polyethulene Bottles," Pharm. Mfg., 2(1):16 (1985).

142. Tensmeyer, L.G., Wright, P.E., Fegenbush, D.O., and Snapp, S.W., "Sterilization of Glass Containers by Laser Initiated Plasmas," J. Paren. Sci. Tech., 35(3):93 (1981).

143. Peeples, R.E. and Anderson, N.R., "Microwave Coupled Plasma Sterilization and Depyrogenation I. System Characteristics," J. Paren. Sci. Tech., 39(1):2 (1985).

144. Peeples, R.E. and Anderson, N.R., "Microwave Coupled Plasma Sterilization and Depyrogenation II. Mechanisms of Action," J. Paren. Sci. Tech., 39(1):9 (1985).

145. Lohmann, S. and Manique, F., "Microwave Sterilization of Vials," J. Paren. Sci. Tech., 40(1):25 (1985).

146. Downes, T.W., "Ionizing Radiation for Sterilization of Medical and Pharmaceutical Products," Pharm Tech Conference 82, Pharmaceutical Technology, Springfield, OR., pages 666-674 (1982).

147. Rangwalla, I.J., Fletcher, P.M., Williams, K.E., and Nablo, S.V., "Electron-Beam Sterilization and its Application to Aseptic Packaging," Pharm. Tech., 9(11):36 (1985).

148. Gaughran, E.R.L. and Morrissey, eds., Sterilization of Medical Products, Vol. II., Multiscience Publication, Montreal, pages 202-223 (1981).

149. Bussey, D.M., Kane, M.P., and Tsuji, K., "Sterilization of Corticosteroids by ^{60}Co Irradiation," J. Paren. Sci. Tech., 37(2):51 (1983).

3

Closure Cleaning and Sterilization

Henry Bondi, with W. P. Olson
Pharma-Technik-Smeja, Princeton, NJ, USA

1. Introduction

To seal a sterile liquid in a sterile container with a nonsterile closure defeats the purpose of aseptic practice. The closure must be sterilized and manipulated to ensure it is not contaminated. At the same time, steam-autoclave sterilization or direct steam sterilization must be performed so as to include maximum elimination of readily extractable solutes so that they do not contaminate the product in the final container. The sterilization system must take into account the need of siliconization of most elastomeric closures. That is to say, any sterilization system for closures must embrace consideration of the reduction of extractables and siliconization where necessary.

2. Attachment of Bacteria to Closures

Bacteria and fungi have a powerful capacity to sorb and then attach themselves to a wide variety of surfaces. The forces that act at long range to bring bacterium and surface into contact are ionic. At intermediate range, London-van der Waals forces can be important (especially in the absence of ionic interactions). Once cell and surface are in contact, short range hydrophobic interaction can occur. See Daniels (1980) and Olson and Greenwood (1986) for discussion of these effects.

A. Ionic interactions

Most particles in aqueous suspension, including bacteria and viruses, are negatively charged when the pH of the suspending water is neutral or alkaline. We may assume that the surface charge of elastomeric closures is negative under most conditions.

Gordon and Millero (1984) have shown that the attachment of Vibrio alginolyticus to a Ca-phosphate solid (hydroxyapatite) varies with salt molarity and valence of the cation. Divalent cations such as Mg form a bridge between negatively charged microorganisms and the negatively charged hydroxyapaptite. Bacterial binding is maximal at the cation concentration that is sufficient

63

to coat the cell or the sorbing surface, whichever has the higher affinity for the cation. Some repulsion occurs at high cation concentrations when both the bacterial cell and the sorbing surface acquire positive charges.

Where the sorbing surface has a positive charge, e.g., anion exchangers and the Zeta-Plus depth filters, bacteria and negatively-charged particles are retained with high efficiency. Local positive charges may occur on the surface of closures due to the inclusion of aluminum and zinc salts in the compounding. Therefore, elastomeric closures may present a mosaic of surface charges, both negative and positive.

B. London-van der Waals interactions

If one assumes a surface energy of 68 ergs/cm² for a bacterial cell, the electrodynamic attractive force between cell and surface (Van der Waals forces) may be calculated as 1.8 x 10⁴ dynes/cm² for both polystyrene and polyethylene. The calculated Van der Waals forces between cell and a Teflon™ surface would be 0.7 x 10⁴ dynes/cm² (Parsegian and Gingell, 1975).

Surface energies of many bacterial cells are reported in van Oss et al. (1975). The interaction energies likely are maximal at distances of 10 to 20 angstroms (Gerson and Zajic, 1979).

The problem of London-van der Waals forces in the retention of particles is exemplified by particle retention of the closures as they emerge from the mold. The environment of a rubber plant, like that of a paper plant, is filled with debris including flakes of mold-release agent(s). All of these particles adhere strongly to the closure which, on release from the mold, develops a high charge which discharges slowly on standing.

C. Hydrophobic interactions

Rosenberg (1981) has shown that a hydrophobic bacterium, *Staphylococcus aureus,* adheres to a smooth surface of polystyrene whereas a bacterium with an hydrophilic surface, *Staphylococcus albus* (now called *S. epidermidis*) does not bind to the surface. Minagi et al. (1985) showed that *Candida tropicalis,* with a more hydrophobic surface than *C. albicans,* adhered better than *C. albicans* to hydrophobic surfaces. Kawabata et al. (1983) sorbed a number of organisms, including *Escherichia coli, S. aureus* and *Pseudomonas aeruginosa,* to polyvinylpyridinium halide particles. Such particles would have been rather hydrophobic.

D. Exudates

Corpe (1979) has reviewed the irreversible attachment of bacteria to different substrata. The review cites polyanionic carbohydrates and proteins secreted by various bacteria to form a film tightly bound to the substratum, and to which the bacterium somehow is attached. Such exudates also can serve to bind cells into a cohesive mass that is difficult to remove from the surface to be cleaned. Many bacteria attach to surfaces via fibrils, and algae attach via specialized basal cells.

E. Summary

Although the molded elastomeric closure may be sterile in the mold, it is not handled in an aseptic manner thereafter and must be assumed to be contaminated microbially. The composition of closures is such that ionic, van der Waals, and hydrophobic interactions between cell and closure seem likely, followed by protein or glycoprotein or anionic polysaccharide attachments in some instances. Consequently, cleansing of the closures to remove adhering organisms and such endotoxin as may be present should include strategies to reduce such interactions. For example, use of a detergent would reduce the hydrophobic interactions, freeing from the closure surface endotoxin sorbed via the lipid A group. Use of a chelating agent such as EDTA sequesters a substantial proportion of the Al and Zn on the closure surface, which cations can bridge the negatively-charged cells and negatively-charged closure surface, and so forth.

3. Closure Washing

A. General considerations

Prior to steam sterilization, a thorough wash of the closures in hot water is essential. Boyett and Avis (1976) attempted the washing of stoppers in 1% sodium lauryl sulfate (sometimes called sodium dodecyl sulfate or SDS), or autoclaving in acidified (pH 1.9) water followed by a water for injection rinse, or a rinsing with acetone. The marker followed as an indicator of closure cleanliness was zinc mercaptobenzothiazole (ZnMBT). Acetone was the most effective, but sodium lauryl sulfate, and 15 or 30 minute autoclavings in acid water were equivalent.

Acetone has the added advantage of killing bacteria, fungi and viruses when applied at 20°C or higher, but poses an explosion hazard and the need of particular care in use to reduce employee exposure. Acidified water or simple water for injection is far less expensive than sodium lauryl sulfate and eliminates the need of rinsing away yet another solute. Therefore, a simple aqueous rinse seems best as a presterilization step. However, the Boyett and Avis data indicate clearly that the hotter the water rinse of the stoppers, the more effective is the removal of soluble extractables.

B. The Upjohn cycles

Smith et al. (1976), at Upjohn, washed closures in 65–70°C water/detergent for 20 minutes, followed by four 3-5 minute hot water rinses and then five rinses with filtered deionized water. Filtered steam then was admitted to the chamber (a rotating drum) during a tumbling drain, and silicone oil was added. Filtered deionized water was added again, to remove unsorbed silicone oil as an emulsion, and was discarded after a 20 minute drum rotation. Note that steam addition during this portion of the process was intended only to warm the closures, to facilitate sorption of the silicone oil, and not to sterilize the closures.

The washing and siliconizing process utilized at Upjohn, also described in Smith et al. (1976), employs a hemispherical-bottom tank with a spray ball for filtered air, deionized water and hot water. A chimney assembly ensures stopper agitation. Aids to cleaning are a detergent, an alkaline phosphate to solubilize extracted waxes and EDTA to chelate extracted metals. The stoppers are rinsed with hot water, followed by filtered deionized water, and then pumped as a water slurry to a double-cone dryer in a clean room.

Details of the washing and rinsing cycles, per Smith et al., are:

Cycle Stage	Activity	Cycle Time (mins)
Wash	Fill kettle with RO water	7
	Filtered air with RO water (agitation)	10
	Filtered air	0.3
	End cycle	
Extract	Steam to jacket (add detergent)	7
	Filtered air with RO water	55
	RO water flush	7
	End cycle	0.3
Rinse 1	Filtered air with RO water	55
	RO water flush	7
	End cycle	0.3
Rinse 2	Filtered air with deionized water	10
	Deionized water flush	7
	End cycle	0.3
Transfer	Filtered air	3
	Start pump	0.3
	Lee valve opens	7
	Lee valve closes	3
	Stop transfer pump	0.3
End cycle		

This series of cycles effectively washes the closures free of particles and a substantial proportion of the solutes that can diffuse to the closure surface, then into the parenteral liquid.

Note that the Upjohn wash cycles are mild and gentle. For example, agitation of the liquid around the packed closures is provided by filtered air. Excessive abrasion and friction of the closures against one another during the washing phase, as likely occurred in Upjohn's old rotating drum system, is not desirable (Anschel, 1977) as it tends to increase particle generation. The new model system developed at Upjohn eliminates this problem by gently agitating the wash solutions with air.

At the time of the writing of the Smith et al. article, water for injection was not required as a final rinse of closures. Upjohn's filtered demineralized water probably met most or all specifications for water for injection. However, WFI presently is used.

C. Solute and particle removal by washing

Danielson et al. (1983) show these extractables to include benzothiazole, cyclo-hexamine, diphenylamine, 9,10-dihydro-9,9-dimethylacridine, benzaldehyde and furfural, among others. Whether any of these leach into a parenteral solution in sufficient concentration to inhibit the growth of a microbial contaminant is not known. As products containing these solutes pass routine USP XXI pre-clinical animal safety tests, the presence of such solutes in minute amounts may be of no consequence, and only an indication of a level of sophistication in analytical chemistry that is far beyond the demonstrated needs of the pharmaceutical community. However, there should be cognisance of the presence of aluminum silicate as a reinforcing agent in some elastomers. Other important extractables can include ZnO, MgO and stearic acid as activators; sulfur and phenolics as curing agents; amines, thiazoles and dithiocarbamates as accelerators; dithiocarbamates, aldehydes and ketones as antidegradants, etc. (Wood, 1980).

The extraction of solutes from filters follows a power series family of curves (Olson et al., 1980), and inspection of the elution curves for solutes from closures (Boyett and Avis, 1976) suggests that the same type of relation applies to leachables from elastomeric stoppers. It appears that the wash cycles also extract particles from closures via a power series function (Bondi, 1985; Grunder, 1983). Where the wash cycle includes a detergent, it is possible that endotoxin sorbed to the closure also might be extracted in a similarly predictable manner.

It has been shown in practice that the extraction of solutes can be enhanced and shortened if the step is performed in a closed system at a temperature of 115 to 123°C for about 5 to 8 minutes. Demineralized water or WFI is used. The used water should be displaced after quick cooling, preferably by an upward plug flow to minimize re-exposure of the closures.

D. The Smeja-Whirl-Flow cycles

Washing systems employing a revolving drum, may be responsible for particle generation from the abrasion of the closures against one another. The ideal washing system employs fluidization and plug flow, wherein wash solutions are pumped from beneath, gently flowing around the closures and washing them without abrasion (Bondi, 1985). The only commercially available system that appears to provide this type of washing action is that of the Pharma-Technik-Smeja stopper washer (Figure 1). An example of the effectiveness of the Smeja system in removing sorbed particles adhering to closures is shown in Figure 2.

Regardless of the techniques employed for closure washing, the wash system must remove soil, organisms, endotoxin and adhering particles from the closures without redeposition of contaminants onto the cleaned closures.

Whether in the "new" Upjohn system or in the Smeja system, closures are dried, siliconized, and steam-sterilized. In this system, all process steps, i.e., washing, rinsing, siliconization, steam sterilization, and drying occur in one process vessel under control of a personal computer. The single-process reactor is

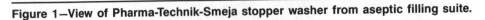

Figure 1—View of Pharma-Technik-Smeja stopper washer from aseptic filling suite.

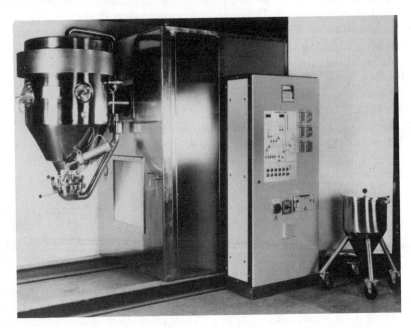

located in the clean room. The stoppers are loaded into the system by means of suction.

4. Closure Sterilization

A. Steam as the method-of-choice

Most readers will correctly assume that sterilization with steam is preferred for elastomeric closures. Ethylene oxide sterilization can be done but is not preferred because ethylene oxide sorbs to elastomers, including closures, and does not penetrate into and through some elastomers with good efficiency (Baan, 1976). Furthermore, ethylene oxide can react with water and with chloride to form ethylene chlorohydrin and ethylene glycol, respectively, of which both are somewhat toxic (McDonald et al., 1977), and likely to leach slowly from an elastomeric closure. Consequently, a washing of the closures, to remove particles and aqueous extractables (including some adherent microbes and endotoxin if present), a necessary step in the preparation of clean closures, could pose problems of toxic residues.

Despite advances in Europe, irradiation sterilization of closures for pharmaceutical purposes is still not common in the United States. The West German rubber stopper manufacturer Pharma-Gummi GmbH has carried out extensive work on the topic and can provide double wrapped bulk packs of closures which have been cleaned, siliconized and gamma irradiated. However, even utilizing this source, the onus still remains with the pharmaceutical manufacturer to determine that the bulk shipped closures are sterile as delivered to the manufacturer's clean room.

Figure 2—Photomicrographs showing particulate contamination levels before and after washing elastomeric stoppers.

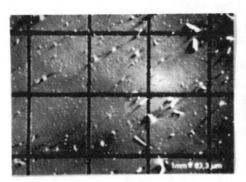 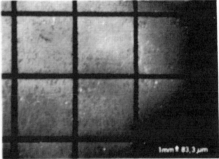

Condition of stoppers, as received, i.e., before treatment (section of filter with particles from 3 stoppers) (1mm = 83,3 μm)

Condition of stoppers after treatment (section of filter with particles from 3 stoppers) (1mm = 83,3 μm)

B. Cycle duration

The first consideration obviously is sterility of the closures. The closures must be essentially free of unbound water which can act as a thermal buffer. If a vacuum is pulled on the closures before the injection of steam, which is the preferred method, vaporization of the unbound water causes the closures to cool and makes necessary a higher temperature, or longer sterilization time, or both. Therefore, free water is drained off, in some systems with gentle tumbling. Usually, the sterilization cycle requires the injection of clean steam (at about 122°C) for the minimal time consistent with a 7 log kill of *Bacillus stearothermophilus*. Usually, 16 to 28 minute of flowing steam is sufficient (Bondi, 1985). By way of contrast, an F_0 of 30 to 60 may be required to achieve the desired level of sterility assurance in a steam autoclave, where the steam does not flow through the mass of the closures (Bondi, 1985). Excessive steaming of any of the closures can result in polymer degradation, resulting in friability and loss of elasticity. Softening and oxidation also may occur (Anschel, 1977).

Table I—Typical Stopper Treatment Cycle*

Action	Description	Time (min)	Temperature (°C)
Loading	Load 30,000 20mm injection stoppers	4	20
Wash	Add demineralized water. Heat with direct clean steam and simultaneously add 5% nonionic detergent, 70°C. Detergent concentration in the reactor: 0.03%	10	20-99
	Agitate the stoppers by steam injection		
Rinse 1	Remove detergent with cold demineralized water (plug flow, bottom to top)	8	99-30
Rinse 2	Cold demineralized water and compressed air	12	30-20
Siliconization	Heat with direct clean steam and metered addition of silicone oil	5	20-99
	Agitate stoppers by means of steam injection of silicone oil	4	99-100
Sterilization	Add clean steam from top to bottom	1	28-105
	Air removal	2	105
	Clean steam	2	121
	Sterilize with steam	16	121
	Pressure release		121
Drying	Evacuate the container	2	100
	Drying (hot air from bottom to top forced by vacuum pump and every 5 minute inversion of the vessel to decant residual water in closure cavities	60	100-70
Leak test	Vacuum timed and recorded	10	70
Unloading	Under laminar HEPA air on the sterile side	5	70

* Cycle parameters in the table are based on cycles developed on the Pharma-Technik-Smeja System, Model WSTB—SST-HTA-RTA-80AE

5. Post-Sterilization Handling

In the Upjohn and Smeja systems, the sterilized closures are deposited into a sterile container under HEPA laminar flow air. With both systems, the closures can be made available in the filling room. Alternatively, in the more common current handling of closures, washed and dried closures are placed randomly into a flat pan that is covered with a suitable autoclave paper held in place with autoclave tape.

6. Problems

The very nature of the formulations of elastomeric closures currently in use poses problems of cleaning and sterilization. The cleaning problems relate to soluble and particulate extractables and, indirectly, to the need for siliconization. The silicone oil acts as a lubricant for closure insertion and as a barrier between the liquid product and the remaining solutes that, in the absence of an elastomeric closure-bound film, might readily disperse into the contained liquid when contact occurs. One approach to this has been the application of a Teflon™ film to the product-contact side of elastomeric closures. Laminates of polyethylene and polypropylene are proposed as alternative solutions to the extractables problem (Knapp et al., 1984).

The cleaning and sterilization problems might be reduced significantly if suitably deformable closures of polypropylene or another heat-tolerant polymer were made (Bondi, 1985). Also, where single-use containers are used, especially single-use syringes, flexibility in terms of which elastic polymers are used as seals is inherent in the system, and one wonders why current rubber formulations need be used where repeated penetration is not a consideration.

7. Conclusions

Where elastomeric closures of butyl, silicone or other rubbers are used, as presently is common practice, unusual care is necessary to ensure:

1. Removal of sorbed particles from the closure surface
2. Elution of solutes that might otherwise migrate into the liquid product
3. Minimal friction between closures during the cleaning process so as to minimize the generation of new particles
4. Avoidance of re-deposition of soil and particles onto the closures when the closures are washed and rinsed
5. Adequate steam sterilization with minimal degradation of the elastomeric polymer.

Where these conditions are satisfied, a sterile closure that contributes minimal particles and solutes to the product can be generated.

8. References

Anschel, J. (1977) Bull. Parenteral Drug Assoc. 31, 302-307.

Baan, E. (1976) Bull. Parenteral Drug Assoc. 30, 299-305.

Bondi, H.S. (1985) Pharm. Tech. Conf. Proceed., 160-165. (The Proceedings are available through Interpharm Press, P.O.Box 530, Prairie View, IL 60069, USA)

Boyett, J.B. and Avis, K.E. (1976) Bull. Parenteral Drug Assoc.30, 169-179.

Corpe, W.A. (1979) In "Adsorption of Microorganisms to Surfaces", (G. Bitton and K.C. Marshall, eds.), pp. 105-144, Wiley Interscience, New York.

Daniels, S.L. (1980) In "Adsorption of Microorganisms to Surfaces", (G. Bitton and K.C. Marshall, eds.), pp. 7-58, Wiley Interscience, New York.

Danielson, J.W., Oxborrow, G.S. and Placencia, A.M. (1983) J. Parenteral Sci. Technol. 37, 89-92.

Gerson, D.F. and Zajic, J.E. (1979) In "Immobilized Microbial Cells", (K. Venkatsubramanian, ed.), pp. 29-57, ACS Symposium Series No. 106, Am. Chem. Soc., Washington, DC.

Gordon, A.S. and Millero, F.J. (1984) Appl. Environ. Microbiol. 47, 495-499.

Grunder, H. (1983) The pulsation whirl-flow process for the treatment of elastomeric closures of vials and infusion bottles, Paper presented to the Parenteral Drug Association, Philadelphia, PA, USA, October. [Grunder is at Ciba-Geigy, Stein, Switzerland]

Kawabata, N., Hayashi, T. and Matsumoto, T. (1983) Appl. Environ. Microbiol. 46, 203-210.

Knapp, J.Z., Dull, H.F., Bjorndall, P.M., Brakl, S.F. and Yuen, P.C. (1984) J. Parenteral Sci. Technol. 38, 128-138.

McDonald, T.O., Kasten, K., Hervey, R., Gregg, S. and Britton, B. (1977) Bull. Parenteral Drug Assoc. 31, 25-32.

Minagi, S., Miyake, Y., Inasaki, K., Tsuru, H. and Suginaka, H. (1985) Inf. Immun. 47,11-14.

Olson, W.P., Briggs, R.O., Garanchon, C.M., Ouellet, M.J., Graf, E.A. and Luckhurst, D.G. (1980) J. Parenteral Drug Assoc. 34, 254-267.

Olson, W.P. and Greenwood, J.R. (1986) In "Fluid Filtration: Liquid, Volume II, ASTM STP 975", (P.R. Johnston and H.G. Schroeder, eds.), pp. 90-99, Am. Soc. Testing & Materials, Philadelphia, PA, USA.

van Oss, C.J., Gillman, G.F. and Newman, A.W. (1975) "Phagocytic Engulfment and Cell Adhesiveness", Marcel Dekker, New York.

Parsegian, V. (1975) In "Physical Chemistry", (H. Olfen and K. Mysels, eds.), pp. 27-72, Theorex, La Jolla, CA.

Rosenberg, M. (1981) Appl. Environ. Microbiol. 42, 375-377.

Smith, G.G., Grimes, T.L., Fonner, D.E. and Griffin, J.C. (1976) Bull. Parenteral Drug Assoc. 30, 53-63.

Wood, R.T. (1980) J. Parenteral Drug Assoc. 34, 286-294.

4

Pyrogens and Depyrogenation: Theory and Practice

Frederick C. Pearson III
Travenol Laboratories, Round Lake, IL, USA

1. Overview of Pyrogens and Depyrogenation

As the name suggests, pyrogens are substances that induce fever when administered to animals by various routes, including the intravenous route. Pyrogens are ubiquitous and can be demonstrated in water, air and raw materials, as well as in some finished parenteral products (Twohy et al., 1984). Although there are many pyrogens, including those of microbial and non-microbial origins, the single most important one in the pharmaceutical manufacturing industry is endotoxin (Pearson, 1985). This material, which is associated with the outer membrane of gram-negative bacteria (GNB), is shed from viable bacterial cells and is also released from bacteria when they die.

In recent years, two major technological advances have been made that provide the necessary basis to deal with endotoxin contamination in parenteral manufacturing, and prevent final container pyrogenicity. The first of these achievements includes the development of the *Limulus* amebocyte lysate (LAL) assay for the rapid and accurate detection of endotoxin in the parenteral manufacturing setting (Pearson et al., 1982). LAL methods have been developed to effectively measure subpyrogenic levels of endotoxin in large volume parenterals (Pearson et al., 1982), small volume parenterals (McCullough, 1982), radiopharmaceuticals (Cooper et al., 1970), plasma fractions (Pearson et al., 1981), and in-process control (Mascoli and Weary, 1979). In addition, LAL can be used to monitor "pyroburden," a term analogous to bioburden, in production waters, raw materials, closures, and stoppers. As will be seen on the following pages, LAL is an effective monitor for the destruction or removal of endotoxin used in depyrogenation validation procedures.

A second major achievement in endotoxin research involves an increased understanding of the molecular biology and biochemistry of endotoxin. Westphal (1975), among others, has prepared and characterized purified endotoxin

75

from phenol water extracts. Other extraction procedures have also been used. In purified form, endotoxin is a white powder composed of lipopolysaccharide (LPS). Purified endotoxins elicit scores of in vitro and in vivo activities, including pyrogenicity (Galanos et al., 1977). These investigators demonstrated that LPS is composed of three distinct molecular portions. The most important of these, Lipid A, is responsible for fever and most of the other biological reactions of endotoxin. Fortunately, a number of depyrogenation procedures can be used, as discussed below. These procedures either remove endotoxin using techniques based on its physiochemical nature, or abrogate its toxicity by altering labile chemical bonds in the Lipid A moiety.

This chapter addresses the structure and chemistry of endotoxins as they relate to destruction or removal of endotoxin (depyrogenation). After a brief overview of endotoxin, the chapter will be expanded in two directions: (1) depyrogenation by destructive process, and, (2) depyrogenation by physical or chemical removal. The material presented in this chapter is not intended to be exhaustive, but is meant to provide access to more specific, detailed information for those involved in routine control of endotoxin in parenteral manufacturing. One must bear in mind that pyrogen control can be a complex challenge that demands validation, use/product compatibility, and, for particular situations, may require multiple or customized depyrogenation strategies.

Throughout this chapter, the terms lipopolysaccharide (LPS) and endotoxin (ET) will be used interchangeably, but one must bear in mind that the substances referred to here are typically purified chemical materials (LPS) purchased from any of various commercial sources. Although a control standard endotoxin (CSE) is usually selected for validation procedures, the real world pyroburden is composed of chemically unpurified "environmental endotoxins" (EET). Endotoxins encountered in the pyroburden do not behave like purified LPS when examined in parallel studies using the LAL assay and the USP rabbit pyrogen assay (Pearson, 1985). There are no extensive studies that report using EET for validation of depyrogenation procedures, but there is little reason to expect that these materials would behave precisely like their purified counterpart.

2. The Chemistry and Biology of Endotoxins

Endotoxin is a family of lipopolysaccharide (LPS) substances associated with the outer membrane of gram-negative bacteria (GNB). These substances are unique to GNB and manifest numerous toxic effects in animals, including pyrogenicity, complement activation, neutropenia, leukocytosis, and coagulopathy. They also interact with a number of cell types. Although LPS is synthesized in the microbial cell membrane, these substances are situated on the cell surface. Most GNB contain LPS with an active Lipid A moiety that has been observed in toxonomically unrelated groups of bacteria. Although this pharmacological portion of LPS is not universal in all GNB, it is common to most GNB and is the primary pyrogen of concern in the parenteral drug manufacturing industry. Both the biological and chemical properties of LPS (Lipid A) have been reviewed recently (Rietschel et al., 1982; Luderitz et al., 1982).

Endotoxins are high molecular weight complexes approaching 10^6 Daltons in solution. These toxins are constantly shed into the environment of the bacterium, much like the daily shedding of superficial layers of human skin. When the bacterium undergoes autolysis, most endotoxin is released from the cell. Unpurified endotoxins contain lipid, carbohydrate, and protein, but highly purified endotoxins do not contain protein and, therefore, are referred to as lipopolysaccharide (LPS) to emphasize their chemical nature.

Figure 1 — General Structure of Lipid A. Lipid A Toxic Region, Common Polysaccharide, and Immunospecific Polysaccharide Chain.

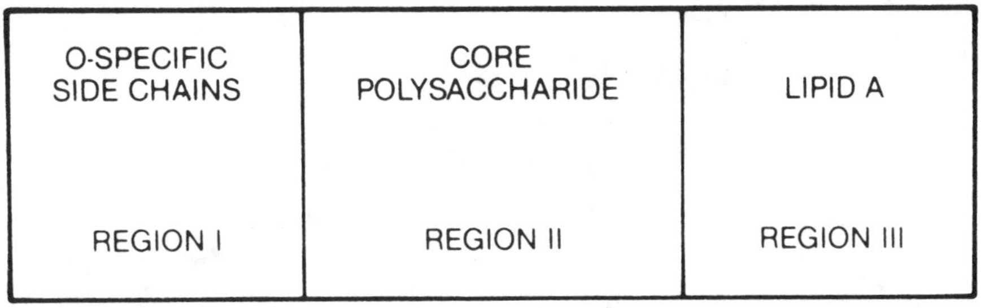

O-SPECIFIC SIDE CHAINS	CORE POLYSACCHARIDE	LIPID A
REGION I	REGION II	REGION III

Endotoxin, as shown in Figure 1, has three distinct chemical regions. The innermost is composed of Lipid A, which is linked to a central polysaccharide core. The core is, in turn, linked to long, whip-like projections, the O-antigenic side chains. These polysaccharide side chains are responsible in large part for the antigenic individuality of gram-negative bacteria and are thus responsible for thousands of individual serotypes. The core portion of endotoxin is remarkably uniform in many rather diverse groups of GNB. Thus, endotoxin contributes to both the antigenic homogeneity and the heterogeneity of these bacteria. It was undoubtedly this combination of endotoxin's novel chemistry and diverse biological properties that led Ivan Bennett, a renowned endotoxin investigator, to conclude that "endotoxins possess an intrinsic fascination that is nothing less than fabulous" (Bennett, 1964).

Scores of biological activities have been found to be induced by the Lipid A moiety of endotoxin. In addition to well known toxic expressions, these activities also include beneficial effects, as can be seen in Table I. Although one of the most often studied effects of Lipid A is pyrogenicity, endotoxin also has the capacity, in sufficient doses, to activate the coagulation system, alter carbohydrate and lipid metabolism, activate complement, induce hypotension, and cause platelet aggregation. In addition to many other pathophysiological aberrations, it can induce disseminated intravascular coagulation, shock, and ultimately, death. To the pharmaceutical industry, however, pyrogenicity remains the most critical aspect of endotoxin's biological activity. Pyrogenicity, like most of the other activities of endotoxin, resides in the Lipid A portion of endotoxin. This unique lipid comprises a simple disaccharide of glucosamine, which is highly substituted with amide-linked and ester-linked long chain fatty acid (Figure 2).

Figure 2—Lipid A

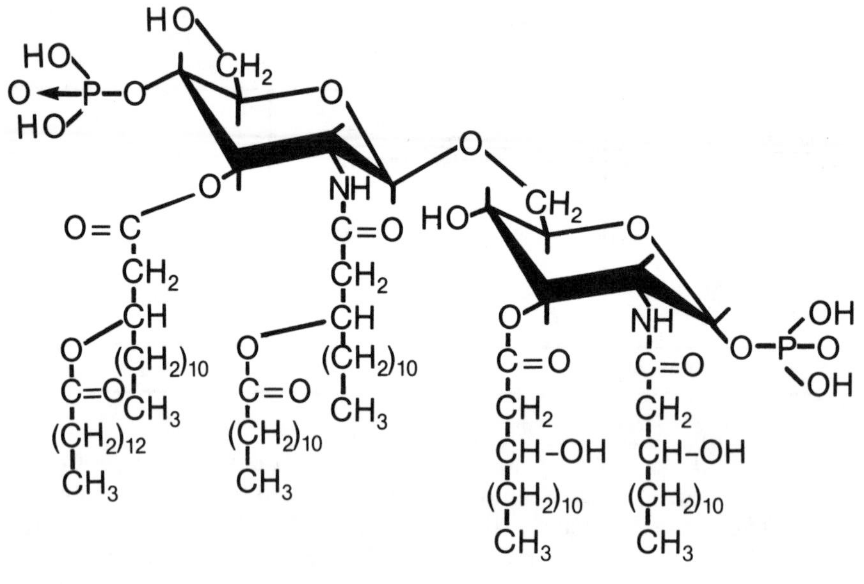

The most common amide-linked fatty acid is a 14-carbon-chain fatty acid, beta-hydroxymyristic acid. Ester-linked fatty acids, which tend to be more variable, commonly include capric, lauric, myristic, palmitic, and stearic acids. These fatty acids are saturated, straight-chained, and have even numbers of carbon atoms in their chains. Removal of the ester-linked fatty acid residues can be accomplished by treatment with dilute base, which abrogates the biological activity of Lipid A. Treatment with 0.25N NaOH for 5 minutes at 56°C results in the liberation of β-hydroxymyristic acid without the loss of pyrogenicity, but extended treatment (for 30 to 60 min) leads to the loss of all the ester-linked fatty acids and a marked reduction in pyrogenicity (Neter et al., 1956). Effective depyrogenation has been reported using 0.1M NaOH at 30°C for 72 hours (Mikami et al., 1982) or 4°C for 16 hours (Kakinuma et al., 1981).

Table I—Biological Activities of Free Lipid A

Pyrogenicity
Lethal toxicity in mice
Leucopenia, leucocytosis
Local Schwartzman reaction
Bone marrow necrosis
Embryonic bone resorption
Complement activation
Depression of blood pressure
Platelet aggregation
Hageman factor activation
Induction of plasminogen activator
Limulus lysate gelation
Toxicity enhanced by BCG and adrenalectomy
Enhanced dermal reactivity to epinephrine
Induction of nonspecific resistance to infection
Induction of tolerance to endotoxin
Induction of early refractory state to temperature change
Adjuvance activity
Mitogenic activity for cells
Macrophage activation
Induction of colony stimulating factor
Induction of IgG synthesis in new-born mice
Induction of prostaglandin syntheses
Induction of interferon production
Induction of tumor-necrotizing factor
Induction of mouse liver pyruvate kinase
Type C RNA virus release from mouse spleen cells
Helper activity for friend spleen focus-forming virus in mice
Inhibition of phosphenolpyruvate carboxykinase
Hypothermia in mice

Commonly, a glycoside link exists between each disaccharide unit. This link is made from the carbon 1 (C1) of one unit and the carbon 6 (C6) of an adjacent unit. Although units can be linked by a phosphodiester bond between C1 of one molecule and C4 of an adjacent molecule, in some cases the C4 phosphate is substituted with 10% to 20% aminoarabinose (Luderitz et al., 1982; Rietscel et al., 1982). The majority of GNB have a complete lipopolysaccharide and are referred to as smooth. In recent years, however, a number of bacterial isolates have been obtained that lack various polysaccharides, including O-specific side chains and core components. Such bacteria, called R-mutants (rough), are incapable of synthesizing various distal portions of core lipopolysaccharide or O-specific side chain polysaccharide. Depending on the extent of the mutation, mutants are designated Ra (the most complete core polysaccharide) through Re (the most deficient, having only KDO). The range of these mutants can be seen in Figure 3. Purified LPS isolated from such mutants has been invaluable in determining the chemical structure of LPS and the associated functions of Lipid A. Because the Re 595 mutant of Salmonella minnesota contains only Lipid A and KDO, it has been used extensively in experiments designed to demonstrate that the biological activity of LPS is associated with Lipid A. Due, in part, to the acid labile ketosidic link between Lipid A and KDO, endotoxin can be inactivated by treatment with dilute hydrochloric acid, as will be discussed later in this chapter.

Figure 3 – Specific Structure of Lipopolysaccharide

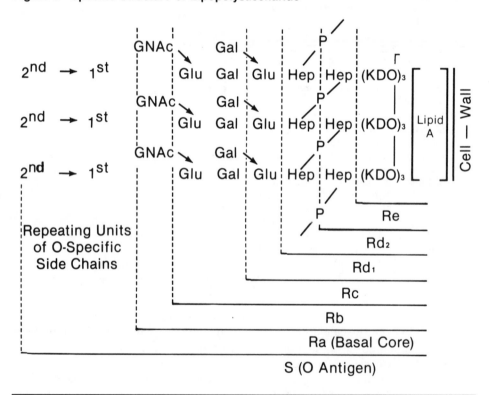

The aggregation state, or molecular weight, of ET is critical to its biological activity, and also affects depyrogenation of fluids by ET removal. Studies have shown that various salt forms of LPS exhibit a wide range of aggregation states and that these have a dramatic effect on pyrogenicity, as well as other biological activities (Luderitz et al., 1982). As can be seen in Table II, pyrogenicity is inversely related to aggregation state; i.e., the more disaggregated an LPS, the more pronounced its pyrogenicity. The aggregation of endotoxin is a function of the Lipid A moiety's interaction to form higher molecular weight aggregates and of the electrostatic nature of cationic components associated with the acidic phosphate and carboxyl groups of the molecule. Thus, substances that either reduce surface tension or chelate divalent cations such as Ca^{++} and Mg^{++} will decrease the size of ET aggregates. Examples of these substances are Tween-20 and ethylene-diaminetetraacetic acid (EDTA), respectively. In the presence of magnesium and calcium, LPS forms bilayer sheets or vesicles with a diameter on the order of 0.1 micron. When endotoxin preparations are reduced by a chelating agent or surfactant, rod-shaped subunits appear, which have a molecular weight of approximately 20,000 Daltons, a diameter of 8 to 12 angstroms, and a length of 200 to 700 angstroms. The importance of these observations with respect to pyrogen removal by microporous filters and ultrafiltration membranes, has been demonstrated by Sweadner et al., 1977.

Table II — Sedimentation Coefficients and Biological Activities of the Lipopolysaccharide of *S. Abortus Equi* in Different Salt Forms

Salt Form	Sedimentation Coefficient (S)	Increasing	Decreasing	Unchanged
Triethylamine	(9.3)	Lethal Toxicity (rat)	Lethal Toxicity (mouse)	Mitogenicity
Ethanolamine	(64)	Rate of Clearance from the Blood	Pyrogenicity (rabbit)	Limulus Lysate Gelation
Pyridin	(72)			
Sodium	(105)	Interation with Complement		
Potassium	(135)			
Putrescine	(230)	Affinity to Red Blood Cells		
Calcium	partly insoluble			

From: C. Galanos et al.)1979), Chemical, physical and biological properties of bacterial lipopolysaccaride; published in Biomedical Applications of the Horseshoe Crab (Limulidae). E. Cohen, ed. Alan R. Liss, New York, p. 319.

These studies have shown that the vesicles and bilayer sheets will pass through a 0.22 micron membrane filter, but will be retained by a 0.025 micron pore size. They showed that the small micellar form will pass through a 0.025 micron membrane filter, but will be retained by a 1,000,000 nominal molecular weight limit (NMWL) ultrafilter. When LPS is reduced to its smallest subunit by a surface-active agent, such as sodium deoxycholate, it will pass through a molecular filter with a NMWL of 1,000,000, but will be retained by a 10,000 NMWL molecular weight filter, as can be seen in Table III. Since endotoxin can be considered to have a molecular weight of approximately 10^6 Daltons in an aqueous environment, this is the approximate molecular weight of endotoxin most frequently found in parenteral solutions.

Table III—Removal of Pyrogens by Microporous and Ultrafiltration Methods

Solution	Endotoxin Conc (g/ml)	Approximate Concentration of Endotoxin (g/ml) in filtrate*				
		0.22 Micron	0.025 Micron	1,000,000 n MOL. WT.	100,000 n MOL. WT.	10,000 n MOL. WT.
Water	10^{-6}	10^{-6}	$<10^{-10}$	$<10^{-10}$	$<10^{-10}$	$<10^{-10}$
0.9% NaCL	10^{-6}	10^{-6}	$<10^{-10}$	$<10^{-10}$	$<10^{-10}$	
5 mM MgCl$_2$	10^{-6}	10^{-6}	$<10^{-10}$	$<10^{-10}$	$<10^{-10}$	
5 nM EDTA	10^{-6}		10^{-6}	$<10^{-10}$	$<10^{-10}$	
0.5% Na Cholate	10^{-5}			10^{-5}	10^{-7}	$<10^{-10}$
1% Na Cholate	10^{-5}			10^{-6}	10^{-7}	$<10^{-10}$
2% Na Cholate 5mM EDTA	10^{-5}			10^{-5}	10^{-5}	$<10^{-10}$
1% Deoxycholate	10^{-5}			10^{-5}	10^{-5}	$<10^{-10}$

* 100 pg/mL(10^{-10} g/mL.) was generally the lower limit of sensitivity of the *Limulus* amebocyte lysate assay used for this study.

3. Depyrogenation by Removal

As can be seen from the above discussion, depyrogenation can be accomplished by ET removal, based on its molecular properties, or by destruction. The former method, reviewed in this section, includes ET removal by washing (dilution), ultrafiltration, reverse osmosis, charged modified filters, hydrophobic microporous membranes, affinity chromatography, distillation, and depth filtration.

A. Dilution

This approach to depyrogenation is based on washing or rinsing materials, such as glassware, until the ET is sufficiently diluted to give non-pyrogenic material (Feldsine et al., 1979). Although these investigators questioned the need for depyrogenation activity in light of glassware manufacturing and handling procedures, validation data were presented demonstrating that washing procedures are effective in depyrogenating parenteral containers. Using a concentrated phenol saline suspension of extract from four GNB, glass containers ranging from 2 mL to 1000 mL bottles were challenged. The USP rabbit pyrogen assay was used as a measure of pyrogenicity with both ET-challenged test containers, as well as positive controls. The data reported clearly support the adequacy and reproducibility of rinsing techniques as a method of depyrogenation. Depyrogenation by rinsing is a convenient method for many objects, such as stoppers, that cannot withstand the elevated temperature associated with dry heat sterilization, e.g., 250°C for 30 minutes.

Water of acceptable quality, such as USP Water for Injection, should be used for rinsing. Such water must contain no more than 0.25 EU/mL (endotoxin units). Prior to developing a depyrogenation protocol, one should consult the USP XXI, Chapter 1211, General Information Section, page 1349, regarding Sterilization and Sterility Assurance, which became effective January 1, 1985. Depyrogenation validation compliance requires challenging articles with a minimum of 1000 EU and demonstrating a three log reduction in ET as measured by LAL. Although this chapter specifically addresses dry heat depyrogenation validation, it serves as a guideline for validating other approaches to depyrogenation. One should also consult the Food and Drug Administration's draft guideline on aseptic filling for further information on depyrogenation validation of containers and closures (Federal Register 50(22) February 1, 1985).

B. Ultrafiltration

Ultrafiltration membranes are rated on the basis of molecular weight exclusion limits, and their effectiveness as depyrogenating filters is due to their action as size-discriminating screens. Thus, endotoxins that exceed the molecular-weight exclusion limit of a given membrane are retained on the surface of the membrane. The basic subunit size of LPS (the monomeric LPS molecule) is about 10,000-20,000 Dalton. It can, therefore, be effectively removed from solution by a 10,000-Dalton ultrafilter. However, the unaggregated monomeric form of LPS is seldom found in aqueous solutions. Normally, LPS molecules aggregate into vesicles, ranging in molecular weight from 300,000 to 1 million Daltons. Therefore, sizable amounts of endotoxin in aqueous solutions can be removed by ultrafilters rated at 100,000 Daltons or even higher (Nelson, 1978). Ultrafiltration as a method for removing pyrogens has been successfully applied to a large number of low- to medium-molecular-weight drugs and solutions. Endotoxin-contaminated antibiotics have been successfully depyrogenated without significant loss of the antibiotic (Sweadner et al., 1977; Takahashi et al., 1983), and the process has also been utilized for large-scale production of electrolyte solutions (Henderson and Beams, 1978; Henderson et al., 1978).

Ultrafiltration has been successfully used to depyrogenate chorionic gonadotropin (Johnson et al., 1980), 5-methyltetrahydrohomofolate disodium (Cradock et al., 1978) and water (Rechen, 1984). Higher-molecular-weight solutions contaminated with aggregated endotoxin of a similar size may also be successfully ultrafiltered, if the endotoxin can be disaggregated through use of such agents as chelators or surface-active detergents (Sweader et al., 1977). The use of ultrafiltration in the parenteral drug industry has been limited to some extent by regulations. These regulations include the USP definition of Water for Injection, which specifies that it must be produced by distillation or reverse osmosis (Tutunjian, 1985). The use of ultrafiltration to remove endotoxin from antibiotics has been reported recently (Takahashi et al., 1983).

C. Reverse osmosis

Reverse osmosis membranes consist of cellulose acetate or polyamide material, with pores small enough to exclude ions. If they can retain large amounts of salts under pressure-filtration conditions, such semipermeable filters are termed "reverse osmosis" membranes. Conventional reverse osmosis membranes (nominally rated at pore sizes around 10 angstrom units) remove endotoxins by simple size exclusion; the pores in the membrane are far too small to pass the pyrogens (Nelson, 1978). At intermediate pore sizes, the ability of these filters to retain pyrogens has been poorly documented and reports have been contradictory. Nevertheless, conventional reverse osmosis membranes are extremely effective for removing endotoxin from water. Their use for depyrogenation has been limited, because very few molecules other than water can pass through the pore structure of the reverse osmosis membrane.

In practical operation, a well-maintained reverse osmosis membrane of high integrity routinely removes 99.5 to 99.9% of the pyrogen load to the system in a single pass, even when the challenge levels are as high as a microgram of endotoxin per milliliter. For this reason, reverse osmosis is currently one of only two methods recognized by the U.S. Pharmacopeia for the production of Water For Injection (WFI), the other being distillation (Nelson, 1985). It is unlikely that reverse osmosis will be used for any product other than water, but in the production of nonpyrogenic water, this approach offers substantial economic benefits over distillation and no reduction in water quality.

D. Charge-modified media and electrostatic attraction

Depth filtration through asbestos-containing filters has also long been for pyrogen removal (Kaden, 1975). The asbestos (chrysotile) fibers' mechanism of removal is ascribed to both mechanical and electrochemical properties, as follows: At pH levels above 2, endotoxin aggregates are negatively charged and behave as anions. As such, they can be removed by adsorption to cationically charged adsorbents, such as asbestos, which has a positive surface charge at a pH below 8.3. In addition to electrostatic attraction, the fine, strongly branched asbestos fibers provide a large surface area that allows the creation of a depth filter. The pores in depth filters are in random and tortuous configurations. Because of this, they retain particles throughout the matrix by such mechanical means as sieving, sedimentation, interstitial impingement, and interception. For this reason, depth filters can retain more particles before clogging than can screen filters of the same rating. They can also retain a substantial quantity of particles that are actually smaller than their flow passages. An asbestos filter with an 1000cm^2 area can eliminate pyrogens from at least 250 liters of aqueous solution containing 0.5 microgram/mL of endotoxin (Wilke, 1954). However, efficiency of pyrogen adsorption is dependent on concentration and molecular size of the dissolved substances. The effectiveness of asbestos filters is lost with high-molecular-weight protein solutions due to "adsorptive" displacement. Of even greater concern is the FDA limit on the use of asbestos for processing small and large volume parenterals (Rossitto, 1979). For this reason, there has been great interest in preparing depth filters from materials other than asbestos, several of which are currently available for commercial use.

Membranes produced from polyamides (nylon), or with amines covalently bonded to their surfaces, will exhibit overall net positive charges in aqueous solutions with a pH below 9, and will absorb negatively charged molecules, such as endotoxins. Charge-modified microporous depyrogenation products utilizing positive zeta potential membranes have been available for several years and have been used successfully for depyrogenating a wide range of pharmaceutical solutions (Gerba, 1980; Hoy et al., 1980; Fiore, 1980). The chemical structure of biologically active pyrogens and the effect of the suspending media on their activity necessitate designing charge-modified filters specifically tailored for the product involved.

Removal of endotoxin by electrostatic attraction to other cationically charged adsorbents is also well documented. Barium sulfate and ion exchange resins have been reported to be effective for reducing pyrogens (Reichelderfer et al., 1975; Nolan et al., 1975; Polmer and Whittet, 1971). However, their performance seems to be highly dependent on the concentration of pyrogens found in the solutions. The ability of positively charged filter materials to remove endotoxin has been reported recently by Carozzone et al., 1985.

E. Hydrophobic attraction to hydrophobic media

Aliphatic polymers (such as polypropylene, polyethylene, polyvinylidene-fluoride, and polytetrafluoroethylene) have a unique specific affinity for binding endotoxin. This property was utilized by Harris and Feinstein to prepare an LAL polypropylene bead assay to detect endotoxins in materials considered to be inhibitory to the gel clot LAL assay (Harris and Feinstein, 1979). However, the electrostatic mechanism does not explain why endotoxin is adsorbed to these polymers, because the polymers lack hydrophilic ionizable groups capable of interacting with the anionic endotoxin. Instead, the nonpolar groups common to these polymers give the membrane surface a hydrophobic quality. Therefore, given that all endotoxins have both a hydrophilic polysaccharide and a hydrophobic Lipid A portion, hydrophobic interaction between the membrane polymer and the Lipid A region is probably responsible for the adsorption of LPS. Robinson et al. (1985) describe a microfiltration process using microporous membrane filters made from hydrophobic materials. This process provides effective microfiltration in a range extending from that of ultrafiltration to the upper boundary of reverse osmosis. According to these authors, a 0.1 micron polypropylene membrane was capable of adsorbing greater than 10 micrograms of LPS per centimeter filter area, over a broad pH range, with a log reduction value of 3-4, a value consistent with the USP XXI guideline for depyrogenation.

F. Distillation

Distillation is the oldest method known for effectively removing pyrogens from water. The mechanism of endotoxin removal is relatively simple. Water is forced to undergo two phase changes, from liquid to vapor and from vapor to liquid. During the first phase, rapid boiling in the still causes the water to evaporate and the water vapor to accelerate. Because LPS is such a large molecule, it cannot accelerate as rapidly as water vapor and is left behind due to inertia. Those LPS molecules remaining in water droplets carried in the steam are dropped by gravity because of their high molecular weight. It has long been known that freshly distilled water collected and maintained in sterile depyrogenated containers is nonpyrogenic. It was the application of this knowledge that allowed initiation of commercial large volume parenteral production in the United States in the years preceding World War II. The use of distillation as a means of depyrogenation has recently been reviewed (Mahoney, 1985).

G. Activated carbon

Depyrogenation of solutions by a method based on physical adsorption of endotoxin to charcoal, particularly activated charcoal, has had a long history and is well documented in the literature (Berger et al., 1956; Gemmell and Todd, 1945; Brindle and Rigby, 1946). Most commonly, charcoal is added to a solution, the solution is agitated and, finally, the carbon is removed via filtration or precipitation. The method has been used successfully to treat a wide range of pharmaceuticals, including saline, dextrose solutions, and antibiotics (Berger et al., 1945). However, activated charcoal has a great affinity for high-molecular-weight, nonionized substances, which in certain situations may limit its application (Gemmell and Todd, 1945). Although activated charcoal can be applied over a broad pH range and is not affected by electrolyte concentrations, its use with solutions that contain low concentrations of active agents is limited, because adsorption of active ingredients can occur. Its principal limitation is the difficulty of completely removing all traces of the charcoal.

Reinhart (1985) describes the use of a sintered activated charcoal filter, which, when used in depyrogenation, lessens the problem of charcoal removal. The filter allows continuous processing of solutions by means of a design that combines adsorption and entrapment (via pore size). The filter itself can be depyrogenated by dry heat and reused. However, with the exception of water and physiologic electrolyte solutions, only concentrated solutions of raw materials and intermediates are likely candidates for filtration by this method. Other solutions would be subject to possible loss of active ingredient by adsorption.

H. Chromatographic removal of endotoxin

Affinity chromatography has been used successfully to remove endotoxin from a number of parenteral products. Methods that have been used include polymyxin B Sepharose, histamine Sepharose, substrate analog Sepharose, LAL Sepharose, DEAE Sephadex, and other ion-exchangers. Each of these will be discussed below. Sofer (1985) recently reviewed chromatographic removal of pyrogens. A procedure for the pyrogen decontamination of Sephacryl S-300 has been published by Sarafin, et al. (1982), and this procedure should be applicable for most chromatographic media.

i. Polymyxin B Sepharose

Several studies have shown that the cationic antibiotic polymyxin B (PMB) can abrogate the biological activity of LPS (Butler and Moller, 1977; Morrison and Curry, 1979). Morrison and Jacobs (1976) described the mechanism of endotoxin inactivation as a stoichiometric binding of PMB to the Lipid A region of LPS. Although these authors claim a 1:1 molar binding between PMB and LPS, in a study by Cooperstock (1974), 100 to 200 times more PMB was required to inactivate LPS, as measured by the LAL test. Novitsky and Gould (1985) recently reviewed this controversy. However, the removal of endotoxin from solution by a method based on its PMB-binding characteristics was recently achieved by Issekutz (1983), who coupled PMB to Sepharose 4B affinity columns and successfully removed from 1–10 μg/mL of several endotoxins from various solutions. The columns retained their binding capacity for at least 18 months and could be regenerated by eluting endotoxin from the columns with 1% sodium deoxycholate. A commercial preparation of polymyxin B in a column format is commercially available. Recently, PMB affinity columns have been used to depyrogenate interferon (Duff et al., 1982).

ii. Histamine Sepharose

Minobe et al. (1983) reported the use of histamine immobilized on Sepharose for pyrogen removal. This adsorbent exhibited a high affinity for pyrogen at low ionic strength, pH around 7.0, elevated temperatures, and relatively low flow rates. The data suggested that as much as 0.9 mg of endotoxin was adsorbed by 1 mL of adsorbent. Immobilized histamine could be regenerated by rinsing with 0.2 M NaOH solution containing 10-30% ethanol. Subsequently, 1.5 M NaCl was used to further wash the columns, followed by 0.5% sodium deoxycholate solution, 0.2 M NaOH, and 1.5 M NaCl.

iii. Substrate Analog Sepharose

Bishop and Desnick (1981) demonstrated the feasibility of pyrogen removal by using affinity purification of alpha-galactosidase A from human sources. This task was accomplished by coupling a substrate analog, alpha-D- galactosylamine to Sepharose, using a spacer arm.

The same basic approach could be used if an antibody were available for the substrate requiring depyrogenation. Although the literature appears to be devoid of attempts to use antibodies against Lipid A or endotoxin, two technical options are now available that could play a role in pyrogen removal. Polyclonal antibody or monoclonal antibody could be coupled to an appropriate matrix to remove: (1) specific endotoxin from a given bacterium, or (2) endotoxin generic to common GNB. Since DNA recombinant products are typically produced from a single strain of bacteria, it would be relatively simple to produce antibody against the specific strain. Braude et al. (1984) and Johns et al. (1983) have demonstrated the ability to produce broad spectrum antibodies against R mutant LPS, which exhibit protection against heterologous endotoxin. These immunoglobulins are directed against the virtually universal antigens of endotoxin and could be coupled to an affinity column for removal of real world endotoxin.

iv. LAL Sepharose

Limulus amebocyte lysate (LAL) is prepared from the only circulating blood cell, the amebocyte, found in Limulus, the horseshoe crab. The lysate prepared from these cells contains several proteins and clots in the presence of minute amounts of endotoxin. Wollman et al. (1982) have shown that the LAL material, when mixed with endotoxin containing colony stimulating factor can remove virtually all demonstrable pyrogen. Furthermore, LAL can be coupled to Sepharose beads and used as an affinity column for endotoxin. The latter approach is far superior, since the former would leave residual foreign protein in the product. While this approach remains somewhat of a technical curiosity, its potential for further application should be investigated and compared to other alternatives for a given situation.

The exact mechanism of depyrogenation by LAL is uncertain. It was suggested by Rickles et al. (1979), that LAL was capable of removing endotoxn from concanavilin A and erythropoietin by adsorption. Simultaneously, another independent report by Nachum et al. (1978) appeared, presumably describing the same phenomenon, but suggesting that the mechanism of depyrogenation was inactivation due to the enzymatic action of LAL. Nachum found that the enzyme inactivating fraction of LAL could be obtained by heating LAL to 60°C for 20 minutes. The LAL was then centrifuged at 5000G for 6 minutes at 5°C to remove the precipitate. The supernatant, which contained the inactivating factor(s), was successfully used to inactivate 80% of several endotoxins tested at 500 ng/mL. Treatment was for 30 minutes at 37°C. Although the method is very interesting, it is reported to be quite costly and difficult to control. A recent report details the removal of contaminating endotoxin from lymphokines including interferon (Biondi et al. 1984).

v. Ion Exchange

Since endotoxin typically has a net negative charge, in part due to unsubstituted phosphoryl and carboxyl groups, it is not surprising that anion exchange resins have been reported to selectively remove pyrogen from solutions. DEAE-Sephadex was reported to bind pyrogen irreversibly from L-asparaginase prepared from E. coli (Grabner, 1975). More recently, Shibatani et al. (1983) reported depyrogenation of urokinase with DEAE-Sepharose CL-6B. While the pyrogen remained associated with the Sepharose, the urokinase was demonstrated in the eluate.

Costin (1980) reported an anion exchange resin that removed bacteria, virus, and endotoxin. The Ambergard filter, developed by Rohm and Haas Company, contains a large pore macroreticular quarternary ammonium anion exchange resin of high porosity. The large pore size of the resin was reported to allow pyrogens to enter the pore cavity and become electrostatically bound (unpublished data presented to the Parenteral Drug Association, 1980).

4. Depyrogenation of Endotoxins by Inactivation

In the previous section, depyrogenation by removal was discussed. In this section, depyrogenation will be addressed from a standpoint of inactivation or destruction of endotoxin as measured by rabbit pyrogenicity and LAL reactivity. Although the traditional method of depyrogenation has been by dry heat, many containers, closures, and drug products are heat labile and require an alternate method of depyrogenation. When alternate approaches are needed, one can develop methods for the removal of endotoxin based on physiochemical properties or destructive processes other than the application of dry heat. Destructive processes include moist heat (steam), the use of acid or base, oxidizing substances, alkylating agents, and ionizing radiation. All methods of depyrogenation predicated on destruction rather than removal of endotoxin are relatively harsh treatments. Because of this, they have limited utility compared to the removal procedures discussed above.

A. Dry heat

The application of dry heat delivered through convection, conduction, or radiation (infrared) ovens has been the method of choice for depyrogenation of heat-resistant materials, such as glassware, metal equipment, instruments, heat-stable chemicals, waxes, and oils. The standard method described in various national and international compendia and reference texts, exposure at not less than 250°C for not less than 30 minutes, is based on the studies of Welch et al. (1945) on the thermostability of pyrogens as measured using the rabbit pyrogen test. The mechanism of endotoxin inactivation is incineration.

The development of the *Limulus* amebocyte lysate (LAL) assay has provided a more quantitative means of studying dry-heat inactivation of endotoxin. Tsuji et al. (1978 and 1979) and Robertson et al. (1979) discovered the inactivation kinetics of LPS from *E. coli, S. typhosa, S. marcescens,* and *P. aeruginosa* to be a nonlinear, second-order process in contrast to the inactivation of bacterial spores, which follow first-order kinetics. They compared the dry-heat resistance of intact and purified LPS to that of spores with the greatest heat resistance. Purified LPS was shown to be twice as resistant as the native (whole cell) endotoxin from which it was derived. Of greater importance was the author's convincing evidence that the general practice of increasing exposure time to compensate for lower process temperature is not supportable for LPS destruction, nor probably for destruction of intact gram-negative cells, particularly at 175°C or less. Akers et al. (1980 and 1982) confirmed these findings and also determined the F-value requirements for destruction of 10 ng of E. coli 055:B5 endotoxin seeded into 50 mL glass vials, using both convection and radiant heat ovens. An F-value is the equivalent time at a given temperature delivered to a product to achieve sterilization. There were linear relationships between oven temperatures and the logarithms of the F-values with both treatments. The use of dry heat depyrogenation has been reviewed by Sweet and Huxsoll (1985).

B. Moist heat

Early investigators studying the thermostability of endotoxin concluded that moist heat applied in conventional autoclaving was ineffective for depyrogenation. Hort and Penford (1911) reported that neither autoclaving nor boiling effectively destroyed pyrogens. Seibert (1923) also found that only "long drastic heating" would destroy pyrogens. Autoclave conditions for "normal sterilization" of solutions were ineffective for depyrogenation. Banks (1984) was able to demonstrate effective depyrogenation by autoclaving at 20psi, for 5 hours at a pH of 8.2, or for 2 hours at a pH of 3.8. More recent studies show that the action of certain depyrogenating agents can be enhanced by autoclaving. Cherkin (1975) found that hydrogen peroxide was more effective in destroying pyrogen when the solution was autoclaved. Autoclaving also helped to eliminate residual peroxide. Similar findings have been reported for other solutions containing acid or base. Recently, Novitsky et al. (1985) confirmed that autoclaving following conventional methods (121°C, 15psi at near neutral pH for 20 minutes) was not sufficient to eliminate pyrogenicity of 100 ng/mL of *E coli 055:B5*. However, autoclaving for longer periods (180 minutes) successfully reduced endotoxin levels to less than an LAL detectable limit of 0.01 ng/mL. Novitsky et al. (1985) also found that activated carbon treatment was more effective in removing endotoxin when solutions containing endotoxin and carbon were autoclaved. For these reasons, there is a renewed interest in the use of pressurized steam for depyrogenation, especially when moist heat enhances the depyrogenating properties of other substances.

C. Use of dilute acids and bases

Depyrogenation utilizing acid or alkaline hydrolysis reduces or eliminates the biological activity of bacterial LPS by inactivation of Lipid A. Lipid A is linked to core polysaccharides by 2-keto-3-deoxyoctonic acid (KDO), an 8-carbon sugar acid unique to bacterial LPS. Acid hydrolysis acts on this acid-labile ketosidic linkage to separate Lipid A from the remainder of the LPS molecule. Because the released KDO and its attached core polysaccharides act as solute carriers for the lipid portion of the molecule, the free Lipid A is insoluble in aqueous systems, and its pyrogenic activity is reduced or eliminated. However, Galanos et al. (1977) demonstrated that when free Lipid A was combined with bovine serum albumin, pyrogenicity was equal to that of intact endotoxin. Further, acid hydrolysis may act on the Lipid A fraction, altering conformation of the molecule and masking necessary functional sites. Alternatively, it may cleave fatty acid molecules at different rates, further effecting lipid solubility and thereby pyrogenicity. Acid hydrolysis, using 0.05N HCl for 30 minutes at 100°C (Tripidi and Nowotny, 1966), or 1.0% glacial acetic acid for 2-3 hours at 100°C (Luderitz et al., 1973), has been used for depyrogenation. Ribi et al. (1984), reported that 0.1N HCl preferentially cleaved the reducing end phosphate group of the diglucosamine backbone of LPS. In the absence of this single phosphate group, toxicity, including pyrogenicity, is markedly reduced, e.g., pyrogenicity is reduced 1000 fold and the chick embryo LD_{50} ($CELD_{50}$) is reduced (see Table IV). Unlike acid hydrolysis, alkaline hydrolysis does not involve loss of pyrogenic activity through

Table IV—Effect of structure of LPS, Lipid A, and Lipid X on some of the commonly used toxicity measurements.

Compound	Source*	Limulus Activity** (EU/mg)	Rabbit Pyrogenicity ADP_{50}***(ug/Kg)	$CELD_{50}$(ug)
Endotoxin	A	2.6×10^7	0.0001-0.0003	0.0031
Endotoxin	B	1.3×10^7	0.0002-0.0007	0.0034
Endotoxin	C	5.0×10^6	0.0015	ND****
Diphosphoryl lipid A (unfractionated)	A	2.6×10^6	0.0005-0.001	0.0088
Diphosphoryl lipid A (purified, TLC-3)	A	8.0×10^5	0.012	0.0064
Monophosphoryl lipid A (Unfractionated)	B	1.0×10^6	2-5	6.7
Monophosphoryl lipid A (purified, TLC-3)	B	1.1×10^5	>10	>20
Lipid X	D	9.5×10^4	>10	>20
Lipid X (O-deacylated)	D	1.4×10^2	>10	>20
Lipid X (dophosphorylated)	D	3.2×10^1	>10	×20

Note:
* Source: A. *S. Syphimurium G30/C21*
   B. *S. minnesota R595*
   C. *E. coli 055.B5 (Travenol Laboratories, Inc.)*
   D. *E. coli MN7*
** EU: Defined as the potency of 0.2 ng of an EC-2 reference standard endotoxin (gel clot method). Source of lysate, Travenol Laboratories, Inc. (sensitivity, 0.13 EU/mL).
*** The approximate dose necessary to cause a febrile response of >0.46°C in 50% of a test population.
**** ND. Not done.

loss of KDO; instead, major chemical and biological alterations of the degraded molecule are reported to result from saponification of fatty acids. Niwa et al. (1969) reported that depyrogenation is enhanced when LPS is subjected to alkaline hydrolysis with 0.1N NaOH in either 95% ethanol or 80% dimethylsulfoxide (DMSO). Effective depyrogenation has been reported by using 0.1M NaOH at 30°C for 72 hours (Mikami et al., 1982), and 4°C for 16 hours (Kakinuma et al., 1981). The application of acids and bases to depyrogenation was reviewed recently by McCullough and Novitsky, 1985.

D. Oxidation

Knowledge of oxidative inactivation of endotoxins can be traced to the beginning of the century when Hort and Penfold (1912) reported that Salmonella typhosa cells lost fever-producing capacity when washed in hydrogen peroxide. Although the mechanism of action of hydrogen peroxide on LPS is unknown, peroxidation of the fatty acids present in the Lipid A region of LPS has been suggested. In 1945, Campbell and Cherkin observed that a gelatin solution was rendered nonpyrogenic after it was boiled with 0.1M hydrogen peroxide for two hours or autoclaved with 0.4M hydrogen peroxide at 116°C for 20 minutes. Taub and Hart (1948) utilized peroxide to detoxify pyrogens in Water for Injection, normal saline, and dextrose-saline solutions. They found that the most effective treatment was boiling in the presence of 0.1% hydrogen peroxide for 2 hours. Under these conditions, the final solution was also free of peroxide. An adaptation of this procedure was successfully applied to large-scale depyrogenation of infusion solutions by Mengel (1951) at a Tel Aviv hospital. Recently, DeRenzis (1981) described the endotoxin inactivation capacity of hydrogen peroxide as measured by a cell-growth inhibitor. When 3% hydrogen peroxide was added to equal parts of cell-growth medium, which was then incubated at room temperature for 24 hours and subsequently dialyzed, the ability of endotoxin to inhibit cell growth was substantially reduced. Gould and Novitsky (1985) clearly demonstrated that the inactivation of endotoxin by hydrogen peroxide is dependent on time, pH, and concentration. Using as little as 2.7% hydrogen peroxide at 65°C for 1 hour, these authors observed approximately a 90% reduction of endotoxin as measured by LAL. When the peroxide was increased to 27%, virtually 100% destruction was achieved within 1 hour. Oxidative depyrogenation using hydrogen peroxide offers several advantages over other methods. Hydrogen peroxide is safe to handle, can be eliminated from solution easily, and appears to inactivate endotoxin under non-extreme conditions (i.e., low concentration of hydrogen peroxide and low temperature). Its chief disadvantage is that hydrogen peroxide may adulterate product. Methods of oxidative depyrogenation using agents other than hydrogen peroxide exist and may offer advantages for specific applications. These include treatment with molecular oxygen (DeRenzis, 1981), hypochlorous acid or hypochlorite (Dean and Adamson, 1916; Charomat and Lechat, 1950), periodic acid or sodium periodate (Neter et al.,

1956; Goebel, 1947), dilute potassium permanganate (Carter, 1930), nitric acid, dichromate, and selenium dioxide (Suzuki, 1953).

E. Alkylation

Several authors have reported that treating endotoxin with alkylating agents decreases pyrogenicity. Schenck et al. (1969) demonstrated a 100-fold decrease in pyrogenicity when endotoxin was treated with acetic anhydride. The same group reported a 100- to 1000-fold decrease when endotoxin was treated with succinic anhydride. The mechanism behind this reduction was thought to be acetylation and succinylation, respectively. However, even though succinylation caused a marked decrease in pyrogenicity, the endotoxin adjuvanicity was not lost. Further studies demonstrated that treatment with phthalic anhydride, a strong alkylating agent, caused a 10,000-fold reduction in pyrogenicity and a 1,000-fold decrease in lethality in mice; however, the ability of treated endotoxin to induce nonspecific resistance was not altered (Elin et al., 1983). Alkylation was thought to occur through nucleophilic substitution in the glucosamine linkage of Lipid A and/or in the ethanolamine of the LPS core region. There is conflicting evidence concerning the ability of succinylation to decrease the pyrogenicity of endotoxin. Westphal concluded that succinylation did not alter the pyrogenicity of endotoxin by reaction with OH groups available on the KDO disaccharide (Westphal, 1975). Ethylene oxide (EtO) is also a strong alkylating agent. A study published by Tsuji and Harrison (1978) showed a 94% reduction following EtO sterilization of E. coli 0127:B8 endotoxin inoculated onto aluminum or glass. The EtO sterilization cycle used involved 12% EtO and 88% Freon™, 50% relative humidity (rH), and 3.5psi for 6.5 hours. Additional work on this method should be encouraged because it could have widespread application for depyrogenation of heat-labile substances and EtO-sterilized medical devices. The use of EtO for depyrogenation has been addressed by Hudson and Nase (1985).

F. Ionizing radiation

Several studies have been reported in which Cobolt-60 ionizing radiation was utilized to reduce the toxicity of bacterial endotoxin. Bertok and Szeberenyi (1983), described the use of a ^{60}Co irradiated endotoxin preparation, Tolerin™, that significantly decreased the endotoxin's lethal and hypotensive effects in a dose-related manner. The ability of endotoxin to activate the complement system was also affected, while immunoadjuvant properties and ability to stimulate nonspecific resistance were retained. Csako et al. (1983) investigated the physical and biological properties of ^{60}Co ionizing radiation. Physical and biological changes were reported to be dose-dependent. A gradual loss of the polysaccharide components (0-side chain and R-core) was observed, and activity tests suggested that destruction of Lipid A was dose-related. Both pyrogenicity and LAL reactivity of the endotoxin were destroyed by increasing doses of radiation. However, because it increases the possibility of unknown chemical changes to drugs and parenteral solutions, use of ionizing radiation in depyrogenating these materials is unlikely. Ionizing radiation would be of far greater use in producing endotoxin that has lost its harmful pyrogenic and toxic properties, but retained beneficial properties, such as adjuvanicity, that increases the body's immune defense. Hudson and Nase (198) reviewed the application of ionizing radiation to depyrogenation.

5. Validation of Depyrogenation Processes

Since the LAL assay has been shown to be a valid test to monitor inactivation or removal of endotoxin, the task of testing for endotoxin has been made simple in recent years. Depyrogenation validation has been reviewed by Novitsky (1984). Two documents are worthy of mention here regarding depyrogenation validation (1) USP XXI Chapter 1211, which addresses Sterilization and Sterility Assurance, and (2) the FDA draft guideline on aseptic filling. The former document provides the following guidance: "Since dry heat is frequently employed to render glassware or containers free from pyrogens as well as viable microbes, a pyrogen challenge, where necessary, should be an integral part of the validation program, e.g., by inoculating one or more articles to be treated with 1000 or more USP Units of bacterial endotoxin. The test with Limulus lysate could be used to demonstrate that the endotoxic substance had been inactivated to not more than 1/1000 of the original amount (3 cycle reduction). For the test to be valid, both the original and remaining amount of endotoxin should be measured." Since USP XXI became official January 1, 1985, and since this paragraph is the only statement regarding validation of depyrogenation in any USP or FDA document, it is recommended as a guide.

The current FDA draft guideline indicates that any properly validated depyrogenation process is acceptable. For glass containers, final rinse water is acceptable if it meets the requirements of USP Water for Injection. Depyrogenation may be accomplished by initial washings with caustic soda followed by Water for Injection. In addition, this document makes provision to depyrogenate glass containers by dry heat. Although parameters of time and temperature are not established, the USP recommends 250°C for 30 minutes, which provides a 6 log reduction in endotoxin activity. As stated above, Chapter 1211 of USP XXI requires demonstration of a 3 log reduction for depyrogenation. The draft guideline simply states that "one method of assessing the adequacy of a depyrogenation process is to simulate the process using containers having known quantities of standard endotoxins and measure the level of reduction." Although the document does not distinguish between the behavior of environmental endotoxin per se and refined lipopolysaccharide standards, this behavioral phenomenon is clearly recognized by the document. The differences between environmental endotoxins and refined endotoxins has been reviewed by Pearson (1985). The FDA is aware of one potential problem where freeze-dried endotoxins are used to assess certain washing processes. It appeared that the freeze-dried material may be much more soluble in the wash and rinse water than other challenge material as well as more soluble than endotoxins that may normally be present on container/closure surfaces. This difference in solubility could result in perceiving the process under consideration as being much more efficient at endotoxin removal than it really is. Therefore, challenge endotoxins should be at least as difficult to remove from surfaces as are endotoxins that would normally be present.

In addition to considering the kind of endotoxin used, one should bear in mind that the nature of the material being used in the depyrogenation protocol is an important variable; e.g., new glass adsorption not only varies among types of glass but also may vary between manufacturers of the same glass type (Novitsky 1985). Endotoxin adsorption is typically fixed, and so the lower the challenge, the greater the total percentage that will be adsorbed. The mode of endotoxin challenge is also important to the percentage of recovery. Some depyrogenation procedures begin with containers having endotoxin in solution. Generally, recovery of endotoxin from an aqueous environment is acomplished readily. Endotoxin recovery from glass is usually more difficult when endotoxin has been air dried. Freeze dried endotoxin is easily recovered. Although endotoxin challenge as reported in the literature has varied significantly, probably a reasonable endotoxin challenge should be a minimum of 1000 endotoxin units (EU).

6. References

Akers, M.J., Avis, K. E. and Thompson, B. (1980). J. Parent. Drug Assoc. 34, 330-348.

Akers, M.J., Ketron, K. M. and Thompson B.R. (1982). J. Parent. Sci. Tech., 36, 23-27.

Banks, H. M. (1934). Am. J. Clin. Pathol. 4, 260-291.

Bennett, I. L., Jr. (1964). In "Bacterial Endotoxins" (M. Landy and W. Braum eds), pp 13, Rutgers University Press, New Jersey.

Berger, A., Ellenbogen, G.D. and Ginger L. (1956). Adv. Chem 16, 168.

Bertok, L. and Szeberenyi, S. (1983). Immunopharmacol 6, 1-5.

Biondi, A., Landolfo, S., Fumarola, D., Polentarutti, N., Introna, M. and Mantovani, A. (1984). J. Immunological Methods 66(1), 103-112.

Bishop, D. F. and Desnick, R. J. (1981). J. Biol. Chem. 256, 1307-1316.

Braude, A.I., Ziegler, E.J., Douglas, H. and McCutchan, J.A. (1977). J. Inf. Diseases 136, S167-S173.

Brindle, H. and Rigby (1946). Qtly. J. Pharm. Pharmacol. 19, 302-339.

Butler, T. and Moller, G. (1977). Infect. Immunol. 18, 400-404.

Campbell, D.H. and Cherkin, A. (1945). Science 102, 535.

Carazzone, M., Arecco, D., Fava, M. and Sancin, P. (1985). J. Parenteral Science and Technology 39(2), 69-74.

Carter, E.B. (1930). J. Lab. Clin. Med. 16, 289-291.

Casko, G., Elin, R.J., Hochstein, H.D. and Tsai, C.M. (1983). Infect. Immunol. 41, 190-196.

Charonnat, R. and Lechat, P. (1950). Ann. Pharm. Franc. 8, 171-181.

Cherkin, A. (1975). Immunochemistry 12, 625-627.

Cooper, J.F., Levin, J. and Wagner, H.N. (1970). J. Nucl. Med. 11, 310.

Cooperstock, M.S. (1974). Antimicrob. Agents Chemothec. 6, 422-425.

Costin, R.C. (1980). Unpublished data. Parenteral Drug Association.

Cradock, J.C., Guder, L.A., Francis, D.L. and Morgan, S.L. (1978). J. Pharm. Pharmac. 30, 198-199.

Dean, H.R. and Adamson, R.S. (1916). Brit. Med. J. I, 611.

DeRenzis, F.A. (1980). J. Dent. Res. 60, 933-935.

Duff, G.W., Waisman, D.M. and Atrins, E. (1982). Clinical Research 30(#2), 565A.

Federal Register 50(22) February 1, 1985, 4799.

Feldsine, P.T., Ferry, E.W., Gauthier, R.J. and Pisik, J.J. (1979). Parenteral Drug Assoc. 33, 125-131.

Fiore, J.V., Olson, W.P. and Holst, S.L. (1980). In "Methods of Plasma Protein Fractionation", (Curling, ed), Academic Press, London.

Galanos, C., Luderitz, O., Rietschel, E.T., and Westphal, O. (1977). Int. Rev. Biochem. 14, 239-335.

Garbner, R.W. (1975). U.S. Patent 3,897,309.

Gemmell, D.H.O. and Todd, J.P. (1945). Pharm J. 154, 126.

Gerba, C.P., Hou, K.C., Babineau, R.A. and Fiore, J.V. (1980). Pharm. Technol. 4, 83-89.

Goebel, W. (1947). J. Exp. Med. 85, 499.

Gould, M. J. and Novitsky, T.J. (1985). In "Monograph on Depyrogenation," Chapter 9, pp 84-92, Parenteral Drug Association, Philadelphia.

Harris, N.S. and Feinstein, R. In "Biomedical Application of The Horseshoe Crab (Limulidae)" (Cohen, ed), pp. 265-274. Alan R. Liss, Inc., New York.

Henderson, L.W. and Beans, E. (1978). Kidney Int. 14, 522-525.

Henderson, L.W., Sanfelippo, M.L. and Beans, F. (1978). Trans. Am. Soc. Art. Int. Org. 24, 178-184.

Hort, E.C. and Penfold, W.J. (1911). Brit. Med. J. 2. 1510-1589

Hort, E.C. and Penfold, W.J. (1912). J. Hygiene 12, 361-390.

Hou, K., Gerba, C.P., Goyal, S.M. and Zerda, K.S. (1980). Appl. Environ. Microbiol. 40, 892-896.

Hudson, C.T. and Mose, R. (1985). In "Monograph on Depyrogenation", Chapter 14, pp. 113-116. Parenteral Drug Association, Philadelphia pp. 113-116.

Issekutz, A.C. (1983). J. Immunol. Methods 61, 275-281.

Johns, M., Skehill, A., and McCabe W. R. (1983). J. Inf. Diseases. 147 (1) 57-67.

Johnson, D.S., Lin, K., Fitzgerald, E. and LePage, B. (1980). In "Ultrafiltration Membranes and Applications" (A. R. Cooper, ed), p. 475. Plenum Press, New York.

Kakinuma, A., Asano, T., Torii, H. and Sugino, Y. (1981). Biochem. Biophys. Res. Commun. 101, 434-439.

Koden, H. (1975). Pharmazie 30, 752.

Luderitz, O., Galanos, C., Lehmann, V., Nurminen, M., Rietschel, E.T., Rosenfelder, G., Simon, M. and Westphal (1973). In "Bacterial Lipopolysaccharides". (E. H. Koss and S. M. Wolff, ed), pp. 9-21. University of Chicago Press, Chicago.

Luderitz, O., Galamos, C. and Rietschel, E.J. (1982). Pharmac. Ther. 15, 383-402.

Mahand, M.W., Fiore, V. and Babineau, R. (1985). In "Monograph on Depyrogenation", Chapter 5, pp. 45-53. Parenteral Drug Association, Philadelphia.

Mahoney, R. F. (1985). In "Monograph on Depyrogenation", Chapter 4, pp. 37-44. Parenteral Drug Association, Philadelphia.

Mascoli, C.C. and Weary, M.E. (1979). J. Parenter. Drug Assoc. 33, 81-95.

McCullough, K.Z. (1982). In "Endotoxins and their Detection with the Limulus Amebocyte Lysate Test" (S.W. Watson, J. Levin, T.J. Novitsky, eds), pp. 91-100. Alan R. Liss, Inc., New York.

McCullough, K.Z. and Novitsky, T.J. (1985). In Monograph on Depyrogenation, Chapter 8, pp. 78-83. Parenteral Drug Association, Philadelphia.

Mengel, E. (1951). J. Am. Pharm. Assoc. 40, 175-176.

Mikami, T., Nagase, T., and Matsumoto, T. (1982). Microbiol. Immunol., 26, 403-409.

Minobe, S., Sato, T., Tosa, T., and Chibata, I. (1983). J. Chromatog. 262, 193-198.

Morrison, D.C. and Curry, B.J. (1979). J. Immunol. Meth. 27, 83-92.

Morrison, D.C. and Jacobs, D.M. (1976). Immunochem 13, 813-818.

Nachum, R., Siegel, S.E., Sullivan, J.D. and Watson, S.W. (1978). J. Invert. Pathol. 32, 51-58.

Nelson, L. (1985). In "Monograph on Depyrogenation," Chapter 3, pp. 28-36. Parenteral Drug Association, Philadelphia.

Neter, E., Westphal, O., Luderitz, O., Gorzynsky, E.A. and Eichanberger, E. (1956). J. Immunol. 76, 377-385.

Niwa, M., Milner, K.C., Ribi and Rudback, J.A. (1969). J. Bacteriol. 97, 1069-1077.

Nolan, J.P., McDeritt, J.J. and Goldmann, G.S. (1975). Proc. Soc. Exp. Biol. Med. 149, 766-770.

Novitsky, T.J. (1984). LAL Update 2(5), 1-4. Associates of Cape Cod, Inc., Woods Hole, MA.

Novitsky, T.J. and Gould, M.J. (1985). In "Monograph on Depyrogeration", Chapter 10, pp. 93-97. Parenteral Drug Association, Philadelphia.

Novitsky, T.J. and Gould, M.J. (1985). In Monograph on Depyrogenation, Chapter 11, pp. 98-100. Parenteral Drug Association, Philadelphia.

Novitsky, T.J., Ryther, S.S. and Gould, M. In "Monograph on Depyrogenation", Chapter 13, pp. 109-112. Parenteral Drug Association, Philadelphia.

Pearson, F.C. (1985). In "Monograph on Depyrogenation", Chapter 1, pp. 1-14. Parenteral Drug association, Philadelphia.

Pearson, F.C. (1985). In "Pyrogens: Endotoxin and LAL Testing, pp. 64-86. Marcel Dekker, Inc., New York.

Pearson, F.C. (1985). Alan R. Liss, Inc. New York. (in press).

Pearson, F.C., Barick, J., Snigley, W., Maglalong, E., Graff, E., Abroson, F. and Garcia, D. (1981). Dev. Indust. Microbiol. 22, 371-380.

Pearson, F.C, Weary, M.E. and Dabbah R. (1982). In "Endotoxins and Their Detection with the Limulus Amebocyte Lysate Test" (S.W. Watson, J. Levin, T.J. Novitsky, eds), pp. 231-246. Alan R. Liss Inc., New York.

Polmer, C.H.R. and Whittet, T.D. (1971). Chem. Ind. 13, 341-344.

Rechen, H.C. (1984). Pharmaceutical Manufacturing, 1, 29-31.

Reichelderfer, P.S., Manischewitz, J.F., Wells, J.A., Hochstein, H.D. and Ennis, F.A. (1975). Appl. Microbiol. 30, 333-334.

Reinhardt, R. (1985). In Monograph on Depyrogenation", Chapter 7, pp. 70-77. Parenteral Drug Association, Philadelphia.

Ribi, E., Cantrell, J.L., Kuni, T. and Omano, K. (1984). In "Beneficial Effects of Endotoxins" (A. Nowotny, ed), pp. 529-554. Plenum Press, New York.

Rickles, F.R., Levin, J. Atkins, E. and Queensberry, P. (1979). In Biomedical Applications of the Horseshoe Crab (Limulidae)", (E. Cohen, ed), pp. 203-207. Alan R. Liss, Inc., New York.

Rietschel, E. T., Schade, U., Jensen, M., Wollenweber, H.W., Luderitz, O. and Greisman, S.G. (1982). Scand. J. Infect. Dis. 31, 8-21.

Robinson, J.R., O'Dell, M.C., Takacs, J., Barnes, T. and Genovesi, C. (1985). In "Monograph on Depyrogenation," Chapter 6, pp. 54-69. Parenteral Drug Association, Philadelphia.

Rossitto, J. (1979). Pharm. Tech. Int. 2, 39.

Sarafin, T.A., Tsay, K.K., Fluharty and Kihara (1982). Biochemical Medicine 28, 237-240.

Schenck, J.R., Hargie, M.P., Brown, M.S., Evert, D.S., Yoo, L.A. and McIntire, F.C. (1969). J. Immunol. 102, 1411-1422.

Seibert, F.B. (1923). Am. J. Physiol., 67, 90-104.

Shibatani,T., Kakimoto, T., Chibata, F. (1983). Thromb. Haemostasis 49, 91-95.

Soter, G. (1984). Biotechnology 12, 1035-1037.

Suzuki, S. (1953). J. Pharm. Soc. Japan. 73, 615-619.

Sweadner, K.J., Forte, M. and Nelson, L.L. (1977). Applied & Envir. Micro. 34, 382-385.

Sweet, B.H. and Huxsole (1985). In "Monograph on Depyrogenation", Chapter 12, pp. 101-108. Parenteral Drug Association, Philadelphia.

Takahashi, S., Yomo, S., Nagsoka, Y., Kawamura, K. and Minami, S. (1983). J. Pharmaceutical Sciences 72, 739-742.

Taub, A. and Hart, F. (1948). J. Am. Pharm. Assoc. 37, 246-250.

Tripodi, D. and Norwoony A. (1966). Ann. N.Y. Acad Sci, 133, 604-631.

Tsuji, K. and Harrison, S.J. (1978). Appl. Environ. Microbiol. 36, 710-714.

Tsuji, K. and Harrison, S.J. (1979). In "Biomedical Applications of The Horseshoe Crab (Limulidae)" ed, Cohen, pp. 367-378. Alan R. Liss, Inc. New York.

Tsuji, K. and Lewis, A.R. (1978). Appl. Environ. Microbiol. 36, 715-719.

Tutunjian, R.S. (1985). In "Monograph on Depyrogenation", Chapter 2, pp. 15-27. Parenteral Drug Association, Philadelphia.

Twohy, C.W., Duran, A.P. and Munson, T.E. (1984). J. Paren. Sci. Tech. 38, 190-201.

USP XXI, Chapter 1214.

Welch, H., Price, C.W., Chandler, V.L. and Hunter, A.C. (1943). J. Am. Pharm. Assoc. 34, 114-118.

Westphal, O. (1975). Int. Archs. Allergy Appl. Immunol. 49, 1-43.

Wilke, H. and Vob, H.E. (1954). Arzneim. Forsch. Drug Research 4, 8-14.

Wollman, Y., Bonak, Y., and Levin J. (1982). Biomed. Pharmacother. 36, 323-325.

5

Sterilization of Small-Volume Parenterals and Therapeutic Proteins by Filtration

Wayne P. Olson
Hyland Therapeutics, Los Angeles, CA, USA

1. Introduction

Large-volume parenterals, such as 5% dextrose in water (D5W), are terminally autoclaved in the final container. When the autoclave system and cycle are validated for overkill, i.e., 10^6 *Bacillus stearothermophilus* spores killed in the coldest portion of the container during the cycle, the probability of survival of any microbe in the final container is sufficiently low that the merit of testing final containers for sterility is questionable (Mascoli, 1981). Ionizing radiation has proven effective for the sterilization of devices but, with the exception of gamma irradiation from, for example, a ^{60}Co source, the penetrating power is insufficient to effectively sterilize aqueous solutions and suspensions. A problem with gamma irradiation of aqueous solutions is that peroxides and free radicals can be generated (Jacobs and Donbrow, 1977); peroxides may cause a pH shift and redox reactions causing degradation of the product, while free radicals may cause cross-linking or other degradative reactions.

There is an ancillary problem with any intravenous drug solution. Particles in suspension, if present in large numbers and large in size (greater than 10 micron diameter), can occlude the small capillaries of the lung. Large particles can be removed by centrifugation, but small particles, such as bacteria, are not fully removed by short-term exposure to a centrifugal force of even 5,000 G. The best solution to the sterilization and particle removal problems is microporous filtration, currently termed microfiltration. In view of the need for

101

particle reduction in injectable drugs and those preparations introduced into the eye, all drug preparations presently are filtered, the large-volume parenterals through 0.45 micron rated pore diameter (RPD) membrane filters and the small-volume parenterals and therapeutic proteins through 0.2 micron RPD membrane filters when possible. Properly set-up systems are reliable and economic in making solutions bacteriologically sterile and relatively particle-free.

This chapter addresses setting up a functional, reliable filtration system: how filters work, how to design a system for a given pharmaceutical application, and how to fix what goes wrong. In the main, the information is intended to be practical and to be used in research, scale-up, and manufacturing.

2. Definitions

A filter is a porous solid that retains particles when a particle-laden fluid passes through it. For practical purposes, we will consider in this chapter only filtration carried out under positive pressure, with one exception: rotary drum filters, which utilize a vacuum on the downstream side. Rotary drum filters are in declining use as they are less efficient than positive pressure systems. Generally, filters are of two types: depth, which tend to trap particles throughout the depth of the filter but often pass some particles, and membrane filters, which tend to trap particles on the surface. In fact, membrane filters actually trap some particles well below the filter surface and may release a small amount of matrix, usually considered as behavior typical of a depth filter. The porosity of a filter is the void volume, or air space in an unwetted filter and is expressed as a percentage of volume. Porosity is often confused with pore diameter or pore size rating, which refer to the diameter of retained particles. The pore size rating of membrane filters used in the pharmaceutical industry are determined by the minimal sizes of the organisms retained 100% by the filters (ASTM, 1983; HIMA, 1982; Rogers and Rossmore, 1970). The term "absolute", applied to a filter, is inappropriate and is deprecated by ASTM Committee F-21 and other filtration standards organizations. The feed to a filter is the fluid from which particles are to be removed. The filtrate is the fluid that has passed through the filter. The filter medium is the porous material used in the fluid-particle separation. Media migration is the shedding of portions of the medium into the filtrate, and commonly occurs with most depth filters. The upstream side of a filter is the side from which the fluid is applied; downstream is the filtrate side. Dead-end filtration refers to unidirectional systems in which all of the fluid in the feed goes directly through the filter. Retentate is fluid that remains on the upstream side of a filter, where it may be recirculated. Circulation of the feed on the upstream side of a filter is called crossflow or tangential flow filtration. Recycle refers either to the initial filtrate from a depth filter, which is returned to the upstream side so as to recapture migrated medium, or to the retentate in a crossflow system (described elsewhere in this Chapter).

3. How Filtration Systems Work

A. Matrix types

The various types of filter matrix systems are: deep bed, filter aids and filter cakes, woven and nonwoven depth filters, asbestos and charge-modified matrices, microporous membrane filters, and ultrafilters. Reverse osmosis (RO) membranes, used in the concentration of some peptides drugs and antibiotics, are also sometimes used in place of distillation in the processing of water.

Deep bed filters are large-diameter columns or flat beds of particles that remove particles from city water and from municipal sewage. These filters are generally comprised of sand and gravel but occasionally exotic materials such as walnut shells are used. The holdup volume in deep bed filters is very large, and the filters operate at one gravity. These limitations are inconsequential with unprocessed water but decrease the economies of manufacturing when used to filter product solutions. Deep bed filters are coarse and are prepared from unrefined materials; they are unsuitable for the preparation of drug solutions. For the description, characterization, and details on the scale-up of deep bed filters, see Ives (1977).

Figure 1 — Diatomaceous earth of freshwater origin. *Photo courtesy of Eagle-Picher Co.*

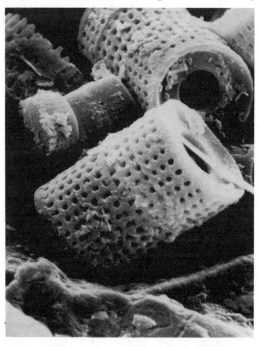

Filter aids and filter cakes are used widely in the pharmaceutical industry. For example, diatomaceous earth (Figure 1) is added (at about 2 to 5 grams per liter) to Cohn fraction IV-1 during the filtration of the ethanolic solution (Cohn et al., 1946; Fiore et al., 1980). The diatomaceous earth provides a continually renewing filtration surface of high porosity as the filter aid forms a cake of increasing thickness on the porous septum (Figure 2). The septum may be a woven or nonwoven cloth, or another filter, e.g., in the form of the Cuno cartridges (Figures 3, 4). The bulk of particles and organisms are removed with such a system. This type of operation is suitable only for batch filtration. Eventually the accumulated cake becomes sufficiently thick that cake resistance becomes significant while the space between filter elements becomes very small.

Figure 2—Filter aid (open particles), as a body feed, forms a cake, entrapping dirt and bioburden (solid particles)

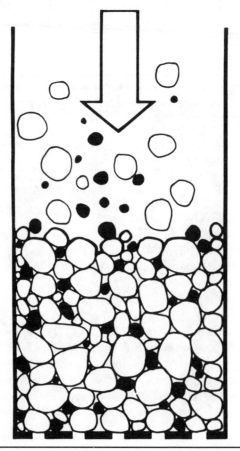

Figure 3—Cutaway of a depth cartridge filter. *Photo courtesy of Cuno, Inc.*

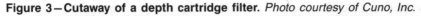

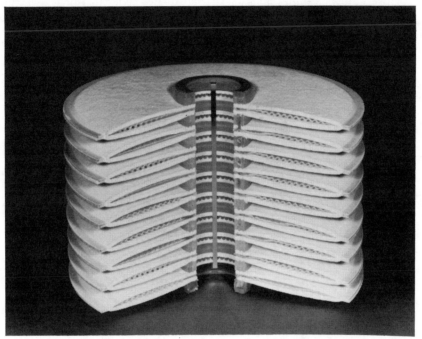

Before filtration with a body feed commences, a pre-coat of a finer filter aid usually is deposited at high velocity onto the septum. Good examples are Hyflo SuperCel (Manville) and the comparable Celatom grade. The pre-coat is suspended in water for injection (WFI) and usually is driven onto the septum under air or nitrogen pressure or with a pump capable of driving slurries, e.g., a diaphragm pump. The desired depth of pre-coat varies with the application and is best determined experimentally; 1mm is commonplace (see Cain, 1979). When filtration of product together with the body feed commences, the initial filtrate is best recycled into the batch tank because some free filter aid may be present. Transparent tubing, e.g., Tygon™, is best used on the downstream side of such filters so that, should breakthrough occur and body feed or pre-coat (or both) appear in the filtrate, it can be seen by the operator before a substantial amount of man-hours are wasted. In the event of breakthrough, a new filtration setup is required.

Figure 4 — Assembled cartridge, less the bell that seals the housing.
Photo courtesy of Cuno, Inc.

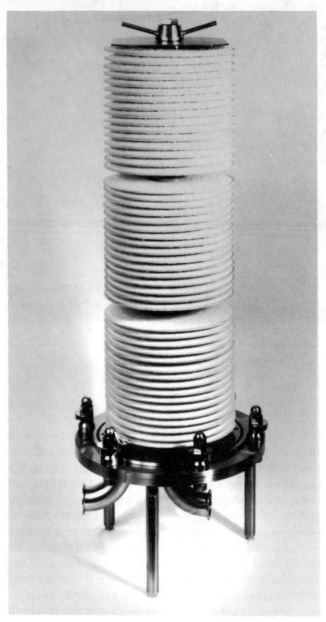

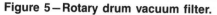
Figure 5 — Rotary drum vacuum filter.

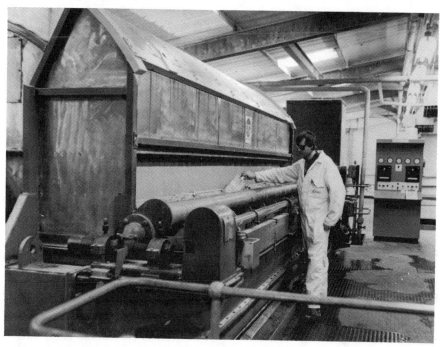

Continuous filtration with cakes also can be done, as with the rotary drum vacuum filters (Figure 5) and other vacuum filters of related design (Dahlstrom and Silverblatt, 1977). The drum rotates into a slurry of diatomaceous earth and the suspension to be filtered. The cake performs the filtration under negative pressure (vacuum) from the downstream side. The spent cake is stripped from the drum with a long knife blade immediately prior to the drum and immersed again into the product-diatom slurry. Dr. Fred Rothstein (Personal Communication) refers to this as "sludge removal"; a step which cannot achieve fine filtration.

Woven and nonwoven depth filters include the silk, cotton and stainless steel woven and sintered matrices. The tightest of the weaves, pore ratings down to about 20 or 25 micron, is Dutch Twill. These cloths are in heavy use in filter presses (Figure 6), pressure leaf filters, and in baghouses they remove particles from industrial exhaust gases. Hot stack gases are filtered through Kynar™ and other heat-resistant synthetics. These media are not truly deep in the sense that they are thick; indeed, they seldom are thick. They are depth media in the sense that they trap particles throughout their depth. The pore size distributions tend to be rather broad and they are used to remove the bulk of particles and organ-

Figure 6— Pharaceutical filter press. *Photo courtesy of Seitz-Enzinger-Noll.*

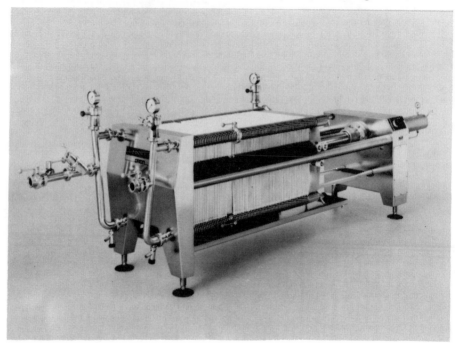

isms from a fluid feed. Borosilicate microfiberglass filters fall in this category. These filters have been very popular in filter presses for the "de-sludging" of pharmaceutical preparations. Oils, heated to reduce their viscosity, are filtered through fiberglass prior to membrane filtration. A membrane filter scavenges the last of the particles and any fibers that might have dislodged from the glass medium.

The relatively thin depth media commonly are pleated and the pleat-packs, together with support structures (core, pleat supports, porous jacket) are married to endcaps that fit into a filter housing. Deadend filtration through such cartridges is done in all industrial-scale pharmaceutical operations. In such cartridges, the nonwoven materials are preferred over the woven materials as the dirt-handling capacity of the former generally is greater and the nonwovens are less expensive to produce.

The CW cartridge series produced by Millipore consist of membrane lacquer cast onto a nonwoven cellulose. Although the membrane portion of the matrix tends to crack at the apices during pleating for cartridge preparation, the membrane portion prevents heavy media migration; fiber release is minimal, but some does occur. The CW cartridges are effective and are in widespread use in the pharmaceutical industry. The AR material produced by Pall (Pall and Krakauer, 1973) consists of titanium microfibrils onto which is cast vinyl acetate. The vinyl acetate polymerizes, bonding the titanium microfibrils into a random pattern like that shown by Meltzer and Lukaszewicz (1979). Double layers of this matrix are pleated and sealed to endcaps to form cartridge filters. The matrix cracks at the apices of the pleats, and most of the cartridges cannot be tested by the bubble-point method (Pall, 1975). This matrix sheds titanium microfibrils in large quantities (Dwyer, 1975). The AR series filters were in widespread use in the pharmaceutical industry in the mid-1970s, but have been replaced by the manufacturer with a nylon 66 membrane filter of high quality.

Asbestos and charge-modified matrices are claimed to possess unusually efficient particle-removal properties attributed to the electrokinetic interaction of particles in suspension (they are usually negatively charged) with a positively-charged matrix (Ostreicher, 1977a; 1977b). Asbestos microfibrils, like the titanium microfibrils of the AR material, are sufficiently thin to fall below the limits of resolution of the light microscope. Asbestos can cause mesothelioma when inhaled (Selikoff et al., 1964; Kang and Salvaggio, 1976), but hard evidence on the effects of intravenously or intramuscularly injected asbestos fibers is not readily available. Titanium microfibrils are known to cause mesothelioma (Stanton and Layard, 1978), and are no longer produced by DuPont. Whether the FDA ban on the use of asbestos filters for injectable products is absolutely necessary has been debated but never resolved. However, the FDA stricture seems to be a conservative step taken properly, under considerable public pressure (Nelson, 1973). When media like this are used in process, whether in filter presses or cartridge form, the initial filtrate is recycled to the upstream side of the filtration system using a system of the type shown in Figure 7. In this manner, the heaviest shedding of particles is recycled to the upstream side of the filter and no product is discarded.

Figure 7—Plate-and-frame press, showing recycle of the initial filtrate so as to retain migrated medium.

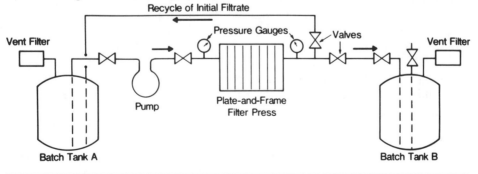

Parenthetically, it is interesting to note that many wineries in Europe still use asbestos pads, and some asbestos appears in the wine, but there is no unusual incidence of related cancers in France or Italy.

The positive charge of asbestos is imparted by Mg(II) on the siliceous core, and the coupling of amino and other positively-charged groups to depth media has simulated the effectiveness of asbestos at mildly acid, neutral, and alkaline pH (Fiore et al., 1980). Viruses and bacteria are trapped with high efficiency by charge-modified media (Hou et al., 1980). The non-asbestos media consist of cellulose fibers, diatomaceous earth, and perlite together with proprietary resins, but the felting is done in the usual manner. The pads or cartridges are used with or without filter aids. Particular attention to extractables and holdup volume are necessary, as discussed later in this chapter.

Membrane filters scavenge the last few bacteria, fungi, and dirt particles from solution. Most of the particle entrapment is on the membrane surface; the particle capacity, before clogging occurs, is modest by comparison with the depth filters. However, the relatively tight range of pore size distributions of the better-made membrane filters provides good assurance of bacterial retention. Disc filters are still in industrial use in Multiplate™ (Millipore) and One-Sevener™ (Nuclepore) systems which place many 293mm diameter (ca. 532cm² or 81in² per disc) in parallel, to upwards of 1.6m² in a single Multiplate housing. These systems can require 45 to 60 minutes for setup. If the system fails the pre-use integrity test, it must be torn down and re-set with new filters. Each disc has long O-ring seals, any of which may fail due to improper seating.

Cartridge membrane filters consist of membranes together with pleat support structures, a core, and a protective cage, all of which are married to endcaps by means of a potting resin (polyurethane, or an epoxy resin, or a combination of both), or by softening the endcaps so that the pleat pack sinks into and is entrapped by the plastic of the endcap. The advantages of the pleated cartridge system are that the O-ring surface, for which an integral bond to the housing is dependent, is small, and 0.7 to 2.1 or more m² (7.4 to 22.2 ft.²) can be put into a relatively small housing (25 to 75cm long) in one or two minutes. The materials of composition for the membrane filter vary enormously. For proteins, cellulose acetate, or a hydrophilic version of poly (vinylidine difluoride) (PVDF or Kynar™) seem best as they tend not to bind proteins. The binding of proteins by a membrane filter reduces the average pore size, causing the rejection of very large proteins late in the filtration process. Polysulfone, especially the membrane filter type cast with unusually high degrees of anisotropy, tend to perform exceptionally well in the filtration of water and simple aqueous solutions but seem unsuitable for the filtration of proteins. The different materials available commercially are not equally suitable in every application. Particulars of various applications are given below.

Different pore types perform well. The polytetrafluoroethylene (PTFE, Polytef or Teflon™) membrane filters are made by stretching PTFE sheets; the filters are used widely in the filtration of gases and solvents, despite the unusual pore geometry (Figure 8). The conventional phase-inversion process creates interconnecting voids bounded by squares, pentagons and heptagons of filter matrix (Figure 9). The Accurel™ process creates interconnecting spherical voids within a polymerized matrix.

Figure 8 — PTFE microporous membrane filter. *SEM courtesy of W. L. Gore, Co.*

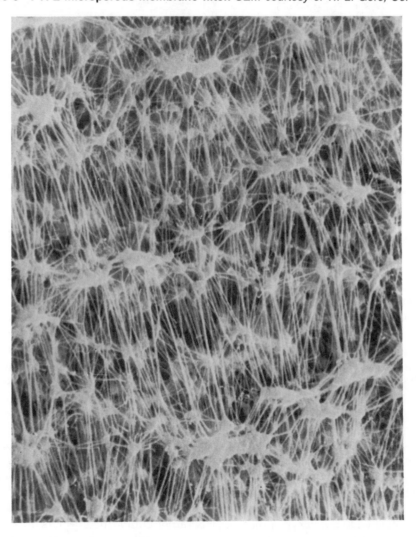

Figure 9 — A microporous phase-inversion filter of cellulose acetate.
SEM courtesy of Sartorius GmbH.

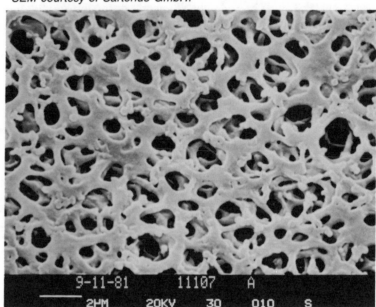

B. Driving liquid through the matrix

Vacuum systems still exist in some process lines, e.g., rotary vacuum drums, but are decreasingly popular because they are slow. The maximum pressure that can be applied is one atmosphere, assuming that a perfect vacuum can be made on the downstream side, a practical impossibility. However, vacuum (or negative-pressure) systems are used with the sterility test manifolds which are still in widespread use. Vacuum systems can contaminate the filtrate with extraneous airborne organisms and particles if any seal in the system fails; the reliability of such systems for sterilizing filtrations is highly questionable. However, the "desludging" applications of such equipment are still legitimate in pharmaceutical use.

Positive-pressure systems are mainly of two types: (a) constant pressure put on a liquid batch tank with a compressed gas such as nitrogen or air, and (b) constant rate supplied by a liquid pump, whether the pump is peristaltic, diaphragm, piston, or centrifugal.

Constant pressure systems are readily implemented and are clean, but are restricted to batch-type processes wherein a liquid-filled tank is pressurized to, for example, 1 bar (about 15psig). Many parenterals are processed in such systems as they are readily scaled-up. The tanks, seals and fittings must be sturdy and tight, or product will leak onto the workroom floor, but the intrusion of external organisms or particles into the system is unlikely.

Constant rate systems invariably invoke the use of a pump and often are necessary when sterile filtration is done in-line with a filling machine. Here the filling rate must be matched by the pump and the filtration system, regardless of other considerations. What happens with such systems is that the differential pressure across the filter does not change appreciably until the filter starts to clog, at which time the pressure differential incrementally increases, causing either a failure in the pump (usually at a shear pin) or in the filter or filter housing unless the membrane filter is changed. Fortunately, systems can be sized so as to avoid this problem.

Figure 10—Crossflow filtration system

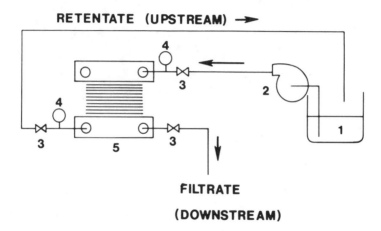

RETENTATE (UPSTREAM) →

FILTRATE

(DOWNSTREAM)

1—feed
2—pump
3—valve
4—pressure guage
5—crossflow cell

Crossflow systems are specialized systems not currently in common use. They involve the sweeping of the feed across a membrane filter as illustrated in the system shown in Figure 10. The feed sweeps particles and macromolecules from the filter surface. For solutions of macromolecules (e.g., hydroxyethylcellulose and most of the proteinaceous suspensions like albumin concentrates and clotting factor VIII concentrates), there is evidence that the shear in the thin channel over a crossflow membrane filter (most often about 0.030–0.040 inch) reduces solution viscosity. The reduction in viscosity reduces the resistance to flow through the membrane filter. Therefore, at very low differential pressures, high fluxes and throughputs of plasma proteins can be achieved (Lindley et al., 1982). An obvious case for crossflow is membrane plasmapheresis, wherein formed elements (red cells, leukocytes, platelets) sweep across the filter surface with approximately 70% of the plasma passing through the filter. The technique makes possible very fine filtrations of thick suspensions that otherwise would prove unfilterable (Lindley et al., 1982). However, the dramatic increase in rate and throughput is at the expense of time, filter area, and the cost of a four to eightfold increase in flow rates required to accommodate the recycle/retentate flow. Dead-end flow rates for factor VIII concentrates (through 0.2 micron RPD mixed esters of cellulose) are shown as filled circles in Figure 11. Open circles show the crossflow rate. The applied pressure was about 10psig.

Figure 11—Crossflow (open circles) and deadend (filled circles) flow rates for high molecular weight proteins through a GS filter.

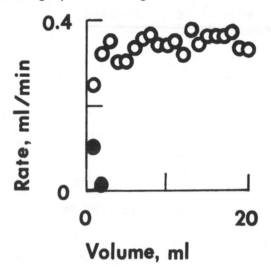

Many observers are of the opinion that the shear of crossflow systems causes the denaturation of proteins. This is not the case; denaturation occurs if air is entrained in the system, in which instance the air/water interface (foam) is the cause of the denaturation. See Olson (1983) for a discussion.

C. Effect of the feed on the system
The volume to be filtered is a critical consideration as can be appreciated from the comments on positive pressure filtration. The volume that reasonably can be filtered before the filters commence to clog to an ineffective degree must be

estimated. The problem is that the feed, the conditions, and the filters all vary from time to time.

Viscosity of the feed has a powerful influence on filtration rate. Viscosity is resistance to flow; a sufficiently viscous solution will not flow through a filter with a very small pore diameter. For example, 0.5% methylcellulose (used as a thickener in some ophthalmic preparations) is all but impossible to dead-end filter through a 0.2 micron-RPD membrane filter, but will filter well through a 0.45 micron-rated membrane filter at low pressure (less than 1 bar or less than 14-15psig).

The viscosity may be the result of a heavy particle burden, in which case correction can be effected by depth filtration. Oils often present problems of this type. An oil may appear optically clear but contain a heavy burden of particles with the same refractive index as the oil. A nonwoven fiberglass pad will usually remove a sufficient proportion of the particles so that effective membrane filtration can be done. A very viscous oil may be difficult to filter through a 0.45 or 0.2 micron-RPD membrane filter, and should be heated to 30 or 40°C to reduce the inherent viscosity.

Some systems, such as liposomes, do not lend themselves to filtration. Although liposomes are deformable, the act of filtration is likely to change the size distribution of the liposomes, and thus is inappropriate. The aqueous phase and the lipoid phase (usually of phospholipids) must be filtered separately, and then aseptically mixed. A similar strategy is applied in the purification of insoluble Zn-insulin.

All the above operations can be carried out using hydrophilic matrices, such as cellulose acetate, nylon, or hydrophilic Durapore™. For membrane filter applications, aqueous systems do not filter well through hydrophobic membranes such as PTFE. Pressures of about 80 psig are required to intrude water into a 0.2 micron-RPD PTFE membrane filter, and this is impractical. However, hydrophobic liquids filter readily, under modest pressure, through PTFE and other hydrophobic filter matrices. Accordingly, the solvents commonly used in pharmaceutical processing are often PTFE-filtered.

Solvents require special commentary. The use of acetone is widespread; however there is both an explosion hazard and a danger of inhalation of significant amounts over time, causing liver damage. Pumps, mixers and any other motors in the workroom must be explosion-proofed and a blowout wall installed, together with a suitable ventilation system and outside-air-source masks for the workers. Highly volatile solvents such as acetone are best transferred and filtered chilled, as low temperatures promote the liquid phase and reduce the vapor. Fortunately, the formation of some vapor is endothermic, and such solvents tend to be self-cooling.

Synthetic macromolecules, e.g. polyethylene glycol, can usually be heated to reduce viscosity for filtration. Most polysaccharides, such as the dextrans, are reasonably heat-tolerant, 30°C being well tolerated. But Methocel™, for example, does not heat well. Alkylated celluloses are solvated by H-binding, and heating of the solution literally strips some of the water away from the molecules, causing them to come out of solution, the so-called "cloud point." Peptides and proteins tend to denature, often irreversibly, at higher temperatures (usually greater than 40°C) and precipitate from solution. Where serious viscosity problems inhibit the filtration of proteins, the alternatives to heat are dilution or crossflow filtration. Even dilution may pose problems. For example, if a solution of fibronectin is diluted with distilled water, it will commence to precipitate as a saline environment is essential to the solubility of such proteins. Similarly, one must take some care with pH. A solution of human or bovine albumin is most viscous at a pH of 4.5-4.8, i.e., around the isoelectric point (pI). The pH of zero net charge on the protein is that pH at which the individual macromolecules tend least to repel one another, hence can aggregate.

D. Vent filters

Ideally, a vent filter is an hydrophobic membrane filter with a RPD of about 0.2 micron. An hydrophobic matrix, such as PTFE, is required so that the medium does not become wetted during steam autoclaving or steam-in-place sterilization. A wetted membrane filter passes air only by diffusion, which is intolerably slow for vent filters. Where vent filters are most needed are on sterile bulk tanks which usually are of thick-walled stainless steel. Thick-walled tanks do not implode when the pressure differential on the sealed tank, outside to inside, is 1 bar (about 15 psig). Therefore, sizing of the vent filters for such tanks is not critical. A small-area PTFE filter allows a slow pump out of the tank unless positive pressure is applied to the vent filter. If the vent filter is pressurized, good outflow of liquid can be achieved without the use of pumps. Nitrogen or air pressure applied via the vent filter cannot compromise sterility.

Many large holding tanks for distilled water, usually in-line with the plant loop, are thin-walled and the vent filters must be sized carefully. Because vent filters are necessary, it is best that the filter vendor size the system and warrant the sizing to be appropriate. The better filter vendors have reliable sizing programs. Considering the expense of 10,000L and larger tanks, it is appropriate that a rupture disc be included in the filter installation so that, if for unforeseen reasons, the filter system should fail to function as required, the tank will not be lost.

The choice of a 0.2 micron RPD PTFE vent filter is not immediately obvious because the efficiency of a filter, rated at 1 micron for particles in a liquid, improves dramatically when the same filter is used to remove particles from air. The improvement is usually an order of magnitude, so the 1 micron PTFE membrane filter will tend to perform like a 0.1 micron membrane filter in the removal of gas-borne particles (Liu and Kuhlmey, 1971). Although this event is accepted within the filtration community, there are no data to show whether a 1 micron-RPD PTFE membrane filter, when intruded with water, would prevent the rapid passage of small organisms, e.g., *Bacillus globigii* spores, which have a diameter of about 0.5 to 0.7 micron. Nor is there any information to indicate whether that apprehension is appropriate.

For most conventional pharmaceutical sterile product and distilled water tanks, the PTFE or polypropylene membrane filters are sufficiently hydrophobic and secure regarding organism penetration that they are the filters of choice. For very large fermentation systems, requiring more than 20,000 SCFM (standard cu.ft./min), it is difficult to envision supplying the air through a membrane system. Usually, large tanks are filled with tightly packed glass fibers downstream of air compressors; the air is supplied through spargers situated at the bottom and sometimes at the middle of the fermentation vessel. The assumption is that blow-through of organisms will not occur, despite channeling of the medium, because there are so many layers. Steam sterilization of the fermentation vessel is straightforward but fully effective steam sterilization of the fibrous vent filter is difficult because the flow of steam follows the path of least resistance, which is not plug flow.

4. System Design for Particular Applications

A. Small systems

Allergens are simple extracts of plant or animal materials that cause allergic responses in man. Most extracts are prepared as simple aqueous or saline homogenates or steepings that are filtered to provide a sterile liquid that can be injected subcutaneously. Some extracts, such as ragweed allergen, are made in oils. By comparison with the balance of the pharmaceutical industry, allergen manufacturers are barely regulated. There are no standards for potency, for example, although the extracts must be sterile and must not contain lethal or powerfully toxic substances. Usually allergens are proteinaceous although they may contain polysaccharides and lipids.

Most allergens are manufactured by small companies or by physicians in the practice of allergy. The batches are small, e.g., 5 to 20L. An example of the filtration system used for such small batches is shown in Figure 12. The extract may be centrifuged to remove the heaviest particle burden, then loaded into the pressure vessel. The pressure vessel is in line with a 293mm diameter disc filter holder which usually will contain (top to bottom) a macroporous depth filter, a microporous depth filter, and a membrane filter or two, e.g., 0.45 micron RPD over a 0.2 micron RPD membrane filter. The 293mm holder is not autoclaved. Downstream of the 293 holder is shown a pre-sterilized self-contained 0.2 micron RPD membrane filter unit. Alternatively, the presterilized unit might be replaced with a 142mm diameter disc filter holder containing (top to bottom) a 0.45, 0.45, and 0.2 micron RPD membrane filters with no spacers between them. The 142mm unit would be autoclaved, preferably with 50mm self-contained PTFE disc filters coupled up and downstream during autoclaving of

Figure 12—Small-scale filtration system employing a stack of nonsterile depth
filters in the 293mm holder.

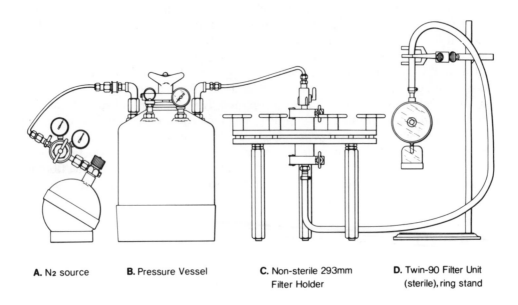

A. N₂ source   **B.** Pressure Vessel   **C.** Non-sterile 293mm   **D.** Twin-90 Filter Unit
                                                     Filter Holder   (sterile), ring stand

the unit, so as to prevent blowout of the filter(s) towards the nonsterile side during the vacuum cycle of the autoclave. This recommendation obtains for any disc filters that are autoclaved and which do not contain backpressure support screens (which infrequently are used). The connection of the 293 holder to the presterilized unit or the autoclaved 142mm unit need not be aseptic as the 293mm unit is nonsterile.

The 293mm unit acts as a depth filter assembly that protects the final sterilizing filter(s). The 293mm unit can be removed from the HEPA laminar flow hood in which the filtration is done, opened, and the spent filter stack removed for replacement, should the system plug. This is a simple and efficient mode of operation.

The hospital pharmacy may require both smaller and larger systems for sterilizing filtration. The smaller lots (e.g., single vials) usually can be sterile-filtered through pre-sterilized Millex™-type of units that fit onto a syringe and are available from several filter manufacturers (see Figure 13). For solution volumes greater than 20L, experimentation is necessary to determine if 293mm discs are sufficient (about 0.5ft² or 500cm²) or if a cartridge system, ranging from 1 to 7ft² in filter area depending on size and manufacturer, are needed.

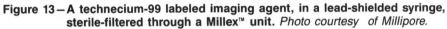

Figure 13 – A technecium-99 labeled imaging agent, in a lead-shielded syringe, sterile-filtered through a Millex™ unit. *Photo courtesy of Millipore.*

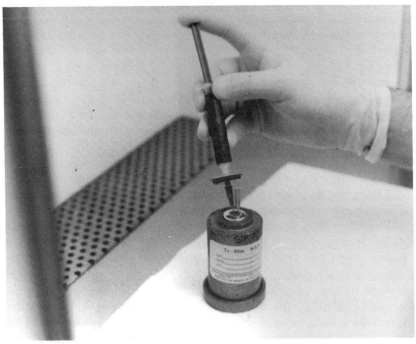

Cartridge systems, especially the self-contained "capsules," are lightweight and easily handled in contrast with 293mm disc filter holders which are heavy and awkward to manipulate.

B. Industrial-scale systems

Biologicals pose more problems than simpler aqueous solutions and, in view of the current emphasis on biotechnology, merit particular attention. These break conveniently into polysaccharides (e.g., heparin and dextrans) and proteins. Proteins are best subdivided into the species of low molecular weight (below 70 kDaltons) and those of higher molecular weight.

Heparin varies in molecular weight according to the source and method of preparation. Solutions at the usual potencies are readily filterable through a 0.2 micron RPD 293mm membrane disc filter with fiberglass depth filters upstream. 200L can be filtered through one or two such discs. If two 293mm systems are used, they must be set up in parallel, i.e., manifolded on the upstream and downstream sides so that the two units function effectively as one.

The same type of system can be used for the low molecular weight dextrans, e.g., 30 kDaltons. However, the high molecular weight dextrans, e.g. 70
kDaltons, are rather viscous and difficult to filter at concentrations significantly
higher than 1%. A s mentioned previously, heating facilitates filtration, but an
alternate strategy is the use of crossflow filtration with a system like MegaFlow™
(New Brunswick Scientific), Prostak™ (Millipore) or Krosflo™ (Microgon).

Those unfamiliar with crossflow microfiltration tend to assume that
depth filtration upstream is not needed since the crossflow tends to sweep particles away from the filter surface. MegaFlow™ and Prostak™ require minimal
depth filtration as the channel height above the membrane filter is sufficiently
high that large particles can be swept across the upstream side and even concentrated, if desired. The KrosFlo system employs hollow fibers in a cartridge
and, according to Microgon, particles up to 80-100 micron in diameter can pass
through the hollow fibers, provided significant bridging does not occur. These
systems, then, are appropriate for the sterile filtration of dextran and heparin
concentrates, even with modest depth filtration upstream.

Proteins, unlike polysaccharides, are sensitive to matrix composition. Cellulose nitrate, mixed esters of cellulose (primarily cellulose nitrate with cellulose acetate) and nylon are least efficient in the filtration of proteins in solution
because these matrices are notorious for binding proteins (see, for example,
Hawker and Hawker, 1975; Olson et al., 1977). Cellulose acetate and hydrophilic
"Durapore" bind little protein but are effective in the retention of bacteria and
fungi, and are the matrices of choice. To obtain satisfactory rates and throughputs, CA or Durapore must be used with solutions of fibrinogen and gamma
globulins. However, nylon and nitrocellulose are satisfactory for the filtration
of albumins, interferons and other proteins of low molecular weight.

Lipids tend to occlude these filters. The fine particles that are β- and
pre β-lipoproteins are deformable and will pass through membrane filters at
sufficiently high pressures, e.g., over 10psig (0.7 bar) for a 0.2 micron RPD Nuclepore membrane filter operated in the crossflow mode (Olson and Faith, 1978).
The lipoproteins are not required in any commercial plasma product, not even
fetal bovine serum. Filtration strategies for the removal of lipids are not well
worked-out. Membranes will work when operated at low pressures (less than
1 bar; usually about 0.7 bar as indicated above), even in the deadend mode. However, it is likely that hydrophobic matrices such as nonwoven polyethylene will
prove most effective, especially if the matrix is substituted with short-chain (ca.
C-8) alkyl groups (see Deutsch et al., 1973; Olson, 1984, and Olson and Greenwood, 1986).

When a large volume of serum (plasma from which the fibrinogen and
fibrin clots have been removed), say 100L or more, or very large volumes of proteins of molecular weight greater than 70 kDaltons (e.g., Cohn fraction IV_4, from
which albumin is precipitated), filter aids should be used. For example, the septum or support (a course filter, such as one of the Cuno Zeta-Plus series) is cov-

ered with 1mm or thereabouts of a fine filter aid such as one of the Celites (Manville Corp.). This is called the pre-coat. The filter aid used in the pre-coat should be suspended in the same fluid as the product that is to follow. In the case of Cohn fraction IV_4, that is 40% ethanol, pH 4.8 and an ionic strength of 0.11 at $-5°C$ (Cohn et al., 1946). The septum is preconditioned because the medium of the pre-coat rinses out such septum extractables which might otherwise find their way into the product filtrate. A body feed of the same, or a more coarse filter aid then is added to the IV_4 feed and stirred constantly. The amount of feed required is a function of the total undissolved solids in the feed; usually, one needs six times as much filter aid as the solids that need to be removed. One to two gram percent filter aid in the body feed can be a successful treatment.

Figure 14 — Depth filter cartridge system between a feed tank and a receiving tank.

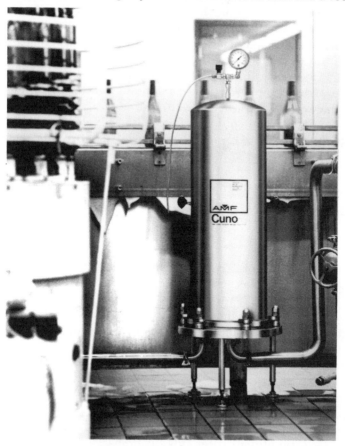

Almost all such filtrations are done under constant pressure, i.e., in a sealed tank under 10 to 15 psig nitrogen providing the force to drive the liquid through a filtration system. A conventional system is shown in Figure 14, See also Figure 7 and Fiore et al. (1980). Constant pressure systems are commonplace in the filtration of proteins because complex mixtures of proteins and preparations of high molecular weight cannot be deadend filtered at elevated pressures; the membrane filters quickly occlude and filtration ceases. Albumin is an exception (Lindley et al., 1982) and can be pumped at constant rate. A constant-rate system is shown in Figure 15. In this instance, the motive force is nitrogen pressure. A pressure transducer downstream of the sterilizing filter provides feedback to the solenoid through which the gas pressure is exerted on the feed tank. Better than a pressure transducer is a flow monitor downstream of the sterilizing filter. Clearly the flow monitor must be sterilizable and compatible with aseptic processing. One such system is MicroMotion™ (MicroMotion Corp.). Such a system also can be driven by a constant rate pump. However, as with all constant rate systems, pressure build-up occurs on the upstream side of the filter that occludes most rapidly. When that pressure becomes sufficiently high, a shear pin in the pump will yield or a seal in the system or the filter will fail. A safety valve in the form of a loop with a check valve (spring setting at about 3 bar) between the pump and the filter provides assurance that the system will not become septic (Figure 16).

Figure 15—Sterile filtration, under nitrogen pressure, in-line with a filling machine.

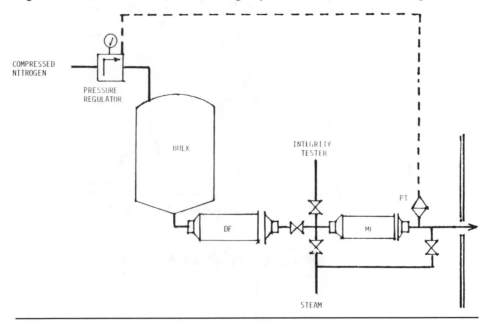

Figure 16 — As in Figure 15, but with a check valve (not shown) or pressure transducer and solenoid on an overpressure recycle line.

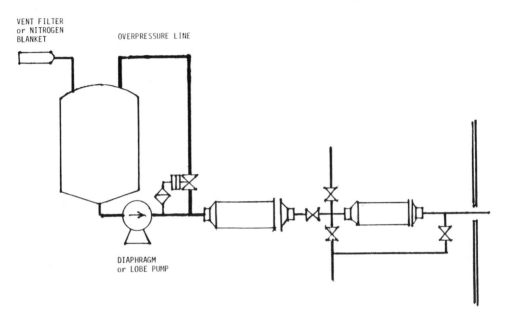

Fermentation products, whether of rDNA or more conventional origin, require extensive cleanup. For example, the flow diagram for penicillin manufacture is shown in Figure 17. Rotary vacuum drums are used in the removal of cell debris, and filter presses (Figure 18, left foreground) remove the bulk of remaining particle debris immediately upstream of the sterilizing filter cartridges. See Inman (1974) for further details of this type of depth filtration system.

At Merck Sharp and Dohme in the U.S., ultrafilters (Dorr-Oliver) are in use in place of rotary vacuum units, and have been shown to be more efficient (Gravatt and Molnar, 1986). Presumably, an ultrafilter with a molecular weight cutoff of 50 or 100 kDaltons would readily allow the passage of most water-soluble organic drugs but would retain cell debris, bacteria and even viruses. In fact, this does not occur because the thin (about 0.2 to 2 micron thick) dense layer of an ultrafilter, which is responsible for molecular sieving, is not intact but contains gaps or "holidays" through which some leakage of macromolecules occurs. These gaps allow the passage of endotoxin monomers and small aggregates, and are the reason that the well-characterized ultrafilters on the market reject only 2.5 to 4 logs of endotoxin and only 2.5 to 4 logs of viruses, whether large or small. Small viruses are intended to include MS-2, a coliphage of about 22nm diameter,

Figure 17 – Penicillin production at Glaxochem. *Photo courtesy of Glaxochem, UK.*

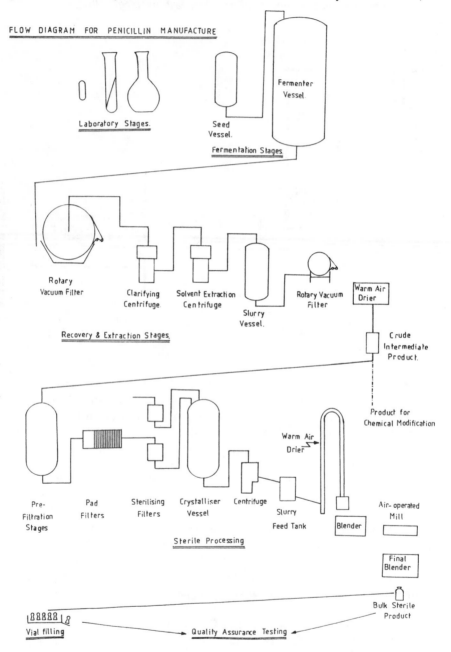

FLOW DIAGRAM FOR PENICILLIN MANUFACTURE

Figure 18 – Filtration of penicillin. *Photo courtesy of Glaxochem, UK.*

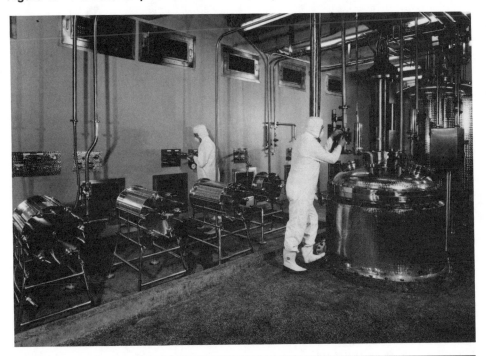

Figure 19 – Channeling in a filter cake.

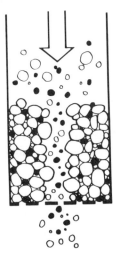

Figure 20—Channeling in a nonwoven depth filter.

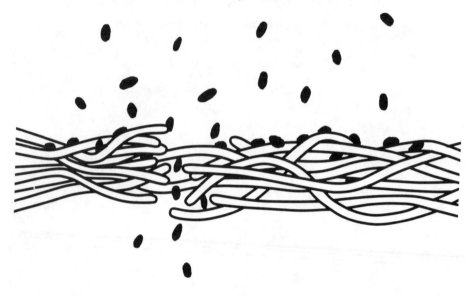

and without a tail. The ultrafilters cannot be used as sterilizing filters because some bacterial passage occurs via the "holidays," and the holiday regions soon become colonized, causing the contamination of the filtrate even if the feed later becomes free of organisms.

A 100 kDalton ultrafilter has been used in the depyrogenation of human chorionic gonadotropin (Johnson et al., 1980) and some are in use for the prophylactic depyrogenation of simple aqueous solutions of drugs (Abramson et al., 1981). But in the main, ultrafilters are used in the diafiltration (molecular washing or solvent exchange) and concentration of proteins (Peine et al., 1982; Mitra and Ng, 1986).

C. Depyrogenation
Although it is always preferable to maintain the lowest possible bioburden and pyrogen content by appropriate good manufacturing practices, some filtration systems also have the potential for reducing bioburden and pyrogens, and hence may be regarded as additional safeguards. For example, hydrophobic membrane filters remove endotoxins from simple solutions, likely by interaction with Lipid A (Sawada et al., 1986). Positively charged depth filters likely bind the phosphate groups on endotoxin (Hou et al., 1980). Unmodified depth filters also may bind endotoxin (Baggerman et al., 1981), and of course, ultrafilters can retain much of the lipopolysaccharides. Additional details on depyrogenation are provided in other chapters of this book.

5. Validation of Sterile Filtration Systems

The various requirements for filter validation have been outlined (Olson, 1979). What follows is applicable primarily to a sterilizing-grade membrane filter, and those tests that also apply to depth filters are indicated.

A. Sterilization of the filter

The membrane filter, usually rated at 0.2 micron RPD, is the sterilizing element in a filtration system. That filter, the last one that the product sees before the product is filled, must itself be sterile.

Ethylene oxide is used widely in the sterilization of self-contained "capsule" type filters made by Millipore, Pall and Sartorius. In the past, Multiplate™ (Millipore) systems, with many 293mm discs in parallel within a single housing, were sometimes sterilized by means of ethylene oxide. However, such practice is rare today. Most in-house sterilization by the user is in the steam autoclave or by steam-in-place.

Thermocouples are placed throughout the sterile receiving tank/filtration system and the system autoclaved, preferably with pre- and post-autoclave vacuum cycles to ensure thorough heating (air trapped in a tank or a filter acts as a thermal buffer). If a cycle of 30 minutes at 121°C is run, movement of the thermocouples to various points within the system soon indicates the coldest spot during the autoclave cycle. The interior of droplines and the surface of water-rinsed filters are usually the coldest; the droplines because of the difficulty of steam penetration, and the filters because they are cooled by the evaporation of water from the surfaces that have been rinsed prior to nondestructive testing. When the cold point(s) are known, thermocouples are placed at the cold spot(s) and elsewhere in the system and in the autoclave, including the drain. Spore strips containing 10^7 *Bacillus stearothermophilus* also are placed at thermocouple positions in the tank and filters. (The plural is appropriate here, as there is one or more liquid filter and a vent filter.) The cycle is run and the thermocouple readings are recorded on a Digistrip™ (Kaye Instruments). The spore strips are recovered and are grown out in soybean-casein digest or in other suitable media. Such testing is replicated several times; an original test and two replicates usually is considered the minimum. No growth may occur from the sporestrips and, for most small volume parenterals, a minimum F_0 of 8 is considered acceptable. That is to say, the equivalent in the lethal time-temperature continuum of 8 minutes at 121°C generally is considered acceptable in the "overkill" approach to sterilization, for a kill of 10^7 of an organism that is very resistant to wet heat. For those working with plasma proteins, the United States Code of Federal Regulations requires an F_0 of 20. The assumption is made that organisms retained in a film or cake of proteins not carefully scrubbed from the interior of a sterile tank or piping, may be protected during autoclaving and may survive an F_0 of 8. This also means that sterilizing-grade membrane filters made available to the human plasma side of the biotechnology industry must be able to tolerate at least 20 minutes at 121°C and likely more.

Kovary et al. (1983) have provided an outline of how one may steam-in-place a sterile receiving tank and the attached filters. The main point of interest raised by their work is that the liquid filter housing (disc filters in this case) must be mounted vertically rather than horizontally and must possess upstream and downstream vents to allow bleeding off of condensate from both sides of the filter (steam is applied from both upstream and downstream sides; otherwise sterility is not achieved). They also preferred to introduce a suspension of *B. stearothermophilus* spores directly into the membrane filter as a test of filter sterilization. This seems appropriate, provided there is no risk of release of the spores into the workplace.

Myers and Chrai (1982) evaluated steam-in-place of cartridge membrane filters in line with sterile receiving tanks. An F_0 of 45 was required for reproducible sterilization of 10 inch cartridges when the filter holders were oriented with the upstream side facing upwards. Other orientations (inverted, horizontal) required F_0s of 60 to 90 to fully sterilize both filter and tank. As with the disc filters (above), upstream and downstream application of steam was found necessary and upstream and downstream drains were necessary to remove condensate that could act as a thermal buffer. Their most important finding was that the filters had to be dry in order to achieve these results, in contrast to Olson (1979) who achieved sterility using water-wet filters in an autoclave and F_0s approximating those of Myers and Chrai. The difference may be attributable to the use of a vacuum cycle prior to the injection of steam when the autoclave was used.

Perhaps the better way to steam-in-place tanks and filters is to draw a vacuum at the top of a tank as steam is introduced both upstream and downstream of the sterilizing filter. In larger systems, e.g., filtration in line with filling, the same principles apply, but monitoring is best done with external thermocouples (which, in separate experiments have been shown to reliably reflect the temperature inside piping) on longer lines of pipe. AdTech now provides a thermocouple system to fit onto filling needles. This system interfaces with the Digistrip so as to provide detailed thermal profiles at the most remote (and difficult-to-monitor) portion of the filtration/filling system.

Depth filters, upstream of sterilizing-grade membrane filters, are usually not sterilized prior to use. The bioburden on such filters is modest and has not been shown to compromise the efficacy or stability of any product.

B. Function tests

A filter must be shown to be capable of performing the function for which it is intended in process. Sterilizing-grade filters must be capable of removing the bioburden normally present in the product. A common bioburden is of the order of 10^7 to 10^8 colony-forming units (CFU) per 10^3L. Soybean-casein digest is exposed to the manufacturing atmosphere, the organisms allowed to grow out, and a sterile filtration is performed in the usual way through depth and sterilizing-grade membrane filters. Samples are recovered from the feed tank and upstream of the sterilizing filter. (The depth filter usually removes 3 to 5 logs of CFU, depending on the level of contamination and the type of depth filter used.) The bulk tank is sampled in the same way as bulk sterility tests (Gee et al., 1985).

Such a function test is different from a microbial estimation of filter pore diameter. That test is done by challenging each square centimeter of membrane filter with 10^7 *Pseudomonas diminuta* ATCC 19146 grown in a standing culture of saline-lactose broth at 30°C for about 40 hour (Leahy and Sullivan, 1978). The filtrate must be sterile; the log reduction value must be at least 7 (HIMA, 1982). A forty hour growth under those conditions provides stationary phase organisms, which are smaller than log phase organisms and which have a smallest diameter of about 0.3 micron. A 72 hour 30°C culture in soybean-casein digest behaves similarly. The measure is that such organisms will pass through a 0.45 micron RPD membrane filter but not a 0.2 micron RPD membrane filter (Rogers and Rossmore, 1970; Gee et al., 1985). The corresponding test for pore size of a 0.45 micron RPD membrane filter is that the filter will retain 10^7 *Serratia marcescens*/cm² filter area. These tests may be done in place of the function test. Certainly the tests of organism retention are more rigorous than the actual function tests. However, most plant managers are reluctant to allow the introduction of flora not presently found in a manufacturing facility. Some filter manufacturers use fluid flow methods based on the Hagen-Poiseuille Law in the estimation of filter pore size (Johnston, 1985). Gas permeability measurements for pore size estimation have been done successfully (Yasuda and Tsai, 1974; Alkan and Groves, 1977 and 1978; Kamide et al., 1977 and 1982), but this is not presently done for the routine testing of filters by any pharmaceutical manufacturer.

It is not necessary to test a sterilizing grade membrane filter with a wide variety of products. Good evidence exists that where the pore diameter rating of a membrane filter is smaller than the minimal diameter of the organisms in the challenge, the conditions of the suspending medium have no discernible effect on organism retention (Levy, 1986).

Although organisms are known that can pass through a 0.2 micron RPD membrane filter (e.g., Howard and Duberstein, 1980), they are not likely to occur in the pharmaceutical manufacturing environment. With the one-time exception of the organism now known as *Pseudomonas diminuta* ATCC 19146 (Bowman et al., 1967), the microbial flora in such facilities does not pass through 0.45 micron RPD membrane filter. Consequently, the 0.3 or 0.2 micron rated filters are used to impart an additional margin of safety. With possibly one exception, the industry does not, and does not contemplate, a 0.1 micron rated membrane filter for the filtration of product. Where rDNA-modified mammalian cells are used in the production of parenteral peptides or proteins, and where such cells are nurtured, in part, with human or animal (e.g., fetal calf) serum, 0.1 micron filtration of the serum is indicated to reduce mycoplasmas to the lowest numbers possible. In fact, this currently is a widespread practice, both in deadend mode with 293mm diameter disc filters and in the crossflow mode using cellulose acetate membrane filter in the Sartorius crossflow cell. Therefore, in order to validate a 0.1 micron RPD membrane filter, the organism of choice is Acholeplasma laidlawii (Bower, 1986).

The standard tests applied to microbiological estimation of pore size are detailed by HIMA (1982), ASTM (1983), and are reviewed in Bower (1986).

The function test of a depth filter consists primarily in the protection of the final sterilizing grade membrane filter. If the depth filter proposed for use fails to prolong the life (throughput) of the membrane filter, that filter is not functional. Very tight depth filters, such as the Pall AB/AR units, are capable of sterilizing when operated under low flux (low flow rate per unit surface area) (Cole and Pauli, 1975) or with a number of units in series, or both. The designations of the AB/AR filters are "absolute" in the literature of the manufacturer. In fairness, however, it must be pointed out that the only reliable sterilizing-grade materials available in the market at the time of the AB/AR introduction were 293mm disc filters, which are difficult to manifold beyond four (about 2ft.²), and the Multiplate™ system which, when employing mixed ester of cellulose filters, could not be autoclaved but could be ethylene oxide-sterilized with a less than fully reliable system. So depth filter-type materials have been made to work as sterilizing filters, but have been validated for organism retention under less than rigorous conditions.

Figure 21—Vent filter test stand that can be used in the workplace.

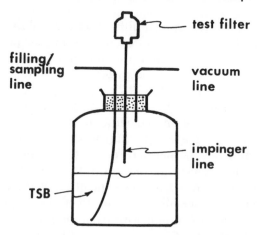

A simple microbial retention test for vent filters, that can be done with safety in the workplace, has been developed (Olson et al., 1981). The test stand is shown in Figure 21. The filter under test is integrity tested after thorough wetting with alcohol (see below for details on the integrity test), then coupled to a glass carboy; the downstream side of the filter is attached to a dropline that extends halfway into the carboy. The system is autoclaved and then soybean-casein digest is sterile-filtered into the carboy to a point 2 to 3cm below the end of the dropline. In the workplace, a vacuum is drawn on the carboy so that any particles, including organisms, that pass through the filter will impinge into the medium. (Bubbling into the medium is less effective than impingement; organisms can adhere to the surface of bubbles that lift from the surface of the medium.) After 4 continuous days of exposure to the filtered room air, the medium will be turbid if organisms have penetrated the filter. If the broth is clear, the filter is assumed to have removed all viable organisms from the impinging air. However, it then is necessary to have a positive control. Therefore, on day 5 the filter is holed, as with a small drill bit, and air flow is resumed. The resulting turbid broth proves that the medium is capable of supporting growth and shows that a non-integral filter element fails the test. Some concentration of the soybean-casein digest occurs during these tests, due to evaporation. The positive control shows that the 20 to 30% concentration of the medium has no dramatic effect on the sensitivity of the test.

C. Correlation of microbial retention with a nondestructive test of filter integrity

To ensure bacteriological sterility of the filtrate from a sterilizing grade membrane filter, some test of the filter, prior to use, is necessary. If organisms are used, the filter will be contaminated and unsuitable for use. Latex beads also would contaminate the filter. The most useful tests are the diffusion test, the bubble point test, and the combined diffusion/bubble-point tests.

When a filter is wetted, usually with distilled water or with saline, the air is displaced from the void volume. A membrane filter becomes a continuous series of water channels connecting both sides of the filter; this is equally true of depth and membrane matrices. When a gas pressure is applied to the upstream side of the filter, some of the gas goes into solution in the liquid and diffuses across the filter from the high-pressure side to the low-pressure side. The flow rate at which the gas moves across the wetted filter is a function of the porosity of the filter (i.e., how much liquid the filter can hold), the thickness of the filter (the distance through which the gas must diffuse), the differential gas pressure across the filter (the gradient that drives the gas diffusion), and the solubility of the gas in the liquid. For example, at a fixed differential pressure, say 10psig, a thin wetted filter will have a higher diffusion rate than the same filter made thicker, as by doubling. A gas diffusion rate provides no information about pore size rating unless the bubble point pressure is met (see below).

Prior to discussion of diffusion of gas through a wetted filter, it is useful to clearly state what is meant by the term "bubble point". If the filter is wetted with a liquid and gas applied upstream with the gas pressure slowly increased, at some point the upstream gas pressure will force gas through the largest pores of the wetted membrane. The pressure at which the largest pores are blown free of liquid is called the first bubble point. As the upstream gas pressure is further increased, the smaller pores begin to unload their liquid contents and contribute to the bulk flow of gas through the filter membrane. In Figure 22 diffusive flow of gas occurs through pore B, while bulk flow of gas is shown occurring from pore A which has a greater diameter.

Figure 22—A is the largest pore in the filter, and water is expelled from A by gas pressure, B remaining water-laden.

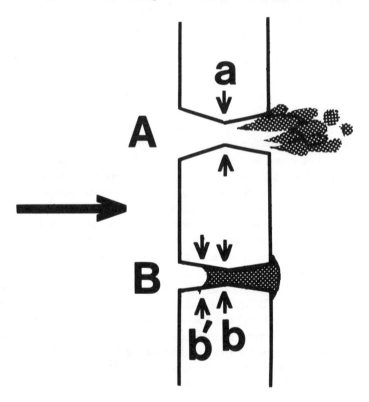

Figure 23—Log-log plot of gas flow as a function of gas pressure upstream of a filter. Curve 2E was taken prior to autoclaving of the filter and 2F after autoclaving.

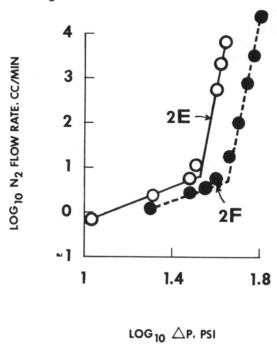

It will be noted (see Figure 23) that diffusive gas flow occurs through the fully wetted filter until the gas pressure reaches a level corresponding with the first bubble point. Thereafter the slope of the line increases dramatically due to bulk flow of gas through increasing numbers of the membrane's pores. Bulk flow is considerably greater than diffusive flow through the same surface segment of the membrane but occurs at higher pressures.

Returning to the diffusion rate portion of the curves, performing a diffusion test at a low pressure, e.g., 5.25psig, provides no useful information about pore size. Even a 1 micron RPD filter would be likely to pass a 5.25psig gas diffusion test. Therefore, this low pressure diffusion test should not be done on sterilizing-grade membrane filters. Rather, the best test shows both mass transfer rates at a variety of gas pressures, the first bubble point, and a measure of pore diameter uniformity. A plot shown in Figure 23 may be taken by hand as in the method described in Olson et al. (1983). The data shows diffusion rates at various pressures, (allowing correction for errors in measurement or gas pressure setting) and the first bubble point. The slope of the final portion of the curve is a measurement of the pore size distribution. A very steep line indicates a very narrow pore distribution, whereas a shallow line indicates a wide range of pore diameters. To perform such measurements manually requires at least one man-hour per cartridge. Where numerous cartridges are required daily, an automated test machine is cost effective.

The only machine that measures diffusion rate, first bubble point and an approximation to pore diameter distribution is the device described by Hofmann (1984). A typical machine plot is shown in Figure 24. Note the resemblance to the plot made by hand.

Figure 24—Automated measurement, from the upstream side of a cartridge membrane filter, of diffusion rate and bubble point. From Hofmann (1984), with permission of the author and the publisher.

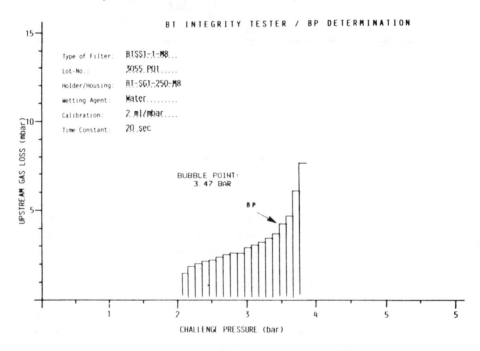

Because bubble point provides a measurement that approximates pore diameter (Washburn, 1921; ASTM, 1970), and the retention of organisms improves as the pore diameter becomes smaller (and bubble point pressure higher, Leahy and Fifield, 1983), it may be possible to show that sterile filtrate is obtained when a contaminated liquid is passed through a filter with a bubble point of, say, 50psig. Therefore the bubble point of a filter can be measured, challenge the filter with organisms, examine the filtrate, and repeat the process with a filter from the same lot but pinholed. The low bubble point will correspond to a contaminated filtrate (see Olson et al., 1981).

A diffusion rate measured at 80% of the bubble point also can be valid (Reti, 1976). However the filter needs to be understood if one is to say that a given gas diffusion rate falls within the diffusion range only and does not extend into the first bubble point or beyond. Machines that measure gas diffusion rates are exquisitely sensitive but lend themselves to error, as a single measurement can be wrong because an additional layer of water has been entrapped in the downstream support structures, or the temperature is lower than usual or the gas is more soluble in the wetting liquid than expected.

The Sartocheck measures diffusion rate indirectly (and with modest sensitivity) and bubble point directly. A valve in the machine releases measured bursts of 80-100psig nitrogen or air (from a compressed gas source) to the upstream side of the filter housing. At a pre-set pressure, no additional gas is admitted to the system. At all times, the gas pressure downstream of the aforementioned valve and upstream of the filter is measured. A pressure decay indicates measurable gas diffusion that appears on the chart record. At the end of this pressure-hold period, bursts of compressed gas are again admitted upstream of the filter until liquid is forced from a number of the largest pores. At that time, the pressure tends to level off or drop. The additional bursts of compressed gas do not increase the pressure between the valve and the filter because equivalent volumes of gas are escaping in bulk flow through liquid-free largest pores in the filter. A machine logic in the Sartocheck™ device then trips, releasing the gas pressure between the original valve and the filter. There are some minor problems with this system, which are mentioned below. A Sartocheck graph is shown in Figure 25.

Bubble point, diffusion, and similar tests are not required of depth filters. However, such tests are required of sterile tank vent filters. While depth filtration may be required of the sparging air for the largest compressed air filters for very large fermentation tanks, hydrophobic membrane filters, amenable to nondestructive testing, are preferred whenever possible.

D. Other critical tests

The filter must not release materials harmful to the patient or damaging to the active ingredient. Therefore any filter intended for product contact must be extraction tested to determine if toxic materials elute. The best test is the initial saline extract of a freshly autoclaved filter, used in acute systemic toxicity testing (USP, 1985). Extraction of an unrinsed filter provides a worst case, as does autoclaving prior to extraction, since all polymeric filters release some soluble matrix after autoclaving.

Figure 25 – Sartocheck chart record.

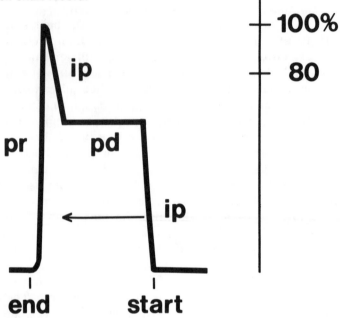

100% – 100% of the bubble point pressure
ip – increasing pressure
pd – pressure decay (pressure hold, airlock)
pr – pressure release at the machien bubble point

Figure 26 – Calcium and Triton X-100 eluted with water from 6 mixed ester filters in a 142mm diameter filter holder.

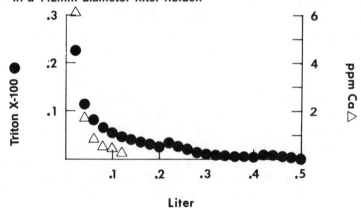

The shape of the extractables curve is shown in Figure 26. This represents the elution of Triton X-100 and calcium from mixed ester Millipore filters (six discs sandwiched into a single 142mm holder, eluted with water). The curve is linear when plotted on logarithmic axes (Olson et al., 1980). Invariably, low molecular weight species, e.g., salts, elute more rapidly than higher molecular weight materials, e.g., soluble polymers of the matrix. Total organic carbon (TOC) is commonly examined as a measure of matrix solubilization and release, or the release of wetting agents, or both. Conductivity measurements provide a measure of inorganic salts. The rinse cycle, prior to filter use, is determined by these tests and the USP test for total nonvolatile solids, which is less accurate and precise, and more tedious than the TOC and conductivity measurements. A rinse cycle should be developed that reduces the total extractables to less than 10ppm, in line with the limits imposed on Water For Injection by USP XXI.

The *Limulus* amebocyte lysate (LAL) test on filter rinses is also performed. The LAL test is accepted widely as a rapid, sensitive, inexpensive test for Gram-negative endotoxin (see the Chapter by Pearson in this book), and is used during process as a measure of the effectiveness of aseptic procedure. Genuine endotoxin can be incorporated into and released from a commercial filter, but this is relatively rare today. More commonly, LAL false-positive materials elute from cellulosic filters. These false-positives may be attributable to beta-glucans in the cellulose or may be highly oxidized cellulose. The evidence for the glucan hypothesis is referenced in the literature. The evidence for oxidized material (with a plentitude of carboxyl groups) is that only a proportion of the LAL false-positive material elutes with water from charge-modified (cation-modified) cellulose/diatomaceous earth depth matrices; much more material elutes when the material is rinsed with saline. All LAL reagents are not equally sensitive to this material, which is active in small amounts, e.g., the Mallinkrodt LAL test is relatively insensitive to the cellulose-source false-positive material.

At the conclusion of these tests, a rinse cycle should be run, autoclaving carried out, and Water For Injection passed through the filter into a clean tank. The filtrate should pass all specifications in the USP for Water For Injection.

Particle release has been observed with membrane disc filters (Olson et al., 1980) but seldom with cartridge membrane filter, which are rinsed and tested prior to packaging. The particles from disc filters are cutting debris. A HIAC automatic particle analyzer can be used to inspect membrane filter rinses for particles but is inappropriate in the examination of filtrate from depth filters. Most depth filters are nonwovens and are fibrous. A relatively rigid fiber of, say, polypropylene, that is 10 micron wide and 150 micron long is registered by the HIAC as a single particle of diameter 10 micron. Therefore, examination of filtrate for fibers should be by the USP membrane filter particle test.

While vent filters do not contact product and should not require extractables testing, depth filters must be tested.

E. Sizing the system

The only reliable way to size a filtration system is by test. Consider for example methocarbamol (Robaxin™ of A.H. Robbins) which is formulated in 50% polyethylene glycol 400 (Yalkowsky and Roseman, 1981). This solution should be relatively viscous from the PEG, have a very low bioburden from make-up water but with some particle burden from the PEG 400 and the product. Likely the best sterilizing filtration system would be in line with the filling machine and might be like the system shown in Figure 15. To size such a system, one might place 5L of solution into a suitable vessel and connect to a positive displacement pump of variable speed. Downstream of the pump is a pressure gauge and downstream of the gauge is a 142mm diameter filter holder. Downstream of the 142 holder is a 90mm holder with an upstream pressure gauge. A sterilizing grade filter compatible with the solvent or cosolvent system (there are no major incompatibilities with PEG) is placed in the 90mm holder and a candidate depth filter in the 142mm holder. The system is run at a low flow rate and the gauge pressures monitored as a function of time. From the particles in the feed, either the depth filter or the sterilizing membrane filter will commence to clog, as manifested by a significant increase in the pressure reading on gauge. If the depth filter is clogging much more rapidly than the membrane filter, use a less dense depth filter, or use more filter area with the depth filter in hand, e.g., shift to a 293mm holder. When the filters clog at about the same rate, one knows the area ratio of a particular depth filter to use with a particular membrane filter. Now the flow rates are increased and the maximum rate feasible with the given filters and areas is noted. This rate then is compared with the feed required to the filling machine. The rate proportion (test stand to rate required for filling) is applied to the filter areas and one adds 50% to allow for contingencies. The scale-up takes into account pressure build-ups to unsuitable levels due to product viscosity. Usually, the highest acceptable level is 50psig as many cartridge filter systems are rated only to that value.

To size a constant pressure system, plot (from 47mm or 90mm systems) mL/min (y-axis) as a function of volume (mL, x-axis) using a 5L pressure vessel as a feed source (see Fig. 12). From the plot, estimate the rate and throughput volume at 80% clog (20% of the initial flow rate). From these values, calculate by simple proportions the area of filter needed to meet throughput requirements and repeat the calculation for the area needed to meet rate requirements. Say, for example, that the volume to be filtered is 50,000mL. Through a 47mm disc (about 10cm² area) at 15psig and 20°C, a cumulative 200mL have been filtered to 80% clog of the filter. Then

$$200mL/10cm^2 = 50,000mL/Xcm^2$$

If the minimal required flow rate is 5,000mL/min and the rate at 80% clog is 5mL/min, then

$$5mL/min/10cm^2 = 5,000mL/min/Xcm^2$$

To each of these solutions, add 50% to account for the variations in feed and conditions. The larger value of the two is used. For the numbers presented, the rate requirement is the determining value (10,000cm² is needed, not including the 50% add-on).

6. What Can Go Wrong

A. Depth filters

Provided care is taken in sizing a system (see above) and in ensuring the identity of the filters used in process, substitution with an incorrect filter type should not cause a problem. However, a frequent problem associated with depth filters is solution bypass caused by improper seating of the filter medium. Bypass also may occur if the system is undertorqued (loose gaskets). Overtorqued systems, causing warping of the cartridges in Cuno-style units, may cause filter rupture, resulting in bypass. Filter presses, if undertorqued, tend to weep product and the event is immediately obvious if the system is equipped with a downstream turbidity monitor.

Figure 27—Poor throughput as a sterile membrane filter clogs rapidly.

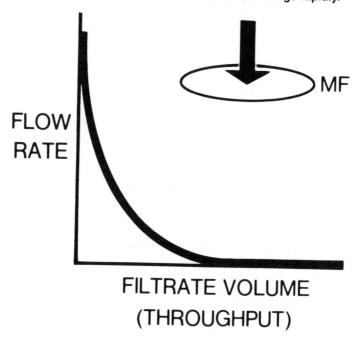

FLOW RATE

MF

FILTRATE VOLUME
(THROUGHPUT)

Figure 28—Improved throughput and rate attributable to depth filtration.

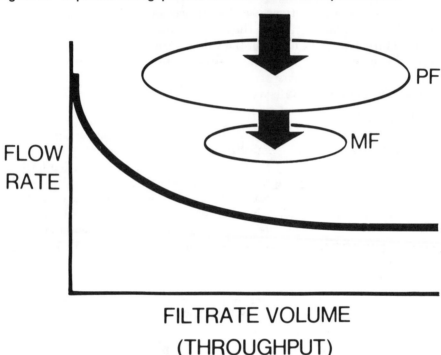

Depth media have a reputation for shedding matrix (media migration). However, it is unlikely that the fibers, or diatomaceous earth, or other particles shed by depth media would clog a downstream membrane filter, as such relatively large fibers and particles are likely to act as a filter aid, prolonging the life of the membrane filter.

In the event of channeling, the filter element must be replaced and filtration recommenced. Channeling can be assumed when reseating of a cartridge does not stop leakage of the pre-coat.

B. Membrane filters

The most frequent cause for operator concern with an otherwise integral filter element at the end of a filtration process is the observation of a low bubble point value. Often, this can be attributed to the surface tension of the product. Proteins have a surface tension close to that of water (Van Oss et al., 1981), but the caprylate in human albumin for injection can lower the bubble point value by as much as 5 psig. Heparin, also a surfactant, reduces bubble point values. To restore the post-filtration bubble point value to approximately the pre-filtration value, rinse the filter with the solution used immediately prior to the pre-use integrity test. Marshall and Meltzer (1976) and SAE (1968) discussed surface tension effects, and Olson et al. (1982) the effect of filter hydrophobicity on the bubble point.

The bubble point value can be lower than anticipated if a fitting upstream of the filter is loose and an upstream monitor (Sartocheck or new Millipore unit) detects a pressure loss at that fitting as the bubble point. Soapy water, applied to fittings with a brush, will reveal loose fittings by bubble formation. If the diffusion rate is monitored by means of a downstream monitor, the same leak may cause the bubble point value to be higher than anticipated due to pressure loss through the loose fitting; a higher-than proper gas pressure apparently will be required to expel water from the largest pores.

The bubble point can be higher than anticipated for several reasons:
  i. Very occasionally the filter has a smaller pore size rating than indicated;
 ii. The filter is partially clogged (a common post-filtration integrity test result and not of concern);
iii. The filter is a membrane filter cartridge potted with a urethane or epoxy resin which renders many of the filter pores near the endcaps hydrophobic. As a result, the hydrophobic pores do not wet with water at room temperature and the diffusion rates and bubble point are as shown in curve 2E of Figure 23. However, after autoclaving or steam-in-place sterilization, steam condenses in the hydrophobic pores reducing the net passage of gas through the filter. The diffusion rate-bubble point curve for the same filter shifts to that shown in curve 2F of Figure 23. Therefore, for a cartridge filter potted at the endcaps, the post-autoclave bubble point is higher than the pre-autoclave bubble point (Olson et al., 1983). Provided the phenomenon is understood, this is not a problem.
 iv. The measurement of the first bubble point is not sufficiently sensitive, hence it actually is made at a pressure differential well beyond the bubble point (Johnston, 1986). It remains to be established whether or not this is important. Consider Figure 23, curve 2E. Assume that the bubble point occurs at a pressure, antilog 1.53psig and the gas flow at that pressure is about 7cc/min. However, the manual or automated measurement method does not have the sensitivity to detect an upstream pressure loss of the filter represented by a 7cc/min bleed (automated) or cannot register the few bubbles or gas volume at 7cc/min (manual). In such instances, the automated or manual method may detect, for example, a gas flow (beyond the bubble point) of 10cc/min. As a problem, this should be rare because automated and manual methods should have the same bias at all times, and a higher-than-actual reading before use also should be reflected in a higher-than-actual reading after use. Note that automated methods (e.g. Sartocheck) provide bubble point values consistently higher than manual bubble points measurements and calculations (see Figure 23).

v. The membrane filter may have been overcooked during autoclaving or steam-in-place sterilization cycles. While poorly documented, this phenomenon may be summarized as the mechanical strength of the polymer failing at some critical temperature. This failure collapses some of the larger caverns in the filter (this relates directly to the membrane filter structure theory of Williams and Meltzer, 1983). The result should be a decrease in diffusion rate and an increase in bubble point value after autoclaving. In practice, the synthetic polymers (nylon 66 and hydrophilic Duropore™) have proven more heat-tolerant than cellulose membranes although this has not diminished use of the cellulose membranes.

Diffusion rates may be much lower than theoretical because the layer of water in the filter is supplemented with a layer of water in the support structures.

A more interesting phenomenon, of increasing concern as lot sizes and filling times increase, is microorganism grow-through. Molander et al. (1965) observed that over a 7 day period L-forms of staphylococci grew through membranes with pore ratings as small as 0.05 micron. Wallhausser (1983) also seems to have observed grow-through of *Pseudomonas diminuta* with a variety of filter types, all rated at 0.2 micron. By way of contrast, Peterson and Hanker (1985) found no penetration of *P. diminuta* through several intravenous filter sets, slowly fed a nutrient broth over 90 days. Simonetti and Schroeder (1984) claimed that no grow-through could occur with a polysulfone membrane filter because the anisotropic filter had extremely small pores on the downstream side, effectively preventing the passage of any intact bacterium. Leahy and Gabler (1984) slowly fed medium to *P. diminuta* on 0.2 or 0.3 micron mixed ester membrane filters; they found grow-through in 12 or 24 hours respectively. These data hint that 24 hours may separate organism passage from grow-through, but also show, in the absence of grow-through for *Escherichia coli* on the 0.2 micron membrane filter, that deadend sterile filtration can be performed for 15 days or more if the microbial contaminants are of the size of *E. coli*. This does not address the issue of pyrogens, which might be circumvented by a strategy of intermittent crossflow as proposed by Microgon Corp. Comprehensive investigation of the grow-through phenomenon has not been carried out.

Particles in the product often are blamed on the filter. Where a membrane filter cartridge is used as the last step in processing prior to filling, the filter is probably not to blame. Rather, the method of cleaning and the environment in which equipment is cleaned is critical. All too often, fibers from protective garments will find their way, in large numbers, into sterile tanks when the tanks are cleaned. Particles from the previous batch, or from the cleaning process (such as fibers from a cleaning brush) in the tank after cleaning; do not compromise sterility after the tank has been autoclaved or steamed-in-place. They do compromise product quality and increase the amount of product rejected during inspection for particulate contamination. Consider, for example, that 80 fibers find their way into a 1,000L tank. The tank is sterilized and sterile-filtered product filled into the tank with the 80 contaminating fibers distributing themselves throughout the solution. When this solution is filled into 100mL vials, the total number of containers filled is 10,000 and the percentage contaminated with the fibers will be 80/10000 or 0.8%. While unacceptable in a perfect world, in reality such a level of particulate contamination may be the best that reasonably can be achieved.

C. Depth or membrane filters

Poor throughput, the rapid clogging to about 20% of the initial flow rate, is a common complaint of many users. Often this occurs because the operator has increased gas pressure (constant pressure filtration) in order to complete the process more rapidly. The effect of this action on flux (flow rate per unit filter area) is dramatic. Reducing the flux by half generally increases the throughput fourfold. That is to say, doubling the filter area while maintaining a constant flow rate, or reducing the flow rate by half, causes the fourfold improvement. This effect is shown in Figure 29.

Figure 29—Flux as a function of throughput for Berkeley, California city water through 47mm diameter membrane filter. Note that the axes are log scale.

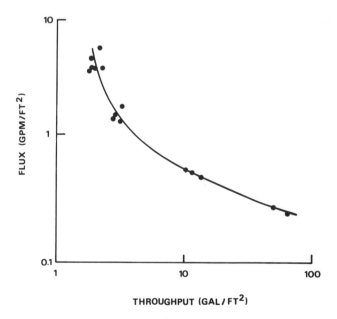

THROUGHPUT (GAL/FT²)

Also commonplace is the situation where an initially low filtration rate increases slowly (Figure 30). Air, not properly bled from a housing, occludes a filter surface (including depth filters) and is displaced only as the bubbles dissolve in the feed, or as the upstream pressure is increased to a pressure above the bubble point, when the air is pushed through the filter by the liquid pressure.

Figure 30 – Squares, cumulative filtrate for trypticase soy broth through a 10 inch 0.2 micron RPD membrane filter cartridge without an air bleed. Circles, as above, with the air bleed but without depth filtration upstream.

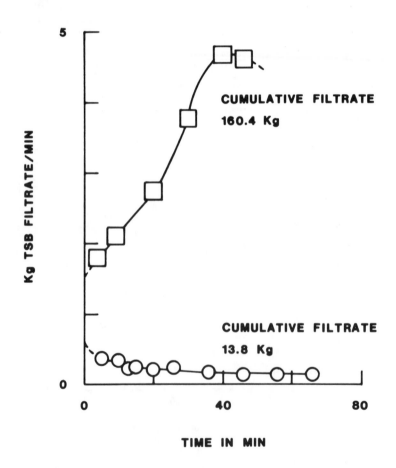

If there is cavitation in a pump upstream of the filter, or there is a leak and air is continually being pulled into an aqueous feed, or a pump seal fails to contain entirely the packing, deformable particles (air in water, lipids in water) can occlude a low-pressure system. Such events can be subtle, and detecting them requires some investigative skills.

A dramatic decrease in flow rate is also possible if the solution contains a preservative or other agent (such as parabens or BHT) which might causing swelling of the filter membrane and a consequent reduction in pore size.

9. References

Abramson,D., Butler, L.D. and Chrai, S. (1981) J. Parenteral Sci. Technol. 35,3-7.

ACS (1978) Chem. & Eng. News Dec. 4, 17.

Alkan, M.H. and Groves, M.J. (1977) The measurement of membrane filter pore size by a gas permeability technique. First Intl. Conf. of Pharm. Technol., Paris 1, 227-239.

Alkan, M.H. and Groves, M.J. (1978) Drug Devel. Industr. Pharm. 4 (3), 225-241.

ASTM (1970) Standard method of test for pore size characteristics of membrane filters for use with aerospace fluids. ASTM Designation F316-70, Am. Soc. Testing & Materials, Philadelphia, PA.

ASTM (1983) Standard test method for determining bacterial retention of membrane filters utilized for liquid filtration. ASTM Designation F838-83, Am. Soc. Testing & Materials, Philadelphia, PA.

Baggerman, C. and Kannegeiter, L.M. (1984) Appl. Environ. Microbiol. 48, 662-664.

Baggerman, C. and Brandsema, C. et al (1981) J. Pharm. Pharmacol. 33, 685-691.

Bower, J.P. (1986) In "Fluid Filtration: Liquid, Vol. II, ASTM STP 975", (P.R. Johnston and H.G. Schroeder, eds.), pp. 51-58, Am. Soc. Testing and Materials, Philadelphia, PA.

Bowman, F.W., Calhoun, M.P. and White, M. (1967) J. Pharm. Sci. 56, 453-459.

Cain, C.W. (1979) In "Handbook of Separation Techniques for Chemical Engineers", (P.A. Schweitzer, ed.), pp. 4,9-4, 14.

Cohn, E.J., Strong, L.E., Hughes, Jr., W. L., Mulford, D.J., Ashworth, J.N., Melin, M. and Taylor, H.L. (1946) J. Am. Chem. Soc. 68, 459-475.

Cole, J.C. and Pauli, W.A. (1975) Bull. Parenteral Drug Assoc. 29, 296-304.

Dahlstrom, D.A. and Silverblatt, C.E. (1977) In "Solid/Liquid Separation Equipment Scale-up", (D.B. Purchas, ed.), pp. 445-491, Uplands Press, Croydon, UK.

Deutsch, D.G., Fogleman, D.J. and von Kaula, K.N. (1973) Biochem. Biophys. Res. Comm. 50, 758-764.

Duberstein, R. and Howard. G. (1978) J. Parenteral Drug Assoc. 32, 192-197.

Dwyer, J.L. (1975) Bull. Parenteral Drug Assoc. 29, 227-237.

Einstein, A. and Munsam, H. (1923) f2Deutsche Med. Wschrift 49 (31), 1012-1013.

Fifield, C.W. and Leahy, T.J. (1983) In "Disinfection, Sterilization and Preservation", 3rd Edn. (S.S. Block, ed.), pp. 125-153, Lea & Febiger, Philadelphia.

Fiore, J.V., Olson, W.P. and Holst, S.L. (1980) In "\Methods of Plasma Protein Fractionation", (J.M. Curling, ed.), pp. 239-268, Academic Press, London.

Gee, L.W., Harvey, J.M.G.H., Olson, W.P. and Lee, M.L. (1985) J. Pharm. Sci. 74, 29-32.

Gravatt, D.P. and Molnar, T.E. (1986) In "Membrane Separations in Biotechnology", (W.C. McGregor, ed.), pp. 89-97, Marcel Dekker, New York.

Hou,K., Gerba, C.P., Goyal, S.M. and Zerda, K.S. (1980) Appl. Environ. Microbiol. 40, 892-896.

Hawker, R.J. and Hawker, L. M. (1975) Lab. Practic 24, 805-807, 814.

HIMA (1982) Microbiological Evaluation of Filters for Sterilizing Liquids, HIMA Document No. 3 Vol. 4, Hlth Industry Manuf. Assoc., Washington, D.C.

Hofmann, F. (1984) J. Parenteral Sci. Technol. 38, 148-158.

Howard, G.A. and Duberstein, R. (1980) J. Parenteral Drug Assoc. 34, 95-102.

Inman, F.N. (1974) Filtration & Separation 11, 377-381.

Ives, K.J. (1977) In "Solid/Liquid Equipment Scale-Up" (D.B. Purchas, ed.), pp. 289-317, Uplands Press, Ltd., Croydon, England.

Jacobs, G.P. and Donbrow, M. (1977) Acta Pharm. Suec. 14, 287-292.

Johnson, D.S., Lin, K., Fitzgerald, E. and LePage, B. (1980) In "Ultrafiltration Membranes and Applications", (A.R. Cooper, ed.), p. 475, Plenum Press, New York.

Johnston, P.R. (1985) J. Testing & Eval. 13, 308-315.

Johnston, P.R. (1986) In "Fluid Filtration: Liquid, Vol II, ASTM STP 975" (P.R. Johnston and H.G. Schroeder, eds.), pp. 5968, Am. Soc. Testing and Materials, Philadelphia, PA.

Kakinuma, A., Asano, T., Torii, H. Sugino, Y. (1981) Biochem. Biophys. Res. Comm. 101, 434-439.

Kamide, K., Manabe, S. and Matsui, T. (1977) Kobunshi Ronbunshu 34, 299-307.

Kamide, K., Manabe, S., Nohmi, T., Makino, H., Narita, H. and Kawai, T. (1982) In "Polymeric Separation Media", (A. R. Cooper, ed.), pp. 3574, Plenum Press, New York.

Kang, K.Y. and Salvaggio, J. (1976) Med. J. Osaka Univ. 27, 47-58.

Kovary, S.J., Agalloco, J.P. and Gordon, B. M. (1983) J. Parenteral Sci. Technol. 37, 55-63.

Leahy, T. J. and Fifield, C.W. (1983) In "Disinfection, Sterilization and Preservation", (S.S. Block, ed.), pp. 125-153, Lea & Febiger, Philadelphia, PA.

Leahy, T.J. and Sullivan, M.J. (1978) Pharm. Technol. 2 (11), 65-75.

Levy, R.V. (1986) In "Fluid Filtration: Liquid, Vol. II, ASTM STP 975", (P.R. Johnston and H.G. Schroeder, eds.), pp. 80-89, Am. Soc. Testing and Materials, Philadelphia, PA.

Lindley,P.D., Olson, W.P. and Faith, M.R. (1982) In "Polymeric Separation Media", (A.R. Cooper, ed.), pp. 173-190, Plenum Press, New York.

Liu, B.Y.H. and Kuhlmey, G.A. (1977) In "X-Ray Fluorescence Analysis of Environmental Samples" (T.G. Dzubay, ed.), pp. 107-119, Ann Arbor Science Publ., Ann Arbor, MI.

Lukaszewicz, R.C. and Meltzer, T.H. (1980) J. Parenteral Drug Assoc. 34, 463-472.

Marshall, J.C. and Meltzer, T. H. (1976) Bull. Parenteral Drug Assoc. 30, 214-225.

Mascoli, C.C. (1981) Med. Dev. Diag. Ind. 3 (4), 8-9.

McGregor, W.C. (1986) In "Membrane Separations in Biotechnology", (W. C. McGregor,ed.), pp. 1-36, Marcel Dekker, New York.

Meltzer, T. H. and Lukaszewicz, R.C. (1979) In "Quality Control in the Pharmaceutical Industry", (M.s. Cooper, ed.), pp. 145-212, Academic Press, New York.

Meyer, M.A. and Klein, E. (1983) Artif. Organs 7, 484-487.

Mikami, T., Nagase, T., Matsumoto, T., Suzuki., S. and Suzuki, M. (1982) Microbiol. Immunol. 26, 403-409.

Milliner, D.S., Shinaberger, J.H., Shuman, P. and Coburn, J.W. (1985) N. Eng. J. Med. 312, 165-167.

Millipore (1976) Preparation of tissue culture media. AB720, Millipore Corp., Bedford, MA.

Mitra,G. and Ng, P.K. (1986) In "Membrane Separations in Biotechnology", (W.C. McGregor, ed.), pp. 115-134, Marcel Dekker, New York.

Mollander, C.W., Weinberger, H.J. and Kagap, B.M. (1965) J. Bacteriol. 89, 907.

Meyers, T. and Chrai, S. (1981) J. Parenteral Sci. Technol. 35, 8-12.

Nelsen, L.L. (1978) Pharm. Technol. 2 (5), 46-49, 80.

Nelson, H. (1973) Size of asbestos fibers blamed for cancer.
Los Angeles Times; Jan. 6.

Olson, W.P. (1979) Pharm. Technol. 3 (11), 85-92,120.

Olson, W.P. (1982) Pharm. Technol. 6 (5), 42-52.

Olson, W.P. (1983) Process Biochem. 18 (5), 29-33.

Olson, W.P. (1984a) U.S. Patent 4,411,795.

Olson, W.P., Bethel, G. and Parker, C. (1977) Prep. Biochem. 7, 333-343.

Olson, W.P., Briggs, R.O., Garanchon, C.M., Ouellet, M.J., Graf, E.A. and Luckhurst, D.G. (1980) J. Parenteral Drug Assoc. 34, 254-267.

Olson, W.P., Eras, M.H. and Parks, R.G. (1982) World Filtration Congress III (Proceedings) Volume II, 484-490.

Olson, W.P. and Faith, M.R. (1978) Prep. Biochem. 8, 379-386.

Olson, W.P., Gatlin, L.A. and Kern, C.R. (1983) J. Parenteral Sci. Technol. 37, 117-124.

Olson, W.P. and Greenwood, J.R. (1986) In "Fluid Filtration: Liquid, Vol. II, ASTM STP 975", (P.R. Johnston and H.G. Schroeder, eds.) pp. 91-99, Am. Soc. Testing and Materials, Philadelphia, PA.

Olson, W.P., Martinez, E.D. and Kern, C.R. (1981) J. Parenteral Sci. Technol. 35, 215-222.

Olson, W.P., VandenHouten, L. and Ellis, J.E. (1981) J. Parenteral Sci. Technol. 35, 70-71.

Ostreicher, E.A. (1977a) U.S. Patent 4,007,113.

Ostreicher, E.A. (1977b) U.S. Patent 4,007,114.

Pall, D.B. (1975) Bull. Parenteral Drug Assoc. 29, 192-204.

Pall, D.B. and Krakauer, S. (1973) Ger. Offen. 2,211,811; Chem. Abstr. 6397n, 79, p. 61.

Pearson, F.C., Bohon, J., Lee, W., Bruszer, G., Sagona, M., Dawe, R.,Jakubowski, G., Morrison, D. and Dinarello, C. (1984) Artif. Organs 8, 291-298.

Pearson, F.C., Bohon, J., Lee,W., Bruszer, G., Sagona,M., Jakubowski, G., Dawe, R., Morrison, D. and Dinarello, C. (1984) Appl. Environ. Microbiol. 48, 1189-1196.

Peine, I.C., Swenson, J.C. and Benedictus, J.D. (1982) J. Parenteral Sci. Technol. 36, 79-85.

Peterson, A.J. and Hankner, D.O. (1985) Med. Dev. Diag. Ind. 7 (6), 150-155.

Que Hee, S.S., Boyle, J. and Finelli, V.N. (1979) Bull. Environ. Contam. Toxicol. 23, 509-516.

Reti, A.R. (1976) Bull. Parenteral Drug Assoc. 31, 187-194.

Rogers, B.G. and Rossmoore, H.W. (1970) In "Developments in Industrial Microbiology, Vol. II". (C.J. Corum, ed.), pp. 453-459, Amer. Inst. Biol. Sci., Washington, D.C.

SAE (1968) Bubble Point Test Method, Aerospace Recommended Practice, ARP 901. Society of Automotive Engineers, New York.

Sawada, Y., Fujii, R. et al (1986) Appl. Environ. Microbiol. 51, 813-820

Selikoff, I. J., Churg, J. and Hammond, E.C. (1964) J. Am. Med. Assoc. 188, 142-146.

Silkey, J.S. and Orton, G.F. (1982) NASA Tech Briefs 7 (1), 52.

Simonetti, J.A. and Schroeder, H.G. (1984) J. Environ. Sci. 27 (6), 27-32.

Southern, J.A. and Katz, W. (1983) J. Biol. Stand. 11, 163-170.

Stanton, M.F. and Layard, M. (1978) Natl Bureau of Standards Special Publ. 506, Proc. Workshop on Asbestos, pp. 143-150, National Bureau of Standards, Gaithersburg, MD, July 18-20, 1977.

Trasen, B. (1981) Pharm. Technol. 5 (11), 62-69.

USP (1985) "The United States Pharmacopeia, 21st rev.", pp. 1198-1199, U.S. Pharmacopeial Convention, Rockville, MD.

Van Oss, C.J., Absolom, D.R., Neumann, A.W. and Zingg, W. (1981) Biochim. Biophys. Acta 670, 64-73.

Wallhausser, K.H. (1982) In "Advances in Pharmaceutical Sciences" (H.S. Bean, A.H. Beckett and J.E. Carless, eds.), Vol. 5, pp. 1-116, Academic Press, London.

Wallhausser, K.H. (1983) Pharm. Ind. 45, 527-531.

Washburn, E.W. (1921) Proc. Natl Acad. Sci. 7, 115-116.

Williams, R.E. and Meltzer, T.H. (1983) Pharm. Technol. f37 (5), 36-42.

Yalkowsky, S.H. and Roseman, T.J. (1981) In "Techniques of Solubilization of Drugs", (S.H. Talkowsky, ed.), pp. 91-134, Marcel Dekker, Inc., New York.

Yasuda, H. and Tsai, J.T. (1974) J. Appl. Polymer Sci. 18, 805-819.

Acknowledgments: Various authors and the following organizations are acknowledged for their permission to use figures in the text: Academic Press, Glaxochem, Parenteral Drug Association and Upland Press.

6

Clean Rooms for Aseptic Pharmaceutical Manufacturing

Douglas Stockdale
American Pharmaseal, Valencia, CA, USA

1. Introduction

The weakest link in the process chain for the manufacture of aseptic parenterals is aseptic filling. Although, in the main, U.S. parenteral manufacturers show fewer than 0.1% contamination during media fills, many large hospitals with LVP and SVP facilities, by way of contrast, show 1 to 4% contamination of media fills. Presumably, media fills are done under conditions representative of product fills and reflect the actual levels of microbial contamination of product. A large proportion of the SVPs are steam-autoclaved in the final container so as to assure sterility; these are not aseptically filled products in the sense of this book. Similarly, some products that cannot be autoclaved at 121°C (due to product degradation) can be heated at 60°C or more, which exposure over time kills vegetative bacteria and viruses but not bacterial or fungal spores. The point is not that microbial contaminants can be killed in the final container, but that for some products microbes cannot be killed with heat in the final container because the product is heat-labile. For such products, the filling step (of all steps in aseptic processing) is most likely to allow the inclusion of microbes in the final container.

Aseptic filling normally occurs in a clean room. For the purposes of this chapter, the terms "clean room" and "aseptic filling room" are considered to be synonyms. This chapter describes the operating practices and characteristics of clean rooms, and where dangers to product sterility exist in the operation of the clean room. Sterilization of equipment, containers and closures, are discussed in detail in other chapters of this book.

2. The Critical Area

By one means or another, preferably via a hot air sterilizing tunnel, the sterile container is delivered to a continuous belt in the filling room. From the time that the sterile final container emerges from the filling tunnel, a tote box or other sterile transport vehicle, the mouth of the final container (sometimes referred to as the "finish") must be under vertical laminar HEPA air until after the filled container has been closed with an elastomeric closure or "stopper". The critical area is the region of the filling room in which the final container is exposed to room air until the elastomeric closure is in place.

3. Meaningful Media Fills

A. Federal Standard 209b and Federal Standard 209c

Existing standards provide one measure of acceptable values for filling rooms. For example, Federal Standard 209b (currently under revision by the Institute of Environmental Sciences) defines particulate contamination levels: a Class 10 area is one which shows 10 or fewer particles of 0.5 micron and larger size per cubic foot; a Class 100 area shows 100 or fewer particles per cubic foot; and so forth. Class limits in particles/cubic foot of size equal to or greater than the particle sizes shown are indicated in Figure 1. The standard (still in revision) provides some information on the means of making the particle measurements. A better source on what the standard means, other than the standard, is Flannery and Walcroft (1986).

B. Validating the clean room

Federal Standard 209b (and its proposed successor 209c) is an external standard. To satisfy the standard for a specified clean room activity, actual data must be obtained both under best possible conditions and under worst-case conditions, condition likely to cause a media fill to fail. Consider the following: we take all possible pains to establish an aseptic filling line. The high efficiency particulate air (HEPA) filtration units over the critical area are tested for leaks in the medium and the frames with cold-generated dioctylphthalate (DOP) particles. Cold aerosolized DOP (or mineral oil for those who continue to believe that aerosols of DOP are carcinogenic) is polydisperse (geometric mean particle diameter of 0.75 micron). The cold DOP generators are sufficiently small and light (about 10 kg) to be placed upstream of the HEPA filters (and downstream of the blowers and any prefilters) in the overhead of a filling room. A generator such as the TDA-5A (Air Techniques, Inc., Baltimore, MD 21207) can aerosolize 100 micrograms DOP/Liter of air at rates of 500 to 7,500 cubic feet per min. Downstream of the HEPA filters, in the clean room and usually about 30cm below the HEPA units, leaks are detected most often with a forward-scattering portable photometer. Such a unit usually contains a quartz halogen lamp and is capable of detecting as few as 5 particles of 0.5 micron diameter and larger/cc of air. Because a DOP generator may produce as many as 5×10^6 particles per cc of air, the theoretical efficiency of such a system is 0.0001%. Consequently, even with polydisperse particles, only a proportion of which are 0.3 micron in diameter, efficient leak testing can be done. The HEPA system must be leak-

Figure 1—Class limits in particles per cubic foot of size equal to or greater than particle sizes shown. *Figure courtesy of the Institute of Environmental Sciences.*

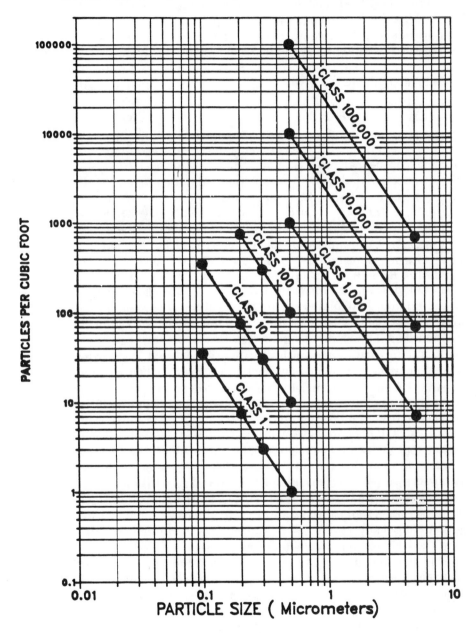

free before additional characterization of the room is done. Multiple media fills, often replicated five or six times, are then performed.

During the media fills, when personnel are in the room, particle levels are monitored in the usual way, e.g., Royco counter. Viable airborne colony-forming-units (CFU) also are measured by means of a slit-to-agar sampler or a Reuters Centrifugal Sampler (RCS); the utility of settling plates is open to question (see the chapter on sterility testing and related tests). The exception for settling plates are the plates adjacent to the filling line in fixed stations and exposed throughout the filling process. These plates likely provide accurate and useful data, especially if they are on the side of the filling line frequented by the operators and are set at approximately the level of the finish of the vial.

If 5 or 6 media fill runs are done in the best possible way and the data are compiled, one then has a baseline from which to measure a system that (hopefully) is effective and meets Current Good Manufacturing Practices (CGMP). Then four media fills might be made with one or more personnel or systems in disorder so that a correlation can be established between a deterioration in the filling environment (as contamination detected by the slit-to-agar and/or RCS, or particle contamination detected by the airborne particle sampler) and the results of the media fills. This is comparable to testing a sterilizing grade liquid filter by performing a bubble point test. The integral filter then is challenged with a bacteria-laden solution and the filtrate is evaluated for bacterial sterility. Unless a failed filter is tested in the same way, there is no proof of the utility of the bubble point measurement, and no means of establishing pass/fail criteria other than those recommended by the manufacturer.

The problem with such a validation is that it is expensive, time-consuming and can be done most thoroughly only at the time of plant startup. Construction is seldom completed before given deadlines, therefore minimal validation consistent with safe practice is done, e.g., three media fills. However, if one elected to do a proper validation of the clean room, some savings could be achieved by reducing the volume of the media fills. The volume of medium filled is less important than the diameter of the bottle mouth, so the container should be identical with that used for product. The volume of the fill must be sufficient that the turbidity attributable to bacterial growth can be seen clearly. The closure also must be exposed to the bacterial growth medium because a media fill takes into account the possibility that the closure has not been sterilized properly. Therefore, the initial validating media fill must include stopper exposure. For a small-volume fill, this may necessitate inverting the stoppered and capped containers during the incubation period. From such a fundamental study, done once during the qualification of a filling room, should emerge a rational basis for the alert and action limits on particles and microbes detected in the clean room. Because no such study has been done, the significance of detected particle and microbial levels as a function of media fill contamination is not known. Alert and action limits are based on best-informed approximations.

The microbial measurements made during filling should be correlatable to contamination in the final container. If sufficient media fills and concomitant microbial evaluations are done, crude but statistically significant data can be accumulated. Only this approach affords a rational basis to control of filling room operation. However, the authors also note that the less complete approach to the characterization of filling rooms has been successful in practice, contamination levels are held below 0.1% throughout the industry and the system seldom goes awry.

4. HEPA Filtered Air Systems

A. HEPA air flow rates

Flow rates through HEPA filters usually are measured with a hot wire anemometer. A HEPA flow rate of 90 feet/min (90 cubic feet/square foot of filter area/min; in the cgs system, 45.72 cm/sec) has been assumed to be optimal per Federal Standard 209b. However, as can be seen from Table 1, the air flow from a person moving about tends to be much higher than 90 feet/min. It seems advantageous to have the HEPA air flow higher, if possible.

Table I—Air Velocities Associated with Clean Room and Other Activities in the Pharmaceutical Plant

Activity	Approximate Velocity (feet/min)*
Laminar HEPA flow	90
Door opening	220
Person walking	320
HVAC vent	440 +
Room air conditioner	760 +

* Adapted from Figure 1 of Gross (1976)

A truly comprehensive overview of the effect of HEPA air flow on sterility in the critical area seems not to have been done. An interesting assumption has been that vertical laminar HEPA flow in excess of 90 feet/min in the critical area causes undue turbulence, leading to the introduction of adventitious organisms from personnel. Unpublished evidence suggests that there is no basis in the assumption, and that HEPA flow rates significantly in excess of 90 feet/min do not contribute to problems of contamination in the final container.

In theory, filter efficiency in particle retention decreases with increasing flux (flow rate per unit filter area). The lower the flux of gas through a filter, the more efficiently the filter will retain particles, including aerosolized bacteria and dust. Although HEPA and all other types of filters work best at low flux, a sufficiently high flux of filtered air is necessary over the critical area to wash particles away quickly. Fluxes in excess of 90 feet/min have not caused problems because the particles in the air fed to the HEPA units are either too large or too small to penetrate the filters with good efficiency. The optimal particle size in air for the penetration of fibrous filters varies from 0.1 to 0.3 micron in diameter, depending on flux of the aerosol challenge to the filter (see Liu and Rubow, 1986 for data). Particles smaller or larger have very poor penetration. This is why HEPA manufacturers test their filters with monodisperse DOP or mineral oil heated to 750°C F (398.89°C) and then mixed with 70°C F (21.11°C) clean air. The DOP or mineral oil vapor condenses to form droplets of about 0.3 micron diameter which is within the optimal range for HEPA filter penetration. Pharmaceutical manufacturers cannot use the hot DOP generator to test HEPA filters in clean rooms because the equipment is cumbersome, heavy, and unsuitable for use in the overheads of cleanrooms between the blower(s) and the HEPA unit(s).

B. Particle levels and sterility

Most filling rooms are monitored, during operation, for total airborne particles by means of Royco, Climet or other suitable counters. As yet, there is no indication that these measurements relate to any level of microbial or particulate contamination of product in the final container. That is to say, an enormous number of measurements are being made that have a rational basis but no data base for validation. For example, Lee et al. (1982) show no correlation of CFU on settling plates with time, a filling room relationship assumed by Whyte (1986). Yet, in a Class 10,000 or Class 100,000 room, airborne bioburden almost certainly is proportional to particles in the air. The difference from the clean room is that clean room garments may shed sterile particles and the sterile product can form sterile particles (aerosols) during filling; in both instances, particle burden has no relationship to the numbers of viable microbes in the air.

When HEPA systems fail, significant problems will occur in the clean room. The failures will occur because an increased proportion of the organisms, fed by the blowers to the HEPA units, penetrate the system at gouges or channels in the HEPA medium or at the seal of the HEPA filter to the frame. Such leaks are best detected in situ with the forward scattering detector mentioned previously.

C. Curtains

Significant eddies form in the critical area if the vortexes from walking personnel disrupt the vertical HEPA flow. In most facilities, the integrity of laminar HEPA flow is maintained in the critical region (which actually is at a level just below the mouth of the final container) by means of flexible plastic curtains. The curtains are overlapping transparent plastic strips, wide or narrow, which are suspended from the sides of the HEPA bank. The curtains ensure the integrity of HEPA laminar air flow until a person disturbs the curtain and the air flow.

D. Vertical v. horizontal laminar flow systems

Filling rooms use vertical laminar flow with wall returns. The bank of HEPA filters usually is about 1 to 1.5 m above the filling line. Because clean room operators stay away from the critical area whenever possible, HEPA flow onto the final container is laminar. Horizontal HEPA flow from a wall bank of filters would seem suitable because the entire room is converted to clean air space, wherein one wall houses the HEPA units and the opposite wall houses the returns. However, such a system is not practical for pharmaceutical manufacturing because personnel and equipment in the room destroy the laminarity of the clean air. Horizontal laminar flow works only in a long hood with the filling/stoppering line close to the HEPA source and personnel-induced turbulence minimized by curtains or plastic walls. A suction system near the forward edge of the filling station reduces turbulence (see Gross, 1976).

5. Personnel Practices

A. Gowning

Within the aseptic process community, the universal understanding is that people shed most of the organisms that present product contamination hazards in the critical area. The organisms are on flakes of skin or on hair or caked cosmetics. Therefore, all, or almost all, skin surfaces are covered with the gown, boots, gloves, mask and goggles. However, this approach is not fail-safe. Some organisms penetrate the woven or non-woven fabrics to emerge into the surrounding air (Whyte and Bailey, 1985) Therefore, proper gowning reduces but does not eliminate organism shed by people in the filling room. Gloving is especially important; operators are present in the room because they can manipulate final containers and closures. The potential exists that a surface of questionable sterility may be touched. For this reason, operators should be double-gloved so that a compromised glove can be removed and replaced without breaking sterility (Stockdale, 1985).

B. Personnel movement

Moving about, even in clean room garments, causes a shed of organisms (Whyte and Bailey, 1985). Movement into the critical area, despite laminar HEPA flow, can cause some level of turbulence and the introduction into the critical area of adventitious organisms. This is the most likely source of transient contamination during filling. The natural tendency of filling room personnel is to touch the vials as they are loaded onto the continuous belt, as they approach the filling needles, or as they approach the closure station. These people, in minimal numbers, must be trained to stay out of the critical area unless and until action is essential.

The numbers and movements of filling room personnel must be kept at a minimum for another reason: walking about on the floor, even in sterile foot coverings, and brushing equipment stirs up particles and organisms sorbed to those surfaces. The HEPA air will not wash from the room microbes adhering to the floor and equipment. Consider the case of driving a dusty car on a relatively clean roadway: even at a speed of 50 mph, most of the dust remains attached to the car's surface. The air flow can clean from the room only those materials that are suspended in the air. The adhering particles and microbes must be killed or removed by the cleaning crew before the filling room is used for process.

6. Filling and Stoppering Operations

A. Filling
The filling of liquid product into a sterile container is complicated by the flow of air around the mouth of the container during the fill cycle. For a bottom fill, the filling needle drives to the bottom of the final container and then commences to fill it. Liquid filled into the container displaces air, reducing the probability of airborne microbes entering the container. By way of contrast, a top-filling machine creates air turbulence at the vial mouth, and the potential for the introduction of adventitious organisms.

Filling heads usually are set onto bulky supports that control the up-and-down movement of the filling needles. Such "towers", in proximity to the filling line, disrupt the laminar HEPA air flow resulting in eddies and turbulence in a portion of the critical area. A design approaching the ideal now is manufactured by AdTech, based on modifications by Gunther Tullmann at Hyland. The filling needles are suspended from a slender post that moves up and down. The bulk of the filling machine equipment is below the finish (aperture) of the final container, and actually below the continuous belt.

The measurement of particles, near the filling needles during operation, may be meaningless. Some sterile product will be aerosolized and the aerosol likely will mask other particles.

B. Stoppering
Most filling operations are labor-intensive not because of the filling process but because most closures are placed by hand. Microbial contamination probably occurs downstream of the filling needles; this is speculation unsupported by data.

Where stoppering is done by hand, the best method would be for the operator to hold the closure in long forceps at arms length, so that the person is as far as possible from the finish and the airflow around the finish. However, this method is impractical. The placement of a small closure, held at arms length, into a moving aperture requires a sustained effort in concentration and hand-eye coordination that is beyond most humans.

One pharmaceutical manufacturer developed a HEPA tunnel in the clean room. The sides of the tunnel were of clear rigid plastic, into which were set rubber gloves at intervals. The bottom of the tunnel was the continuous belt and several inches of open space on either side of the belt. A long, narrow HEPA unit was the roof of the tunnel. This was, in effect, a clean tunnel within a clean room also supplied with HEPA air in the critical areas.

The better solution is automatic stoppering, with minimal contact between the machine and the final container before the closure is in place. The stoppering machine disrupts vertical laminar HEPA air flow but, unlike a human, can be cleaned sufficiently that few or no microbes are shed from the machine surface. Because most stoppering machines are rotary, the tendency is to carry the final container through 180 to 300° of the machine rotation. If the closure is not in place immediately as the container reaches the machine, proximity time may be of consequence in maintaining microbial and particulate cleanliness in the final container. Hence the best designs insert the stopper at first contact.

7. Robotics

The replacement of operators with machines has obvious economic advantages but also eliminates the primary source of microbes (humans) in the filling room. Automation and robotics achieve this objective and the difference between the two seems to be that a robot tends to simulate the action of the human hand and can perform multiple functions, whereas a portion of an automated system is dedicated and performs a single function in a small number of movements. An example of robotics in the aseptic filling room is a check weighing system. The in-line computerized check weigh system places containers on a tare weigh cell for weighing prior to filling, and then repositions them to proceed to the fill station. After filling, the system moves the filled vial to the check weigh cell. The computer compares the target and actual weight and. if necessary, adjusts individual filling heads to deliver the appropriate weight of product. The robotic function is a reject station. If any container exceeds predetermined acceptable limits, the container is automatically rejected by means of an arm that moves the reject off-line.

8. Future Developments

The most immediate means of reducing the risk of microbial contamination of the final container is to package by form-fill-seal. The problem with form-fill-seal is the rate of cooling for heat-labile products. There also is the matter of the closure; the industry is accustomed to an elastomeric closure through which a sterile needle is inserted to withdraw product. There might be problems in placing such a closure with a form-fill-seal system. A possible alternative is that all containers are made for single use.

As form-fill-seal and related technologies become the method of choice for parenterals packaging, the importance of clean rooms will diminish. The environment requiring control and measurement will become the environment within the packaging machine rather than that of the room. As the packaging methods advance, we should expect major decreases in the percentage contamination. As detailed in another chapter of this book, zero contaminated units out of 20,000 units filled has been achieved by manufacturers using form-fill-seal technology. The problem, a pleasant one for all quality control managers, will be how to measure the efficiency of microbial exclusion from such a system without going to the absurd lengths of a 10^6 final container medium fill.

ACKNOWLEDGMENTS: The author gratefully acknowledges the assistance and information provided by the following individuals and organizations in the development of this chapter: Gary Seeger, W.L. Gore and Associates, Flagstaff, AZ; Air Techniques, Inc., Baltimore, MD; Mark Preziosi, Hyland Therapeutics, CA; and David Cutler, AdTech, Lansdale, PA.

9. References

Cadwell, G.H., Jr. (1978) J. Paren. Drug Assoc. 32, 182-187.

Flannery, J.L. and Walcroft, J.P. (1986) In "Fluid Filtration: Gas, Volume I, ASTM STP 975", (R.R. Rabin, Ed.), pp. 390-401, Am. Soc. Testing & Materials, Philadelphia, PA.

Gross, R.I. (1976) Bull. Parenteral Drug Assoc. 30, 143-150.

Gross, R.I. (1978) J. Paren. Drug Assoc. 32, 174-181.

Lee, M.L., Kantrowitz, J.L. and Ellis, J.E. (1982) J. Paren. Sci. Tech. 36, 237-241.

Liu, B.Y.H. and Rubow, K.L. (1986) In;ff1 "Fluid Filtration: Gas, Volume I, ASTM STP 975", (R. R. Raber, Ed.), pp. 1-12, Am. Soc. Testing & Materials, Philadelphia, PA.

Olson, W.P., VandenHouten, L. and Ellis, J.E. (1981) J. Paren. Sci. Tech. 35, 70-71.

Stockdale, D.P. (1985) Pharm. Tech. 9(5), 39-40, 44, 47.

Whyte, W. (1986) J. Paren. Sci. Tech. 40, 188-197.

Whyte, W. and Bailey, P.V. (1985) J. Paren. Sci. Tech. 39, 51-60.

7

An Introduction to Aseptic Filling of Sterile Powders

Gerry Prout
Parenteral Society, Swindon, United Kingdom

1. Introduction

The aseptic assembly of a sterile powder drug presentation is one of the most difficult processes in the pharmaceutical industry. It is generally recognized that the major source of contamination in such products is derived from the personnel involved in product manufacture.

However, there are many other aspects of the production of sterile powder drug presentations which need to be addressed to ensure the required level of assurance of sterility for such products. In this context, it is inevitable that the final degree of assurance of sterility will not be greater than the level achieved during that part of the process where the level of assurance is lowest.

It has been established that contamination includes both viable microorganisms and non-viable particles (1); the sources of such particles being numerous (14, 15). Consequently it is necessary to consider all appropriate parameters commencing with facility design and progressing through construction, commissioning, validation, routine operation and revalidation (16).

The design of the facility should be undertaken with a full understanding of what is required of the facility and the equipment and personnel contained within it. It is also fundamental that the support services are adequately specified and suitable for their intended purposes.

Since personnel occupy a focal role in the process, unless the facility is operated robotically, it is essential that they should understand the nature of the process and its associated problems, and that they should be fully trained in all aspects relevant to their job function and performance (17).

The process of aseptic filling of a sterile powder drug product is, above all other processes, dependent upon a quality assurance program, since it is essential that quality is built into the product as only limited confidence can be placed on the results of end product testing.

161

The nature of the process is that aseptic filling of a sterile powder drug product requires the sterilization of the powder itself and of all components to a required level of sterility assurance and the subsequent amalgamation of drug and components into a drug product in a specially controlled environment.

The essential factors in this program include:

   Powder sterilization
   Component sterilization and depyrogenation
   Aseptic filling
   Aseptic container sealing
   Environmental monitoring including:
      Room pressure differentials
      Frequency of air changes
      Room temperature
      Room humidity
      Viable micro-organism levels
      Non-viable particulate levels
   HEPA filter efficiency
   Air distribution patterns
   Room cleaning programs
   Operator training
   Basic microbiology
   Hygiene gowning
   Clean room comportment

Recent proposals have clarified the essential differences between products sterilized in their final containers, terminally sterilized, and those prepared aseptically and although the guideline deals almost exclusively with liquid products, the principles described are useful for powder products.

As early as 1974 the difficulties of aseptic assembly of a sterile dry product were recognized (3). As a result of the legislative pressures and moves to adapt quality assurance and GMP approaches from an existing quality control philosophy those difficulties have increased rather decreased. However technology has advanced since that time, particularly in container sterilization monitoring and control techniques and in starting material production technology and these advances have, to some extent, compensated for the increase in effort required to ensure that the filled product is suitable for its intended purpose.

2. Scope and Definitions

The scope of this chapter is to describe the legislative requirements, production methodology, validation procedures and quality assurance and quality control measures to ensure that a sterile dry powder product will meet its published specification and be suitable for its intended purpose. Some areas are outside the scope of the chapter such as original product research, formulation and product development. The most important factor in this, and every other pharmaceutical operation is the requirement of the commitment to quality of the product to serve the needs of the patient. All other considerations are of secondary importance.

The definitions of words used in the text have been derived from a variety of sources (2, 4, 5).

APA: Aseptic processing area

APR: Aseptic processing room

APS: Aseptic processing suite

Batch (Lot): A defined quantity of material intended or purported to be uniform in character, produced by a defined cycle of manufacture

Batch (Lot) Number: A distinctive combination of numbers or letters which specifically identifies a batch (lot) and which ensures traceability

Calibration: A documented series of activities to demonstrate that a measuring device produces results within specified tolerances compared with those produced by a reference standard device over a declared range of measurement

Critical Area: Any area where sterilized product, starting material, container or closure may be exposed to the environment

Critical Surface: Any surface with which previously sterilized product, starting material, container or closure may come into contact

Dedicated Facility (equipment): Any room or suite of rooms (or equipment) with attendant services (equipment) used only for the manufacture of one product or closely related group of products

Diluent: A liquid used to reconstitute a process simulation powder or microbiological medium

Finished Product: A medicinal product which has undergone all of its stages of manufacture, including packaging

Good Manufacturing Practice (GMP): Part of Quality Assurance aimed at ensuring that products are consistently manufactured to a quality appropriate to their intended use; GMP incorporates both production and quality control activities

Monitor: Carry out repeated measurements or observations on characteristics of a process or situation to determine whether it is continuing as intended

Packaging Components: Packaging materials which come into contact with the product

Processing Stages: The separate activities involved in the manufacture of a medicinal product

Process Simulation Trial: A test of the ability of the manufacturing process to combine starting material, containers and closures to produce a simulated product under routine operating conditions

Quality Assurance: The sum total of organized efforts made with the object of ensuring that products will be of the quality required by their intended use

Quality Control: Part of GMP concerned with sampling, specification, testing, organization documentation and release procedures which ensure that the necessary and relevant tests are carried out and that materials or products are not released for supply or sale until their quality has been judged to be satisfactory

Revalidation: Repetition of a validation process or part of it

Standard Operating Procedures (SOP): A written authorized procedure which gives instructions for performing operations not necessarily specific to one product

Starting Material: Any substance, excluding packaging material, used in the manufacture of a medicinal product

Sterility: The complete absence of living organisms

Validation: A systematic program of activities to demonstrate that a process will reproducibly and consistently meet the claims made for it.

3. Personnel

In most pharmaceutical operations and particularly those concerned with aseptic assembly of medicinal products, there is a requirement for the involvement of personnel. Much has been written about validation of processes. Most papers deal with the equipment and mechanical processes involved and many ignore the fact that personnel are required to perform many activities. It is undoubtedly true that more recently this fact has become increasingly recognized and that the impact of personnel on the aseptic assembly of sterile powder drug product manufacture, is profound. The influence of personnel on quality must not be underestimated.(4) It is also true that human error accounts for many mistakes, omissions and acts that may result in product defect potentially harmful to the patient (6).

It is not only essential to have personnel available to carry out the various tasks but also that the selection and training of personnel is carried out in an effective and orderly manner. (18)

There are a variety of ways in which this can be achieved, but as with all aspects of aseptic processing, there is a necessity to start at the earliest stage.

Before recruitment there should be a specification for the role which describes what the person will be appointed for and expected to do. Selection of the right person for the appointment is essential. All too often either the person is expected to modify their personality or ability, or the role has to be altered to enable the person selected to fit into it.

There is increasing awareness of the essential nature of good training both on and off the job. This training should be carried out by appropriately qualified and experienced trainers and there should be assessment of whether the training has been successful (5). Training should be carried out on a continuous basis. Corporate commitment to a flexible pragmatic program is essential. Technological change can affect the program as can changes in product types. However, training correctly selected personnel is much less difficult than attempting to re-educate misfits.

Personnel should not only be selected with great care and be effectively trained in the respective procedures comprising their job function, they should also know the basic elements of microbiology and why personal hygiene and cleanliness is of great importance. They should be encouraged to inform the microbiologist or medical staff of any condition which may cause shedding of unusual numbers or types of micro-organism and should not be permitted to work in aseptic production units if they have lesions on exposed surfaces of the body.

It is commonsense that the number of staff within an aseptic processing area should be limited to the minimum number required to efficiently carry out the designated tasks. In situations where it is necessary for untrained staff to enter the aseptic processing area, there should be close supervision to ensure that the internal environment of the area is not compromised. The human factor in the aseptic assembly of sterile powder drug products should be "quality aware" and this quality attitude and awareness can be achieved only by good selection and training not only how to do the job but also the reasons why their performance is critical.

4. Gowning

Since it is recognized that some eighty percent of viable and non-viable particulate contamination in an aseptic processing area originates from personnel, it is essential that a barrier to such shedding will prevent the dispersion of the particulate material throughout the area. The risks to product can be reduced by correct facility design, good operator selection and training, and other parameters. However, the primary barrier in aseptic processing areas is the clothing worn by operators. Such clothing must act as a filter and must be of low linting characteristics.

Most modern cleanroom garments are made from continuous filaments of synthetic fiber woven into a fabric. While not as conducive to operator comfort as fabric made from natural fibers such as cotton, these synthetic fiber garments achieve their function of low linting. When these garments are ripped or damaged, they lose their low linting property and should be replaced. Generally, polyester fabrics are more acceptable than nylon. Modern weaving technology enables fabrics to have minute interstitial spaces while still being capable of carrying moisture across the fabric.

It is accepted that at rest, the average person will generate and shed up to 250,000 particles greater than 0.5 micron per minute; figures of over 1 million are not difficult to achieve with even moderate movement (13).

Gowning for entry into aseptic processing areas must be carried out under controlled conditions. The methods used should ensure minimum shedding of particulate contamination into the surrounding area (7). Each aseptic processing area requires its own gowning procedure to minimize environmental contamination. The eventual system selected should take into account the individual characteristics of the gowning facility to ensure that best advantage is made of them.

5. Quality Assurance

Quality Assurance, as defined in section 2 of this chapter, assumes singular importance in the context of aseptically assembled sterile powder drug products (5). It is evident that to provide assurance of sterility of such products, special precautions are required during the processes involved in their production.

Quality Assurance is the foundation upon which a system of current good manufacturing practice can be constructed. It cannot be over-emphasized that quality cannot be tested into aseptically assembled drug products. Quality must be designed and built into the product. Individual companies will wish to select their own pathways but in all cases, corporate commitment to the quality objective is mandatory.

For the quality assurance approach to be effective, the concept must be transformed into an organizational reality (8, 9, 10), with every person in the organization aware of his/her respective role in the manufacture of the product required by the customer. For the approach to realize full effectiveness, the quality assurance executive or director should be invested with sufficient independence and authority to allow the role to be performed effectively.

It will be the main responsibility of the person appointed to provide the organization with an effective quality assurance system to include an internal audit function.

The effectiveness of a quality assurance function can be assessed in purely financial terms in the reduction of rejects, waste levels and post production inspection and testing rates. Approximately ten percent of total sales values on a global basis are attributable to quality failure costs. Quality conscious companies are generally self motivated to produce what the consumer requires at a satisfactory quality level. The selection of the correct quality assurance system can result only as a consequence of good management decisions.

6. Quality Control

A. General

The Pharmaceutical Industry has recognized for a considerable period of time that final testing of drug products is insufficient. It was shown that strict attention to all stages of research, development, manufacture and distribution was required to provide the level of safety and efficiency demanded.

It became increasingly obvious that the control of quality had to be more dependent upon control before and during manufacture and less dependent upon final product testing.

Quality control philosophy as a means of determining the quality of a product suffers from serious shortcomings. First the data obtained is retrospective; second the most important factor for determining quality often became the quality of the sampling regimen. Quality Control also has limitations with respect to the techniques used during testing; furthermore there is a finite limit on the number of tests carried out.

One needs to define the necessary and relevant tests which will provide the most convincing evidence of the suitability of the product. Quality Control, in isolation, can result in the acceptance of a batch which contains a proportion of defective product; therefore its role has become that of monitoring that the quality assurance program for a process or product is achieving its intended aims.

B. Starting materials

The acquisition of starting materials for the manufacture of aseptically produced sterile powder drug products should form part of the Quality Assurance program.

In this context starting materials refers to the active drug, excipients, containers and closures. The quality of the finished product is a direct consequence of the quality of starting materials. It is essential for quality control testing of starting materials to be carried out at a pre-determined frequency to ensure compliance with specification.

Each company should have a scientifically based logical argument to support its policy with respect to selection, testing and acceptance of starting materials. This policy should ensure that the product manufactured from approved starting materials is suitable for its intended purpose and does not compromise the welfare of the recipient. It is necessary that this policy is in compliance with compendial and legislative requirements.

C. In-process control

Many of the aseptically produced sterile powder drug products are antimicrobial agents. It is therefore essential to control not only the environmental factors to give an acceptable assurance of sterility, but also the uniformity of contents of the product dispensed into the container. Where uniformity of dose from container to container is required, the assessment of content uniformity is based on two parameters, namely weight of contents and potency of contents (11, 12).

It is required that the maximum and minimum product potency limits include all tolerances to account for sampling errors, assay variables, product overages, and variations in the manufacturing process. (11) Hence the fiducial limit of error of the potency must be determined; the lower limit must be not less than 95 per cent and the upper limit not more than 115 per cent of the content declared on the product label.

A more realistic approach requires that the content uniformity lies between 85 per cent and 115 per cent of the label claim (12) These requirements can still be achieved if no more than one container in thirty has contents outside the specified range, but within the range 75 per cent to 125 per cent and the relative standard deviation is less than 7.8 per cent for the thirty containers, when calculated using the formula.

$$\text{Relative Standard Deviation (RSD)} = (100s)/X$$

where X is the mean of the values obtained from units tested and expressed as a percentage of label claim and

$$s = \frac{(xi - X)^2}{(n - 1)}$$

where n is the number of units tested and xi represents the individual values of the units tested (x_1, x_2, x_n) expressed as a percentage of the label claim.

The validation of fill weights is an unusually difficult subject and will be dealt with in the section on validation in this chapter.

In-process control should also be used for checks of the closure system during production to ensure that microbiological security is being maintained.

To minimize the probability of ingress of particulate matter during processing, particulate levels in the environment should be monitored especially in the more sensitive areas, such as zones where either product or open components are exposed. Where possible and practicable, monitoring should be carried out on a continuous basis with warning and action limits clearly specified. These limits can be established during validation and on the basis of historic records during routine production. Particle levels may be measured using any suitable technique. The individual manufacturer may choose from a wide range of equipment available. Most frequently employed today are automatic devices using forward light scattering techniques which are easily fitted with audible or visual alarms to inform personnel when pre-set particulate contamination levels are reached. Using this type of equipment, it is possible to determine the levels of a wide range of particle sizes, the levels being recorded at pre-determined intervals. Suitable particulate standards for operations encountered in sterile powder drug production can be found in several official or semi-official documents (5, 19).

It must be recognized that it may not always be possible to comply with certain particulate standards at the point of fill when filling is in progress due to the release of particles from the product.

Viable particles should be evaluated as part of the in-process quality control system using any appropriate one or combination of methods available for qualitative, semi-quantitative, and quantitative estimation of viable particles in the environment. There is a lack of official standards for viable particle warning and action limits, although there are guidelines (5) as well as parallel industrial requirements. (20) As with non-viable particulate monitoring, each manufacturer should establish warning and action limits, which will vary from critical to non-critical areas. Recently various statistical methods have been used to evaluate environmental trends which are almost certainly more relevant than single units of data. These techniques include cumulative frequency distribution, (21) cumulative summation techniques, (22) negative binomial distribution (23) and control charting (24).

Qualitative methods available for microbiological quality control include the use of settle plates, contact plates and swabs. The latter two techniques can be semi quantitative when used in a disciplined consistent manner.

Quantitative methods are based on air entrapment techniques. In these techniques, air is drawn past a capture medium such as an agar surface, or a membrane filter. These techniques include slit samplers, centrifugal air samplers, liquid impingement techniques, membrane filtration, cascade impactors and sieves. For routine quality control, the determination and selection of microbiological monitoring methods and the sampling regimen used must form part of the standard operating procedures; otherwise less than useful reliance can be placed on the results obtained. Close adherence to written operating procedures by the personnel involved in aseptic manufacture is essential and personnel movements should be moderated to restrict the amount of particulate dispersion produced.

D. Finished product testing

It is necessary that all products should be defined in an appropriate specification. This specification will cover not only the microbiological characteristics of the finished product but also the chemical (purity) and physical requirements for the product. For finished product testing to be meaningful, an acceptable system of sampling must be in operation, otherwise the results obtained may not be representative of the batch as a whole. The sterility test is the most frequently used finished product microbiological test despite its undoubted shortcomings. Various methods are available for the test but the two major techniques involved are direct inoculation of product into microbiological media and membrane filtration. Wherever possible membrane filtration should be used. Descriptions of the test are to be found in all of the major pharmacopoeia (25, 26, 27). The statistics of the sterility test are such that with 0.1 percent of units within the batch being contaminated, the probability of accepting the batch as sterile is 98 percent. With ten percent of units within the batch being contaminated, the probability of acceptance as sterile is still as high as 12 percent. The sterility test is further discussed elsewhere in this book.

It is frequently not recognized that the same statistics apply not only to the test for sterility but also to all other quality control tests. It is for these reasons that quality assurance assumes great importance in the sterile product field.

7. Production

A considerable number of different methods are available for production of a sterile powder drug product. Very few of these methods have been described in

the literature (6) and most publications are primarily concerned with validation methodology. There is similarly a lack of official guidelines, with most
authorities demanding that the user of a particular method must demonstrate
its effectiveness.

The multiplicity of product presentations and manufacturing methods
can lead the manufacturer into problems and misunderstanding.

Many sterile powder filling operations are carried out on a continuous
or semi-continuous basis as a result of the development of the tunnel sterilizer.
Batch processing is also used.

Ideally, serious consideration should be given to a total operation which
includes on-line powder production, glassware and stopper washing and sterilization, powder filling, container stoppering and sealing.

Once the production method has been defined and installed, the system
should be validated using an appropriate method (4, 16). The manufacturing
method for each product should be described in the manufacturing process specification in a stepwise manner, with provision being made for each critical step
to be checked by a recognized competent person.

Product yield should be compatible with input quantities of all starting
materials. In-process quality control should monitor trends through the entire
production cycle.

The aseptic processing area is the final point at which airborne particulate or microbiological contamination can occur.

The production facility should be designed and constructed in a manner
which facilitates the application of Good Manufacturing Practice and which
minimizes the possibility of cross contamination.

In powder filling operations, product can be filled by either weight or
by volume. The former operation, weight filling, is usually operated by position-
ing an empty container over a load cell which monitors the quantity of powder
added to the container. An intermediate hopper may also be used to pre-weigh
the quantity of powder being dispensed. This system of weight filling generally
gives tighter weight variation tolerances. The second filling option, filling by
volume, using an auger system or "slug" of powder contained within depressions
on a filling wheel. This equipment is usually simple to operate but weight variation may become a problem if the particle size and bulk density of the powder
change.

Weight control for the aseptic filling of sterile powers is a major problem
and accurate on-line weight checking is being developed in conjunction with
microprocessors to provide systems of optimal economic performance.

This stage of the production cycle is the most critical since both container
and product are exposed to the environment for a finite period. However, studies
have shown that the probability of contamination by either viable or non viable
particles can be calculated and theoretical levels of sterility assurance determined. (14, 15) This is the final stage at which airborne contamination can occur.

Stoppering of product containers usually occurs on-line immediately after filling and equipment is either in-line or rotary. These units can usually be operated under unidirectional air flow. To ensure efficient operation the containers and stoppers must be restricted to very narrow tolerances. Particulate contamination may be generated in the stopper feed bowls and hence stopper design and siliconization are important. Non vibratory stopper feed systems are available. Stoppers can be inserted manually, particularly on low volume lines, but this process increases the risk of microbial contamination.

It is preferable that the application of aluminum collars and over-caps should be carried out well away from the stoppering process since the application of the collars and overcaps almost inevitably produces significant quantities of small metal particles.

All subsequent manipulation should be performed outside the aseptic room.

8. Particulate Contamination

Particulate contamination in sterile powder drug dosage forms is frequently difficult to observe. In many cases, the powder is colored and particles of similar color may not be evident. In those cases where the powder is white, particles, such as lubricant from rubber gloves etc., may also be white or the powder may coat the particle as a result of electrostatic attraction of fine product particles to the contaminant particle.

Generally the size of the contaminating particle is not of a dimension to be detected visually in the powder. Examination for particulate contamination requires special techniques. In all cases, reconstitution of the powder with a particle free diluent is essential.

Microscopic methods are frequently used after the reconstituted drug has been filtered through a membrane filter of appropriate porosity. Using this method it is possible, although not always easy, to identify the nature of any contaminating particle or particles.

Other methods involve the use of light scattering devices for detection of the particles. These devices are a convenient way of counting and sizing the particles but identification is usually not possible by these methods.

It is a pharmacopoeial requirement (12) that solutions constituted from solid dosage forms should not be significantly less clear than an equal volume of diluent contained in a similar vessel and examined similarly, and that the solid material dissolves completely, leaving no visible residue as undissolved matter. The solution so constituted should be essentially free from particles of foreign matter that can be observed on visual examination. The medical relevance of particulate matter below visual proportions has been under discussion since 1963. Many conflicting reports have been made with pharmacopoeial statements are open to subjective assessment. Clearly much more work is required before official standards can be established.

9. Validation

Basically there are three methods by which the aseptic drug powder filling process can be validated. These methods have been adequately described. (4, 16) All suffer from shortcomings and none are truly process simulation tests, in that they are dependent upon additional manipulations.

It must be acknowledged that the powder filling process, while aiming at the same end result, is different from the liquid fill validation system in this respect. It is possible to validate the process without the use of media but it is then necessary for all other aspects of the operation to be thoroughly validated and to ensure that design of the facility does not give rise to opportunistic contamination

In some cases the filling operation is run with the exception that powder is not filled into the product containers. At the end of this activity, microbiological growth medium may be added to the product containers. The possibility of contamination occurring during this latter manipulation must not be overlooked and results obtained must be examined carefully.

Where the validation program uses a process simulation test with media, there are two approaches, one using a liquid medium and the second a dry powder medium. The former approach can be carried out in two ways, either the liquid can be sterilized in the product container before presentation to the filling equipment, or the liquid can be filled into the container using a modified filling unit.

For the dry powder approach, the powder can be filled into empty vials with subsequent addition of a diluent or the powder can be added to the vials when they already contain a sterile liquid diluent.

For small volume containers, the addition of normal fill weight of microbiological growth medium and either the previous or subsequent addition of appropriate diluent will lead to hyperosmotic solutions in which many microorganisms will not grow. Additionally the growth medium will require pre sterilization and may well have different flow and or compaction properties when compared with the product powder.

For example l gram of trypticase soy broth powder dispensed into a 15mL container will lead, even when the container is filled to capacity with diluent, to a solution which is 2.2 times the normal concentration, and when 10mL of diluent is added, to a solution 3.3 times the normal concentration.

In an ideal situation, the quantity of powder dispensed in process simulation tests should equal that of normal product quantity. Where the powder dispensed in a process simulation test is not a microbiological growth medium, it must be ascertained that the powder does not have innate antimicrobial properties and it should be easily soluble in the diluent to be used.

There have been numerous statements regarding the number of containers which should be filled during validation programs and the permitted level of contamination. Statistically, frequent small numbers of containers are of greater value than one large number. However, this approach is often difficult because of production demands on the filling equipment.

Aseptic powder drug processors should determine for themselves the number of vials to be filled to give statistical validity to the test. This number can be determined using the equation:

$$P = 1 - (1 - A)^N$$

Where P = Probability of detecting non-sterility.
A = Acceptable contamination rate (expressed as a percentage).
N = Number of containers filled in test.

Using this formula, it can be calculated that for an acceptable contamination rate of 0.1 per cent, it is necessary to fill 5000 containers to give a slightly better than 99 per cent probability of detecting contamination. For the same acceptable contamination rate, it is necessary to fill some 2500 containers to give a better than 90 per cent probability of detection of non sterility. The acceptable level of contamination permitted in process simulation test is still the subject of some disagreement since several authorities permit different levels (32, 33, 34). It would seem reasonable that a 0.1 per cent level of non sterility is acceptable for these process simulation tests although ideally a zero level should be obtained and recent studies (14, 15) have indicated the improbability of contamination occurring when Good Manufacturing Practices have been followed.

For the test to be valid it is necessarily to qualify liquid and powder media for their growth promotion properties, and not only compendial organisms should be used to demonstrate either positive or negative growth promotion properties. The use of environmental isolates in this situation is considered to be of greater value.

It is necessarily to carry out validation work, in terms of process simulation studies before permitting routine production of the drug product and three successful process simulation tests are considered to be a suitable level for qualification of a new facility.

Revalidation should occur when any major change in standard operating procedures or equipment takes place and each company should continuously appraise their validated systems according to a schedule of either internal or external audits or on a planned annual basis.

Diagrammatic approaches to the validation program are shown in Figures 1, 2, and 3, while a complete schematic for a dry sterile powder drug filling is shown in Figure 4.

Figure 1—Dry sterile powder filling process simulation

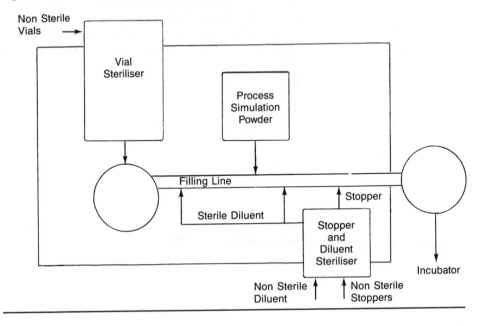

Figure 2—Dry sterile powder filling process simulation

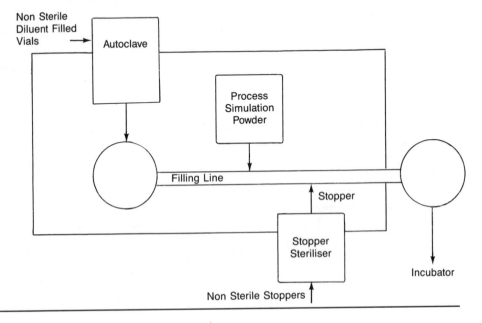

Figure 3 – Dry sterile powder filling process simulation

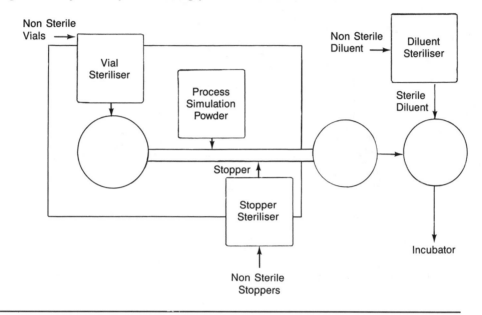

Figure 4—Schematic for validation of sterile process

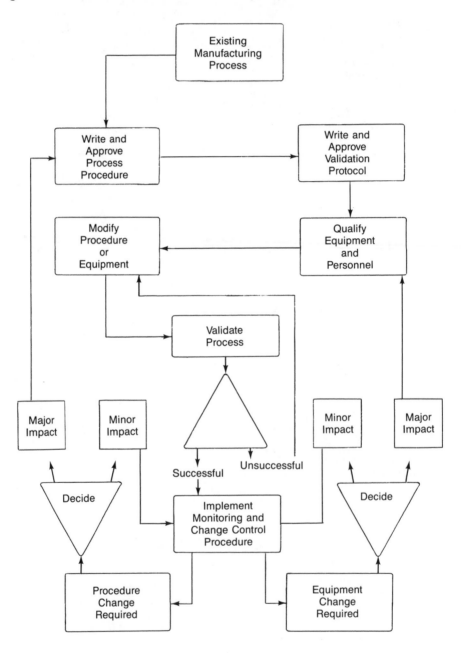

REFERENCES

1. Hammer, H. F., "Problems of Particulate Matter in Sterile Solid Products for Injection", Bull Parenteral Drug Assoc., 28 (5) 205 1974

2. Draft Guideline on Sterile Drug Products Produced by Aseptic Processing January 1985, Prepared by Center for Drugs and Biologics and Office of Regulatory Affairs, FDA Division of Drug Quality Compliance (HFN - 320) Office of Compliance, Center for Drugs and Biologics 5600 Fishers Lane, Rockville, MD 20857, USA

3. Rohde P.A., Brabander W.J., and Tylec F.W., "Challenging the Sterility of a Sterile Powder Filling Line", Bull Parenteral Drug Assoc., 28 (5) 241, 1974

4. Technical Deport No. 6 (1984) Validation of Aseptic Drug Powder Filling Processes, Parenteral Drug Association Inc, Philadelphia, PA 19107, USA

5. Guide to Good Pharmaceutical Manufacturing Practice, (1983), Her Majesty's Stationery Office, London, United Kingdom.

6. Begg D.I.R.,"Validation, An Inspectors View", Manufacturing Chemist 55 (12) 31 1984

7. "Gowning for Aseptic Areas" (Tape-Slide Presentation), Parenteral Drug Association Inc, Philadelphia, PA 19107, USA

8. "A Guide to Quality Assurance", British Standard BS 4891 (1972), QA Division, British Standards Institute, Linford Wood, Milton Keynes, UK.

9. "Quality Systems", British Standard BS 5750 (1981), QA Division, British Standards Institute, Linford Wood, Milton Keynes, United Kingdom.

10. Cooper MS (1972, 1973, 1979) In "Quality in the Pharmaceutical Industry" Parts 1, 2 and 3 Academic Press, London.

11. "Compendium of Licensing Requirements for the Manufacture of Biological Medicinal Products" (1977), Her Majesty's Stationery Office, London, UK.

12. The United States Pharmacopoeia, XX, 1985. p xlvii and General Chapter (905) p 1277 U.S. Pharmacopoeial Convention Inc., Rockville MD, USA.

13. Whyte W., and Bailey P.V., "Reduction of Microbial Dispersion by Clothing", J. Parent. Sci. Tech., 39, (1) 51, 1985.

14. Whyte W., Bailey P.V.,Tinkler J., McCubbin I., Young L.,and Jess J,. "Evaluation of the routes of bacterial contamination cccurring during aseptic pharmaceutical manufacture", J. Parent. Sci. Tech., 36 (3) 102, 1982

15. Whyte W., Bailey P.V.,and Hodgson R., "Monitoring the causes of clean room contaminaion" Manuf. Chem. Aerosol News Sept, 65, 1979

16. Prout G. "Validation and Routine Operation of a Sterile Dry Powder Filling Facility", J Parent. Sci. Tech., 36 (5) 199, 1982

17. Deluca P.P., "Micro contamination Control : A Summary of an Approach to Training", J Parent. Sci. Tech., 37 (6) 218, 1983

18. Snyder J.F., "Successful selection of Professional People", J Parent. Sci. Tech., 38 (2) 64, 1984

19. "Clean Room and Work Station Requirements, Controlled Environment", Federal Standard 209 b, 1973, General Services Administration, Federal Supply Service Standardisation Division, Washington DC 20406, USA.

20. "NASA Standards for Clean Rooms and Work Stations for the Microbially Controlled Environment, NHB 5340.2, 1967, National Aeronautics and Space Administration, Washington DC 20546, USA

21. Dixon W.J., Massey, Jr., F.J., in "Introduction to Statistical Analysis" 3rd ed.,1969, McGaw-Hill, York.

22. Russell, M P., Purdie, R.N., Goldsmith J.A., Phillips, I. "Computer Assisted Evaluation of Microbiological Environmental Control Data" J. Parent. Sci. Tech., 38 (3) 98, 1984

23. Lee M.L.,Kantrowitz J.L., Ellis J.B., "A application of the Negative Binomial Distribution to a problem in Microbiologically Clean Area Testing". J. Parent. Sci. Tech., 36 (6),237 1982.

24. Grant E.L. in "Statistical Quality Control", 3rd ed., 1964 McGaw.Hill, New York.

25. The United States Pharmacopeia, XX, 1985 p. 1156 et seq., U.S. Pharmacopeial Convention Inc., Rockville MD, USA

26. The British Pharmacopoeia 1980 vol. II, Appendix XVI p. A186 et seq., Her Majesty's Stationery Office, London, United Kingdom

27. European Pharmacopoeia 1971 vol. II, p. 53 et seq., Maisonneuve SA, Paris, France.

28. Wegal S., "Short time sterilisation of glass material under ultraclean conditions", Bull. Parent. Drug Assoc., 28 (4) 122 1974.

29. Elias T.F., Webb B.H., Taylor F.D., "A laminar flow approach to in line vial sterilisation", Bull. Parent. Drug Assoc., 31 (1) 33 1977.

30. Willing W.G., "Short term hot air sterilisation by the laminar flow process", Pharm. Tech. Intl., 2 (1) 23 1979.

31. Garvan J.M., and Gunner B.W., "Intravenous fluids", Med. J. Australia, 2, 140, 1963.

32. "Sterility and Sterility Testing of Pharmaceutical Preparations and Biologicals", WHO/BS731062 and WHO/PHARM/73.474 (1973) World Health Organisation, Geneva, Switzerland

33. "Good Manufacturing Practices for Drug Manufacturers and Importers", Cat No. H42-21-1982, Health Protection Branch, Health and Welfare Canada, Ottawa, ON, Canada

34. "Code of Good Manufacturing Practices for Therapeutic Drug Product", Australian National Biologic Standards Laboratory, 1983; Canberra, ACT, Australia

8

Evaluation of Closure Integrity

Michael S. Korczynski
Abbott Laboratories, Abbott Park, IL, USA

1. Introduction

Methodologies used to evaluate the integrity of closure systems are constantly evolving. Various well documented methods such as dye testing of entire batches of ampules and evacuation tests or autoclave "pressure drop" stress tests have been used to test the integrity of containers such as ampules and vials. Less published information is available related to the evaluation of container/closure systems. In recent years companies have placed greater emphasis on introducing new container/closure systems for the delivery of a variety of parenteral solutions. The growing complexity in the design and number of parenteral delivery systems has necessitated the further development of physical and microbiological closure integrity tests.

Maintenance of sterility of a container/closure system is achieved by design and manufacturing factors that take into consideration a number of variables. The closure and container configuration that protects the contents from intrusion of microorganisms during assembly, shipment, and storage will permit the product to remain sterile during its shelf life. The closure system must be (a) designed in a manner that provides security to the container contents, (b) capable of being processed and affixed to the container in a sterile manner, (c) capable of maintaining the contents of the container sterile throughout the stability life of the product or until expiry of the product and (d) capable of withstanding practical hospital or pharmacy usage without an introduction of microorganism into the fluid contents.

2. Relationship Between Physical and Biological Closure Integrity Testing

Qualification of a container/closure system as a microbial barrier requires the review and assessment of numerous engineering, physical, and microbiological data. The validity of closure integrity should be based on a well conceived design configuration balanced by supporting physical and micro-biological data

181

that confirm that microbial ingress will not occur. The proof that a container/closure system is indeed a microbial barrier should not be based on the results of any one particular test. A review of composite of physical and biological data may be required.

Engineering and micobiological personnel must work together to examine the closure design to determine whether any potential pathways exist that would allow ingress of microorganisms. Once the design concept is accepted as feasible, challenges to the design concept may be made by conducting an assortment of dye and/or pressure tests or other appropriate physical tests. In the initial stage of development, the type of closure capping or insertion application and associated forces must be considered. The manufacturing process must permit appropriate sidewall and/or sealing surface contacts to occur in the case of rigid container systems such as glass. If plastic and rubber components are used in the closure system, the process must assure appropriate fit to preclude outward or inward leakage. The adequacy of a closure system's integrity should include an evaluation of overall design, sealing qualities and characteristics, functionality, product contact, materials of composition, size of the container and closure, and process conditions.

Microbiological testing may be reserved for validating the final closure design established by physical testing means or may be used to challenge the design concept as it progresses to the final design.

If a correlation between physical properties of the closure system and results of microbiological testing are desired, parallel studies may be conducted. Specific manufacturing procedures, test designs, and stressing conditions to be used should be established prior to testing. Physical, functional, and microbiological data should be generated from samples that have been exposed to the same manufacturing and stress conditions. If possible, samples from the extremes of the proposed design specification ranges should be obtained and evaluated. If this is not possible, a statistically based representative sample is satisfactory.

Very little information exists in the literature concerning the evaluation of closure systems by either physical or microbiological methods. Due to the heterogeneity of closure and container systems that exist in the pharmaceutical industry, standardized procedures are not available. The situation has become more pronounced since the advent and wide usage of plastic container systems.

While physical and microbiological tests may not be standardized, physical tests for the most part will yield a quantitative measurement that permits one to compare or evaluate process and design changes upon the integrity of the closure system. When conducting physical tests on closures, the type of equipment to test the closure and fixtures to hold the container or closure are limited only by the ingenuity of the laboratory or engineering personnel and the availability of the equipment. The selection of the physical method is independent of the end use of the product. However, the microbiological test method selected should have a relationship to the intended end use of the product. For example, if the closure is not going to be in contact with an aqueous environment during use of the product, the closure does not need to be immersed in a microbiological suspension to evaluate integrity. Perhaps exposing the closure to an aerosol microbial challenge more closely resembles shipment and storage conditions. Table I includes factors that might be considered at various stages of closure development and during routine manufacturing.

Table I—A Proposed Scenario of Closure Integrity Selection and Testing

Closure Selection	Developmental Testing	Routine Monitoring
Selection of appropriate design related to end-use of the product.	Evaluate preliminary design by dye leakage, and/or pressure leak tests or other appropriate physical tests.	Assure maintenance of specified engineering and microbiological operating conditions.
Appropriate fit and tolerance designs to assure sterility of the fluid pathway or contents during processing and prior to usage.	Confirm integrity by microbial challenge studies.	Physical inspection of container, closure and visual examination of contents.
	Evaluation of closure properties following exposure to shipping conditions.	Assessment of potential shipping and storage conditions.

3. Physical Testing

During initial integrity evaluation of a closure system, a number of physical tests may be used. (1) These tests may also be used to release test final product. These physical tests may include pressure testing of ampules and vials, dye immersion tests, and electronic spark testing of an evacuated container, visual examination for glass cracks, and loss in cap torque force for screw cap types of closures. An assortment of pressure tests for the container itself and the closure system may be used.

A. Pneumatic pressure tests

Pressure tests are generally conducted on plastic semi-rigid or flexible containers. Pressure may be applied to the outer container while the container is immersed in water to determine whether air bubbles are emitted from the container proper or its closure system. Similarly, forced air pressure or other inert gas pressures may be used and applied to the container proper or its container/closure system by a small bore cannula. While the container or closure is subjected to the flowing pressure, the unit is immersed in water or other solution. The container is examined for the presence of gas bubbles emanating from the container or closure while pressure is being applied.

B. Closure blow-off tests

A bottle or container may be cut or sectioned from the bottle leaving the area above the shoulder container area and closure system intact. Pressure is then applied to the closure to determine how much pressure is required to cause the seal to fail. This study leads to quantitative pressure blow-off values that may be used to compare different manufacturing procedures and closure designs. Gaseous pressure applied to the underside of the closure may establish whether changes have occurred within the closure resulting in a change to the closure sealing surface. This procedure may also indicate whether the durometer or hardness of the closure has changed during processing, thereby influencing the fit of the closure in the container.

C. Torque values

Torque testing of closure systems generally applies to screw cap type closures. A number of physical events occur during the capping of a rigid or semi-rigid container system. These parameters include such events as sidewall pressure and vertical pressure applied to the closure. If a metallic cap is applied to the container, roller shape must be taken into consideration. The determination of whether closure torque has changed may indicate whether the primary closure and container thread alignment has changed or the closure has unseated in some manner during sterilization. The torque values that are applied before sterilization processing and after sterilization processing may be compared to establish the influences of the manufacturing and sterilization process upon integrity of the closure.

Table II includes a summary of some of the most frequently employed physical tests used to evaluate the integrity of closure systems.

Table II – Some physical methods for evaluating container/closure leakage

Vacuum Retention	Air is evacuated from the container and leakage is detected by vacuum loss.
Pneumatic Pressure	Headspace in the container is pressurized to observe leakage. The containers may be immersed inverted in an appropriate solution to more readily observe bubbles leaking from the closure area.
Vacuum Chamber	Container with closures may be placed inverted into a vacuum chamber and observed for leakage.
Dye Immersion	Immersion in dye solution with or without pressure. May be important to consider the charge associated with the dye.

D. Specification variabilities

During the testing or design evaluation of a manufactured product, the best evaluation plan would include testing of the design specification extremes. The same logic applies to the testing of the design of closure systems. It would be ideal if, for example, a rubber stopper closure system with the smallest outer diameter dimensions and the container with the widest inner diameter dimensions were selected for microbial integrity testing. With certain closure systems it may be ideal to test containers with the least internal pressure, lowest torque value, or least pressure blow-off value. However, under practical conditions of assembling and manufacturing, it is frequently extremely difficult to obtain and generate sufficient samples for statistical calculation purposes that are representative of a very narrow range of physical and engineering parameters. Therefore, frequently closure container assembly equipment is set-up at conditions that may yield a large group of samples at the lower range of the acceptable specifications for purposes of special closure studies. The overall impact of dimensional tolerances upon interference, clearance, and sealing surfaces must be considered prior to final manufacturing of the closure.

E. Rigid container systems

Rigid container systems such as glass containers were among the first type of containers subjected to integrity evaluation by microbiological methods. The microbial immersion test originated to evaluate whether mold or microorganisms could enter fissures within glass containers or fine cracks near the closure area. The test eventually evolved into usage as a closure integrity test for rigid containers. The test is very stringent because in actual use it would be unusual for the closure to experience a submerged condition, even for a brief period.

F. Flexible plastic containers

These containers are becoming widely used throughout the health care field. Frequently flexible plastic containers used for intravenous or irrigation solutions are comprised of an inner primary container within a secondary overwrap package. The overwrap may be used to provide an additional barrier to gas transfer through the primary container and may act as a dust cover during handling procedures. The secondary overwrap is frequently comprised of a flexible plastic composition or a foil barrier.

Combinations of foil and plastic overwraps also exist. When considering actual shipment and handling, the secondary package affords some protection to the inner primary container. The secondary barrier or overwrap not only minimizes physical trauma to the primary container during handling and shipment, but prevents dust and particulate debris from contacting the primary container. Therefore, while in most cases secondary packages are not designed to assure container or closure integrity, the overwrap greatly minimizes the insult to the primary container during in-use shipment and handling. The question arises, is it necessary to test the entire package, both primary and secondary packaging, during physical and biological integrity testing, or to evaluate only the primary container? The consensus among the pharmaceutical industry would probably support the premise that, while the secondary package adds a large measure of integrity assurance to the primary container, the primary container must independently demonstrate container and closure integrity properties. In evaluating the closures of flexible plastic containers, some variation of the shipment test previously described may be used, or alternatively an aerobiological challenge as described in the microbiological testing section.

4. Test Methods Related to Product Use

As previously mentioned, the microbiological immersion system was developed to respond to an early identified need in the manufacturing of glass containers. This is no longer the case with plastic containers, and the classical immersion test does not apply to actual conditions of use for plastic containers.

The design of closure integrity tests should include parameters that simulate the stresses the closure will experience during processing as well as conditions that may be experienced in transport, storage and in use. The container/closure system that is aseptically processed may not experience the thermal dynamic conditions of an autoclave cycle as an entire entity during processing. However, once placed in a clinical setting, the container/closure system will be subjected to central supply storage and handling, and other hospital environments. Such conditions include atmospheric changes and generally do not include the wetting or submersion of the closure system prior to use. Conditions related to potential pressure deferential conditions experienced by shipment, especially by air, should be considered. These conditions require development of appropriate methods of closure integrity evaluation.

5. Microbiological Testing

A. Microbial immersion test

This is a simple and straightforward test. The containers are filled with a culture media, such as soybean casein digest broth, and sterilized. Following cooling, the containers are immersed into a suspension of a motile microorganisms such as *Pseudomonas aeruginosa*. If the closure rather than the entire container is evaluated, the containers may be inverted and immersed into the microbial suspension. This method generally requires construction of a special rack system to assure that the weight of the entire container is not supported by the inverted closure. Figure 1 is a schematic illustration of the immersion testing system. Generally the closure system is immersed into the microbial suspension for durations of one day or less. Increased immersion time increases the probability of contact and passage of the motile microorganism through or around the closure system or any hole or fissure in the container and may be an unrealistic challenge.

Several technical procedures should be followed when utilizing this method. The microbial count per milliliter should be determined at the beginning, middle and end of the container/closure immersion time. In certain cases

Figure 1—Illustration of a Container/Closure System Microbiological Immersion Test

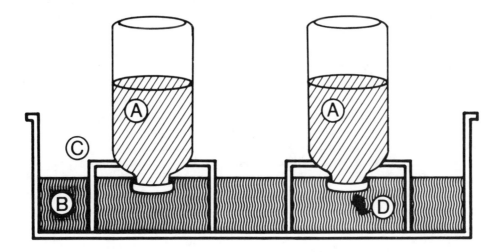

Legend:
A—Culture medium   C—Container rack system
B—Microbial suspension   D—Closure/container system being evaluated

where product is still within the container during the test, the contents may be tested by filtration using a 0.22 micron bacterial retentive filter. The filter may then be immersed into the bacteriological recovery media and incubated for a minimum of seven days. In the event the container contents contain a potential bacteriostatic agent, the filter must be subjected to an appropriate rinsing procedure such as three independent rinses of 10mL of sterile peptone solution. (1)

Consideration must be given to using proper ventilation during this study. The test should be conducted in a well ventilated area with limited personnel traffic. A chemical fume hood or specialized exhaust system that covers the microbiological suspension bath should be used. At the end of the immersion time, the containers should be disinfected with several applications of 10% hydrogen peroxide or an appropriate commercial disinfectant. A special ultraviolet decontamination box may be developed to reduce the microbial count on the exterior of the containers and closures. It is advisable to wear gloves, gown, mask and respiratory system during the removal of containers during disinfection. The challenged containers and closures should be incubated at 30–35°C for a period of seven days. The challenged containers and closures may also be incubated at room temperature if microbial growth occurs at ambient conditions. Consideration should be given to venting the bottles with a sterile needle containing a vent filter if an obligate aerobic microorganism is used in the test.

B. Shipment simulation testing

This test may also be used to evaluate the integrity of closure systems. The container is placed within a shipping carton and oscillated on a reciprocating shaker at a specific number of oscillations per minute to simulate transit conditions. During the test the container is reoriented in several directions. Following the shipment simulation, the containers and closures may be subjected to either physical evaluation or microbial integrity testing.

Another system that may be considered is to place bacteriological culture media within the containers or actual product be used and then ship the cartons to a transcontinental destination followed by return shipment of the carton and contents to the original testing laboratory. The product should be packaged in the same manner that will be used with the actual commercial product. Following receipt of the returned containers, the containers may be incubated for 7–14 days at 30–35 °C. Alternatively, the product may be exposed to an immersion type microbiological test following trans-shipment. If the immersion test is conducted in addition to the shipping test, it should be viewed as an extremely rigorous test of the closure system's integrity.

C. Microbial aerobiology test

This test can be used to evaluate the effects of atmospheric or environment microbial and pressure conditions upon the closure system. This test involves the generation of a nebulized cloud or aerosol of microorganisms in a confined vessel or chamber. Upon stabilization of the microbial aerosol within the chamber, various pressure dynamics may be used to potentially increase the opportunity for microorganisms to penetrate protected areas of the closure system. The number of microorganisms used per liter of aerosol can be determined and equated to the number of microorganisms that might exist under in-use conditions. Generally, manufacturing conditions or in areas where two or three personnel are conducting manipulative tasks outside of an aseptic area, microbial counts may remain well under thirty microorganisms per cubic feet of sampled air. During the aerobiology test, approximately 1.0×10^3 microorganisms per cubic foot of chamber environment may be used. Therefore, the test not only utilizes pressure dynamics but may employ a concentration of microorganisms that exceeds in-use microbial conditions by a several hundred-fold factor.

An aerobiology test may be performed by utilizing the shell of a sterilization vessel or perhaps a suitable stainless steel mixing tank that will tolerate pressure differentials and that has been converted to meet the specialized needs of an aerobiology vessel. Figure 2 illustrates an example of an aerobiology chamber equipped for evaluation of container/closure systems. The microbial aerosol is generally nebulized into the vessel under pressure. The containers with closure systems or the devices that are exposed to the aerosol should be arranged in a pattern that does not inhibit aerosol contact. The vessel should not be fully loaded.

Figure 2 — Illustration of a Microbial Aerosol Test System to Evaluate Container Closure Systems

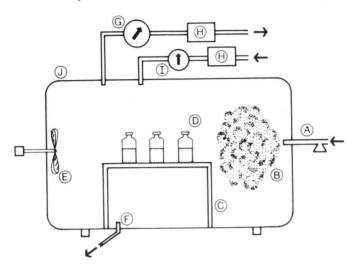

Legend:
A — Microbial nebulizer
B — Microbial aerosol cloud
C — Rack on tray
D — Containers being evaluated
E — Fan system
F — Air sampling line
G — Vacuum guage
H — Bacterial retentive filter
I — Pressure gauge
J — Pressure/vacuum vessel

The microbial aerosol cloud must maintain viability during the course of the study. Certain microorganisms may exhibit die-off at various relative humidity ranges. Proper relative humidity may have to be maintained in the chamber during the study. Also certain microorganisms may be selected that are not readily dessicated in the test system. The mean diameter of the aerosolized particle should approach submicron conditions to assure that the microbial cloud will remain suspended. At the initiation of aerosolization, droplet nuclei may form that result in droplet impingement on the surfaces of the vessel and the surfaces of the container system. It facilitates evaluation if the containers of the closure system being evaluated contain sterile culture media. Care should be taken to assure that microorganisms that are impacted on surfaces during the test are not subjected to excessive drying. This may be accomplished by the use of an agar layer on surfaces or premoistened surfaces containing broth or another suitable diluent such as glycerol. During the aerobiology test, various pressure dynamics may be used to simulate various pressure altitude conditions encountered in a non-pressurized aircraft or trans-shipment through high altitudes.

Several excellent publications on this subject appeared in the 1960's (see literature citations). These references contain information describing various nebulizer systems as well as experimental designs for assessing generated aerosols with small particle size ranges.

D. Sterility testing

This is another microbial method to determine whether the closure has maintained the sterility of the container contents. Most parenteral industry technical personnel are aware of the statistical limitations associated with the sterility test (6). While the sterility test should not be relied upon during the design development of a closure system, there are situations whereby sterility testing may have applications after routine manufacturing of the closure system. Appropriate physical and functionality tests should be routinely incorporated to evaluate any possible effect of manufacturing or commodity changes upon integrity of the closure system. The values obtained from these physical evaluations should be consistent with the range of values obtained when the closure system design was finalized. Also prior to finalizing the closure design, appropriate microbiological tests as previously described may have been employed to demonstrate closure integrity. Knowing that closure integrity evaluation has occurred using a combination of physical and microbiological evaluation methods, sterility testing may continue to be used as a lot release test. Also during the shelf-life it should be ascertained whether the container/closure system maintains the contents of the container sterile. If initial closure design studies have proven that the closure maintains the contents of the container sterile, and subsequent physical testing demonstrates closure integrity during the product shelf life, sterility testing of the container contents following expiry may be considered an additional evaluation to further supplement the associated physical testing data and the successful historical actual use record of the product.

6. Shelf-Life Stability

During the design of a container/closure system, it must be considered whether the closure will maintain sterility during the shelf life of the product. While the manufacturer can design studies to evaluate shelf life conditions at various durations or time intervals following manufacturing, such studies are not designed to include misuse or abuse during storage by the customer. In recent years the subject of appropriate shelf life storage studies have been the subject of discussion and deliberation within the pharmaceutical industry.

The central issue of the discussion has involved whether physical or biological testing are appropriate for testing closures at product expiry. Proponents of physical tests believe the physical evaluations of the closure system will determine whether or not microbial ingress will occur. Others believe that the microbial integrity is a biological issue and the only appropriate manner to determine whether microbial ingress will occur is to use a microbial challenge. Rather than present the varying viewpoints associated with the merits and disadvantages of physical and biological testing, a model testing system is presented for consideration.

Prior to introduction to a new container/closure system, the proposed container should be evaluated for integrity by a combination of physical measurements and tests. Also, various microbiological studies should be conducted to ascertain that the closure system will not permit an ingress of microorganisms. Immediately following manufacturing, designated as t_0 time, a combination of physical tests should be conducted. These tests may include analysis of glass container defects such as cracks or splits through the glass wall, stopper dimensions, stopper defects such as splits, tears, or non-filling in the sealing contact surface, overcap seal strengths, and general material identification.

Concomitant with the physical testing at t_0, microbiological tests may be conducted, including any one of the previously described tests based on the end usage of the container. The t_0 physical data information will be maintained as baseline data to be compared to the testing that occurs following shelf life storage for a defined period. Rather than wait for prolonged storage conditions to occur, samples of the containers may be placed on accelerated stability stations using a combination of high temperature and short time durations. Following storage under accelerated conditions, the container and closure systems may be subjected to either physical and/or microbiological tests. Testing of accelerated aged samples should not be totally substituted for evaluation of container/closures at expiry to assure maintenance of closure integrity during the label claim duration of storage.

Testing of the container and closure at expiry primarily may involve the use of physical tests to establish whether the performance and physical tests initially conducted on t_0 samples can be reproduced on testing aged samples. If the t_0 and aged sample physical test data demonstrate equivalent results relative to closure integrity then microbiological methods become optional. If physical characteristics or testing results from aged or expiry samples have appreciably changed since the t_0 testing time, microbiological testing is advisable. For example if closure systems change due to ultraviolet effects generated by fluorescent lighting or sunlight, the closures may have experienced some degradation due to oxidative effects. The question becomes one of whether the closure still maintains the sterility of the container contents. Tests similar to those conducted at t_0 time should then be repeated.

Tests that most closely represent conditions that might be encountered in storage should be considered to evaluate product at expiry.

An example of microbiological evaluation that represents storage conditions would be to place culture media in the container and store the container under shelf life conditions. Appropriate control samples would have to be included to permit periodic analysis of the culture media for microbial growth support or bacteriostasis testing. This method is somewhat subject to challenge because the microenvironment within the container may not be sufficiently aerated to permit the growth of obligate aerobic microorganisms that may have ingressed into the container. Even though the statistical validity of conducting a sterility test on a limited sample size is questionable, the sterility test of products stored for a prolonged period may permit the determination of gross recontamination of the closure system. Also, during shelf life storage studies the influence of the container solution upon the stopper should be considered. Certain solutions with solvent vehicles may influence the physical and functionality features of the closure. Chemical stability analysis of the container solution following prolonged aging may indirectly determine whether serious closure degradation has occurred.

Various strategies that may be considered when conducting shelf-life evaluations of closure systems are presented in Table III.

Table III — A Proposed Scenario for Shelf-Life or Aged Product Testing

Microbiological testing options might include, immersion testing, long term media fill and storage, sterility testing, or any test that is germane for the specific product and its associated manufacturing and usage conditions. Physical testing options could include vacuum leak test, pressure hold test, dye immersion testing, and/or resealability evaluation.

1. T_0 time microbiological test correlated to a t_0 time physical test(s); t_{AGED} time physical test conducted, no microbiological test required if t_0 and t_{AGED} physical testing values from t_0 and t_{AGED} samples are equivalent.

2. T_0 time physical test; t_0 time and t_{AGED} time microbiological tests conducted independently of, and without correlation to physical testing results.

---

7. Monitoring Aseptic Filling Operations

During aseptic processing in which container components are sterilized as separate entities prior to filling, the integrity of the closure system is related to the basic design and associated sealing characteristics of the closure, and the process reliability of the aseptic processing manufacturing line.

Maintenance of the integrity of aseptically assembled closures is not assured simply by conducting various post processing tests. It is extremely important to control the manufacturing environment during processing.

Other means to assure that the container and closure system is initially sterile is process validation of the filling line. In 1979 a survey of the industry (7) indicated that a wide disparity existed both in the number of samples used in product media fills, and the acceptance level. Since that time, the industry has progressed to the point whereby at least 3,000 units per media run are used to permit a 95% confidence level in the resulting data (8).

An on-going or routine microbiological monitoring program should exist to assess the microbial count associated with various manufacturing areas and components. Microbial and particulate air monitoring should be conducted in various manufacturing areas near to the product filling and assembly areas. While monitoring near product fill and container capping areas is of particular importance, consideration should be given to obtaining data in the overall aseptic processing area to obtain a data base relative to typical average microbial load, and potential seasonal variation associated with microbial count. Defined action level limits should exist for surface and air counts taken in various areas and a program should exist for taking corrective action in the event the defined action level is exceeded. A detailed description of an environmental control program has been presented elsewhere (9). The important factor is that a microbiological environment provides an index or profile of microbial intrusions into the aseptic filling operation. Microbial intrusions may be related to particular manufacturing events or procedural changes. Cross matching events to periods when microbial counts are high could in fact permit corrective action to be taken to reduce the possibility of similar events occurring in the future.

8. References

1. Aspects of Container/Closure Integrity. Technical Information Bulletin No. 4. Parenteral Drug Association, Philadelphia, Pennsylvania, 1983.

2. Sterility Tests. United States Pharmacopeia XXI, page 1156, Pharmacopeial Convention, Inc., 1985.

3. Demmeck, R. L., and M. T. Hatch, 1969. Dynamic Aerosols and Dynamic Aerosol Chambers, In, Introduction To Experimental Aerobiology, Semmeck and Ackers (Ed.), Interscience, Chapter 9, page 177-193.

4. Porter, F. E., Crider, W. L., Mitchell, R. I., and Margard, W. L., 1963. The Dynamic Behavior of Aerosols, Ann. N. Y. Acad. Sci., 105 (Art. 2): 45-87.

5. Green, L. H. and Green, G. M., 1968. Direct Method for Determining the Viability of a Freshly Generated Mixed Bacterial Aerosol, Applied Microbiol., 16:78-81.

6. Bowman, F. W., 1972. Sterility Testing, in, Industrial Sterilization, G. B. Phillips and W. S. Miller (Eds), Duke University Press, page 35-47.

7. Korczynski, M. S., 1979. Validation of Aseptic Process by Media Fill—Survey Report and Discussion, in, Proceedings of the Second PMA Seminar Program on Validation of Sterile Manufacturing Processes: Aseptic Processing, page 186-213. Pharmaceutical Manufacturers Association, Washington, D.C.

8. Technical Monograph No. 2, Validation of Aseptic Filling for Solution Drug Products. Parenteral Drug Association, Inc., Philadelphia, Pa., 1980.

9. Korczynski, M. S., Peterson C. L. and Schawel, K., 1975. An Approach to Establishing Parenteral Solution Sterilization Cycles, Parenter. Drug Assoc. Bull, 290:146-152.

Supplemental Reading

a. Medical Device Sterilization Monographs Microbiological Methods for Assessment of Package Integrity, Report No. 78-4.11, Health Industry Manufacturers
Association, 1030 Fifteenth Street, N.W., Washington, D.C. 20005, June 1979.

   This monograph reviews various methods associated with evaluation
of different types of disposable device packaging materials. Typical microorganism used in such challenges are discussed. Various tests for evaluating
single sheets of materials are included. Methods describing the use of a multi-
sample chamber, evaluation followed by a aerosolization of a microbial liquid
or talc is described. Several key references related to aerobiology are included.

b. Aseptic of Container/Closure Integrity—Technical Information Bulletin No.
4, Parenteral Drug Association, Inc., 1983.

   This bulletin primarily contains a summary or overview of physical
methods to determine closure integrity. These methods include vacuum retention, vacuum chamber, internal pressure, dye immersion and seal force testing. Limited information is presented concerning microbiological evaluation,
although four categories of tests are included; (a) static-aerosol challenge, (b)
static-immersion challenge, (c) static-ambient challenge, and (d) dynamic-
immersion challenge.

c. John T. Connor, In-Process Verification of Closure Seal Integrity, J. Paren. Sci.,
37:14-19, 1983.

   A device coupled to a vial capping machine is described that determines the total force required to crimp a cap onto a vial and simultaneously
determines closure integrity. The device is called a Seal Force Monitor. A force
transducer is used to measure varying forces during capping. The applied force
is sensed as a voltage variation and stored in electronic memory.

d. Ronald Lee Nedich, Selection of Containers and Closure Systems for Injectable Products, Am. J. Hosp. Pharm., 40:1924-7.

   Various formulations and characteristics of containers and closures
are discussed. Evaluations which are frequently used to determine which components are selected include functional evaluations, physiochemical screening, and biologic screening tests.

9

Blow/Fill/Seal Aseptic Packaging Technology

Frank Leo
Automatic Liquid Packaging, Woodstock, IL, USA

1. Introduction

Sterile plastic packaging has gained wide acceptance by the pharmaceutical industry during the past ten years. The logical extension of pre-made plastic packages was the form/fill/seal technology for aseptic strip packaging of sterile medicinal products. More recently, the industry has begun adopting the blow/fill/seal system where container production is an integral part of the packaging operation in which there is an uninterrupted sequence of aseptic steps conducted in an unbroken sterile environment.

Historically, much of the technical challenge as well as the cost of manufacturing solution medications can be traced to the processes required to prepare sterile containers and closure systems. Ironically, a great proportion of these strenuous and costly efforts have been directed toward bringing a container back to the state of cleanliness and sterility that existed at the moment it was originally molded or formed, but which was lost quickly because of handling, processing, transporting and storage.

The concept underlying blow/fill/seal technology is that the packager of pharmaceutical products can maintain and take advantage of that original cleanliness by combining the processes of container and seal fabrication with those of filling and sealing the container.

The focus of this discussion is blow/fill/seal technology for production of sterile-liquid packaged pharmaceuticals. Illustrations and descriptions are based on the proprietary technology developed by Automatic Liquid Packaging, Inc. (ALP), but it should be noted that the principles of aseptic processing and maintenance of a sterile environment are generic, applicable to the development or evaluation of any such closed-environment, closed-circuit packaging system. (See Figure 4 for a typical blow/fill/seal apparatus.)

A. Development of blow/fill/seal technology

Early applications for form/fill/seal pharmaceutical packaging in the United States were based for the most part on flexible pouch technology and systems.

Figure 1—Different forms of sterile packaging possible from blow/fill/seal packaging systems. *Courtesy of Automated Liquid Packaging, Inc.*

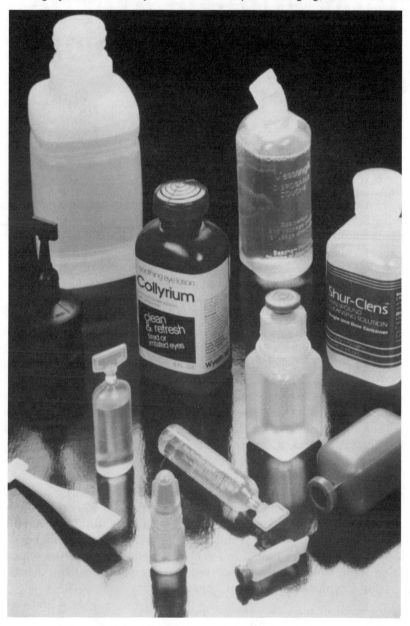

Sterile-environment adaptations of flexible strip packaging techniques developed to meet the needs of non-sterile product packaging were created to meet the growing hospital demand for unit-dose oral medications. Transparent film and opaque foil strip packages were created to individualize unit dose medication, at the same time preserving product integrity and identity from manufacturer to bedside.

Figure 2—Different forms of sterile packaging possible from blow/fill/seal packaging systems. *Courtesy of Automated Liquid Packaging, Inc.*

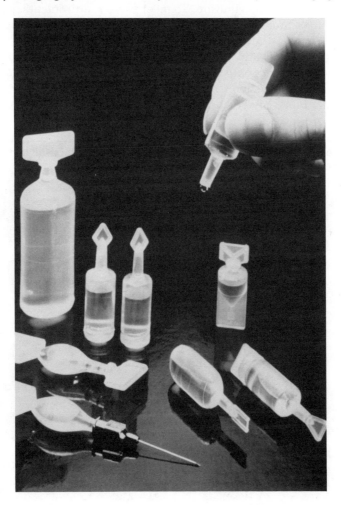

Along with the need for product integrity and the perceived advantages of unit-dose packaging, the medical profession, hospitals in particular, were concerned with the control of rapidly escalating costs. Had the pharmaceutical industry been forced to utilize conventional premade containers rather than form/fill/seal packaging technology, the cost of medications would have risen dramatically. The adoption of form/fill/seal technology made possible the delivery of product in unit-dose containers at a reasonable cost.

There was parallel development in continental Europe, although originally propelled by long-standing social laws in many European nations, some dating to the early 1930s, that required production of unit-dose (or prescription-size) packages for retail distribution. To meet these requirements, pharmaceutical manufacturers produced small-quantity trade units using relatively expensive containers made of aluminum, steel, glass and rigid plastic.

During the 1950s and 1960s, mass-produced blister packaging for unit-dose oral medications came into being to meet demands for product-dosage delivery at reasonable cost. The more recent adoption of blow/fill/seal technology has made it possible to satisfy requirements even more economically.

Figure 3 – DIfferent forms of sterile packaging possible from blow/fill/seal packaging systems. *Courtesy of Automated Liquid Packaging, Inc.*

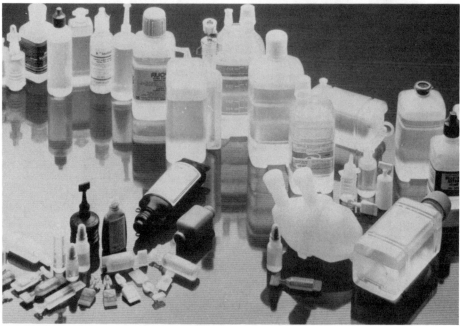

B. Definitions

The term blow/fill/seal in this context refers to the technology and related equipment and procedures in which the formation of the container, its filling with liquid pharmaceutical material, and the subsequent formation and application of a seal for the container are achieved aseptically in an uninterrupted sequence of operations without exposure to nonsterile environments between operations. (See Figures 1 through 3 for examples of the types of packages that can be produced by the blow/fill/seal method.)

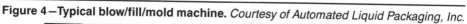

Figure 4—Typical blow/fill/mold machine. *Courtesy of Automated Liquid Packaging, Inc.*

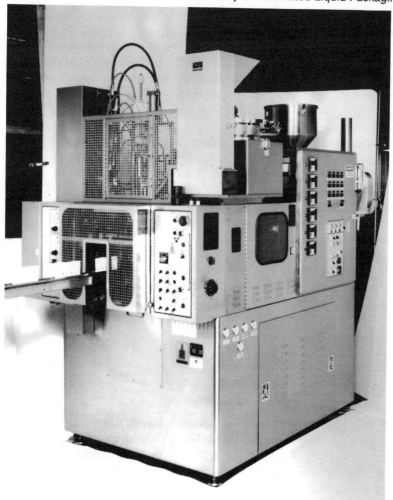

2. Regulatory Considerations (Conventional Aseptic Processing)

Familiarity with the currently proposed FDA guidelines for aseptic processing as applied to conventional aseptic processing is required in order to consider the differences between blow/fill/seal aseptic packaging technology and conventional technology. The draft document of the proposed FDA guidelines was published to help pharmaceutical producers meet current good manufacturing practice (CGMP) for drug products according to the requirements of Title 21 Code of Federal Regulations (21CFR), Parts 210 and 211, and for CGMP as related to biological products regulated under 21CFR Parts 600 through 680. (See "Sterile Drug Products Produced by Aseptic Processing," Federal Register, February 1, 1985).

A. Aseptic processing

The FDA guidelines describe aseptic processing as a procedure in which the drug product, container and closure are subjected to sterilization processes separately, then brought together. Because there is no further processing to sterilize the product after it is in its final container, it is critical for the maintenance of product sterility that the containers be filled and sealed in an environment of high quality.

In aseptic processing, as defined by the FDA, there are more variables than for terminal sterilization, making it more difficult to attain a high degree of assurance that the end product will be sterile. The potential for error is greater for aseptic processing than for terminal sterilization in which there is but a single sterilization step at the end of the packaging procedure.

In contrast, before aseptic assembly, different parts of the final product may have been subjected to different sterilization processes, such as dry heat for glass containers, steam under pressure for rubber closures, and filtration for a liquid dosage form. Each requires thorough validation and control. Each has the possibility of error. Furthermore, any manipulation of the sterilized dosage form, containers and closures immediately prior to aseptic assembly involves the risk of contamination; therefore each must be carefully controlled.

As we review the FDA Guidelines, it will become quite evident that this document was prepared for conventional sterile-fill operations. In review, specific comparisons are made between blow/fill/seal and conventional sterile fill, and the ability of the blow/fill/seal process to circumvent conventional operational pitfalls.

B. Environment control

Section 211.42 of 21CFR requires, among other things, a separate or defined area of operation to prevent contamination. Where there is aseptic processing, this section requires that where appropriate the air supply is to be filtered through high-efficiency particulate air (HEPA) filters under positive pressure.

Section 211.46 requires, where appropriate, that there be provision for equipment to control air pressure, microorganisms, dust, humidity and temperature. It also requires that air filters, including prefilters and particulate matter air filters, be used on air supplies to production areas when appropriate.

C. Area separation and control

Two areas of particular importance requiring separation and control in aseptic processing and in which different degrees of air quality are required for each area, according to the FDA guidelines, include the aseptic core area and the preparation area.

i. Aseptic Core Area

The area in which the sterilized dosage form, containers and closures are exposed to the environment is cited as the most critical area. Activities include manipulations of sterilized materials and product prior to and during the filling/sealing operations. This area is called the "aseptic processing" area.

This area is critical because after it, there is no further processing of produce in its immediate container, making the container vulnerable to contamination. The environment here must be of the highest quality.

Particles must be eliminated. When they enter a product, they can either contaminate it physically or serve as vehicles for microorganisms. Air in proximity to exposed sterilized containers/closures and filling/sealing operations is acceptable if its particle count is no greater than 100 (size range of 0.5 micron and larger, i.e., Class 100) per cubic foot when measured one foot above the work site during filling/sealing operations.

The air should also have incidence of no more than one viable organism per 10 cubic feet. Other gases, e.g., nitrogen or carbon dioxide, in proximity to filling/sealing operations should meet the same standards. Additionally, compressed air should be free from demonstrable oil vapors. These areas should have a positive pressure of at least 0.05 inches of water relative to adjacent less-clean areas.

ii. Preparation Area

The second area where it is important to control the environment is that in which unsterilized product, in-process materials, and container/closures are prepared,e.g., where components are weighed and mixed, and where components, in-process materials, drug products and the drug product contact surfaces of equipment, containers and closures (after final rinse of such surfaces) are exposed to the plant environment.

Air and other gases here are generally acceptable with a particulate count of no more than 100,000 (size range of 0.5 micron and larger, e.g., Class 100,000) per cubic foot. This quality is maintained by sufficient air flow and positive pressure differentials.

D. Containers and closures

Section 211.94 "Drug Product Containers and Closures" of 21CFR, requires that containers and closures be clean, sterilized and depyrogenated. For aseptic processing, preparation of the containers and closures must be more than mere cleaning to remove surface debris. Both containers and closures must be sterile and, in the case of some products, non-progenic.

The FDA guidelines note that any properly validated process is acceptable, with the following aspects being of particular importance.

i. Pre-Sterilization

Pre-sterilization of glass containers involves a series of wash and rinse cycles to remove debris. Final rinse water must be of high quality, e.g., meet the requirements of USP Water For Injection. Depyrogenation may be accomplished by initial washings with caustic soda followed by rinses with Water For Injection. Dry heat may be used to sterilize and dypyrogenate glass containers, as well as for sterilization of equipment used in fluid handling and filling.

ii. Depyrogenation

Plastic containers, especially if washed with water, may be a source of pyrogens. They may be sterilized with ethylene oxide gas, but there may be potential for residues of ethylene oxide and ethylene oxide degradation products to remain on the container surfaces.

iii. Rubber Stoppers

Rubber-compound stoppers are another potential source of microbial and pyrogen contamination. They are usually cleaned by multiple cycles of washing, rinsing and leaching, prior to a final steam sterilization. The final rinse should be with USP injection-grade water.

E. Time limitations

Section 211.111 of 21 CFR deals with the time limitations of production. The FDA guidelines point out the requirement of establishing a time limit for the completion of each phase of production to assure the quality of the drug product. That is, a limit of total time for product filtration and filling operations to prevent contamination of filtrate by microorganisms growing through the filter over a period of time.

F. Aseptic assembly validation

This same set of FDA draft guidelines describes the "sterile media fill" approach to validation of aseptic assembly processes. This method uses microbiological growth nutrient media in the simulation of sterile product filling operations.

The nutrient media should be manipulated and exposed to the operators, equipment, surfaces, and environmental conditions to closely simulate the same exposure that the product itself will undergo. Following exposure, the sealed media-filled containers are incubated to detect microbiological growth.

Three separate runs are generally required as a minimum control. At least 3,000 units are recommended to determine, with a 95% probability, a contamination rate of one in one thousand. The frequency of revalidation will depend on factors such as facility and equipment modification, personnel changes, and testing anomalies. A generally acceptable revalidation-run frequency is at least twice yearly for each personnel shift applied to each filling/sealing line.

The FDA considers this guideline to be a priority because of the frequency of compliance problems in aseptic processing. The agency notes a high degree of industry unfamiliarity with FDA expectations for aseptic procedures, and a lack of uniformity in sterile manufacturing processes between firms.

While the guideline states "principles and practices" generally acceptable to the FDA, "not legal requirements," the ultimate result may be to require that firms rewrite procedures or establish monitoring programs to meet FDA standards.

3. General Equipment Design

There are no formal regulatory codes for the design of aseptic processing equipment. There are, however, well-established principles which should be observed.

A. Ease of cleaning

It must be possible to maintain the equipment in a sanitary condition, either by in-place cleaning or through ease of dismantling for manual cleaning, as the initial sterilzation cycle is based on the use of "clean" equipment.

B. Initial sterilization

Equipment must be able to withstand the temperatures and pressures necessary for initial sterilization. Equipment should be free of cracks and crevices that might not be contacted by the sterilizing media.

Sterilization temperatures may reach 300°F, with consequent metal expansion. Gaskets and seals must withstand these elevated temperatures. The pressure of 300°F steam is 52 psig, for which the equipment must be designed. Moving parts must be arranged to allow for both initial sterilization and maintenance of the sterile condition.

C. Sterility maintenance

The equipment should be closed or positively sealed to maintain its sterile condition during operations. Product zones should be under positive pressure to prevent contamination from surrounding environments.

After sterilization at 300°F, operating temperatures may drop to 50°F, creating a sequence of expansions and contractions, with changes of clearances between parts.

D. Proficient operation

Equipment must operate efficiently and economically, and should be designed for ease of maintenance. Operating costs should be reasonable, including power requirements, time to clean and maintain the unit, and other operations. Design should simplify routine preventive maintenance.

E. Cleaning

Design should allow for effective in-place cleaning and sterilization, mandatory considerations for sterile equipment used in aseptic processing. Design must also consider the corrosive and erosive effects of chemicals and sanitizers used for cleaning, with particular attention to seal and gasket materials. Interior surfaces should be nonporous so as to resist entrapment of contaminating particles.

F. Safety

Equipment design should conform to existing safety codes, as well as accepted safe practice. While there are no codes specific for aseptic processing equipment and systems, other industry codes and standards can be adapted as guidelines for good engineering practice.

4. Design of Aseptic Systems

There are numerous ways to organize and equip an aseptic processing system. In most cases, there will be one system that is optimum for the handling of a particular product.

Regardless of the system, sterile packaged product is the major design concern. The physical characteristics of the product must also be considered, including factors such as viscosity, heat sensitivity, and volatility.

The physical and chemical stabilities of the product are important during and immediately after processing, as well as during storage. Product end use, formulation and more must be kept in mind when designing the total processing system.

5. Technology of Bottle Pack Blow/Fill/Seal Packaging

It is with blow/fill/seal packaging that the producer has packaging size and style flexibility along with the economic advantages of process integration and sterile product that is relatively free from particulates. In the following description of the ALP method for blow/fill/seal packaging of sterile pharmaceutical products, it will be shown not only how the technology works, but how it both meets and overcomes problems inherent in ordinary aseptic-process packaging as covered by the FDA guidelines for 21CFR.

A. Process overview

In the blow/fill/seal aseptic packaging system, plastic containers are manufactured from a thermoplastic granulate, filled, and sealed in the same automatic machine without the need to move the container from place to place. Chief materials for the containers are high-, medium- and low-density polyethylene, as well as various blends of polypropylene and polyallomers.

In operation, a plastic tube is extruded from melted granulate (see Figures 5 and 6). Then, by a plastic-forming process called blow-molding, compressed air is blown into the tube, pushing out the warm plastic walls until they conform to the shape of a surrounding mold. A mandrel unit then adds a metered amount of product liquid into the container. The mandrel is then raised vertically, and the top dies of the mold weld the upper part of the plastic container to form an impervious seal. At this point, the mold opens, and the finished, filled container is removed. The total production cycle from start to finish is about 9 to 19 seconds, depending on container size and complexity.

Figure 5—Plastic granulate is melted, then converted into a continuous plastic tube by extrusion.

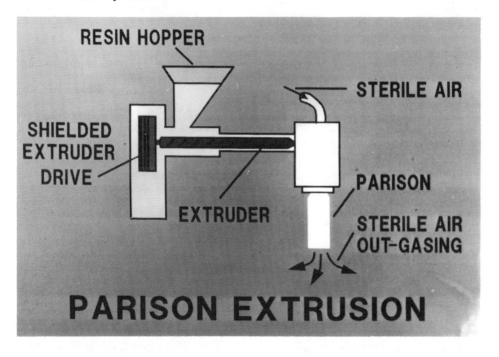

B. Polyolefin packaging grades
Manufacturers of polyolefin materials produce special grades to use for pharmaceutical packaging. These are nontoxic, odorless and tasteless, and therefore physiologically safe. However, before these materials can be used for pharmaceutical packaging, there must be documented confirmation on record of their physiological safety; namely, they must conform to United State Pharmacopeia (USP XXI) Sec. 661, Physical Tests: Plastics.

Only these types of plastics are used in pharmaceutical operations. They account for the familiar plastic containers that are used as packages for infu-

Figure 6 — Cutaway showing the sections of the mold in which the extruded tube will be shaped into the final container and seal.

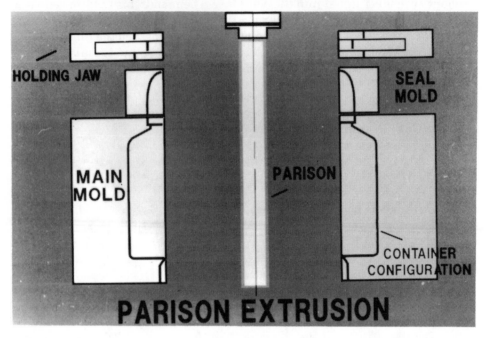

sions, injections, enemas, eye, ear, and nose drops, and other pharmaceutical specialties.

C. Sterilization of the plastic container

The significant contribution of a blow/fill/seal aseptic packaging system is that production and distribution of pharmaceutical materials with complete sterility is possible during the extrusion, forming, filling and sealing operations. The single-apparatus approach in which the container is aseptically filled immediately after it is blow-mold formed, circumvents the contamination hazards inherent with conventional sterile fill when packaging containers are moved from place to place, submitted to washing, blown out, steamed, irradiated, and more, prior to the filling and sealing operations.

The extrusion process itself is at temperatures of 170°C to 230°C, with holdup times of several minutes at pressures of up to 350 atmospheres gauge. This melts and heat treats the plastic granulate to produce a sterile extruded tube of plastic material in a warm, thermoplastic state, from which the sterile packaging container is formed.

This fact was confirmed by test series conducted for ALP by Geneva Laboratories of Elkhorn, Wisconsin. The final packaged media sterility was confirmed for each test series, where the starting raw resin granulate was inoculated with bacterial growth spores. The tests were made using an ALP Blow/Fill/Seal Machine No. 301-181 and associated equipment, with validation by Geneva Laboratories.

i. Bacterial Inoculation of Resin

The "challenge" inoculum was a certified spore suspension of *Bacillus subtilis (globigii)*. The raw resin granulate (Alathon 20)™ was inoculated to a CFU (Colony Forming Unit) level of approximately 106/pound of resin. The media fill used for the test was trypticase soy broth (soy casein digest media USP). This media was steam sterilized, and, with the inoculated resin, transported to the ALP facility in Woodstock, Illinois.

The growth media was transferred to the bulk mixing tank, and the inoculated resin was poured into the extruder hopper. The media fill operation (blow/fill/seal) proceeded for about two hours. The media-filled containers were returned to Geneva Laboratories where they were incubated. Complete macroscopic readings were taken at the end of 7 and 14 days of incubation.

Final analysis showed that of the 638 containers incubated and assayed, only one was contaminated. The content of this container was Gram stained to determine its Gram and morphological characteristics, which were shown to be dissilimar to the resin inoculum organism, *B. subtilis*.

Details of this test are given in Table I.

ii. Endotoxin Inoculation of Resin

In a "challenge" similar to the bacterial-inoculation test, three separate samples of Alathon 20 resin were inoculated with *E. coli*-derived endotoxin in concentrations of 75,000 Endotoxin Units (EUs), 150,000 EUs, and 300,000 EUs, respectively. The inoculated resin was delivered to the ALP facility where it was used to extrude (blow/fill/seal) containers filled with purified water.

The filled containers were returned to Geneva Laboratories where they were agitated on an orbiting shaker, then opened and the contents submitted to LAL (*Limulus* Amebocyte Lysate) testing. No evidence of endotoxin was found in any of the 15 containers tested. Verifiable endotoxin reduction was on the order of 300 times.

Details of this test are given in Table II.

iii. Test Conclusions

Based on these tests, it can be seen that the single process of extrusion which is used on the blow/fill/seal machine eliminates the risk associated with container handling, storage, cleaning, sterilizing, and depyrogenating; i.e., one process handles all.

Table I—Methodology of *B. subtilis* bacterial challenge to the ALP Bottle Pack Blow/Fill/Seal Aseptic System

Objective: To determine the efficacy of the aseptic filling processes of the Bottle Pack Machine when challenged with an inoculated plastic resin and bacterial growth media.

Equipment: ALP Bottle Pack Machine No. 301-181 and associated equipment.

Testing Laboratory: Geneva Laboratories, Inc., Elkhorn, Wisconsin

*Procedure:*The systems challenge was divided into three sections:

1. *Preparation of Inoculated Resin*
1.1 Certified spore suspension of *Bacillus subtilis (globigii)* chosen as challenge inoculum.
1.2 Using direct recovery study, the exact CFU population of the inoculum vial was determined to be 5.4×10^6 CFU per 0.1 ml. of inoculum.
1.3 Forty pounds of plastic resin (Alathon 20) was inoculated at 1.3×10^6 CFU per pound of resin.
1.4 Working bioburden level determined by direct recovery of spores from a half-pound sample.

2. *Aseptic Media Fill*
2.1 Two 20-liter containers of trypticase soy broth were prepared from Gibco certified dehydrated powder concentrate.
2.2 The prepared (but not sterilized) media was filtered within six hours of preparation.
2.3 Sample tubes were drawn from the filtered media for growth studies to validate the trypticase soy broth lot.
2.4 The media and sample tubes were sterilized together by steam sterilization.
2.5 The two 20-liter containers of media and inoculated resin were transported to the ALP plant at Woodstock, Illinois.
2.6 Just prior to machine startup, the growth media was transferred to the bulk mixing tank, and the inoculated resin to the extruder hopper.
2.7 Media fill progressed for approximately two hours; bottles of media were boxed in consecutively numbered cases.

3. *Incubation and Evaluation*
3.1 Upon completion of the filling operation, the media-filled containers were transported to Geneva Laboratories.
3.2 A complete macroscopic reading of all containers was completed ate the end of seven days.
3.3 All cases were returned to their incubators to complete a full 14-day incubation period.
3.4 Final macroscopic readings were taken at the end of 14 days.
3.5 Containers from cases 1, 2, 17 and 18 were opened and media tested to assure that the product containers had not in-induced any bacteriostatic/fungistatic effects.
3.6 The average mass of an empty test bottle was determined, from which the inoculum challenge level per bottle was determined.

Test Results: Only one contaminated container was noted from among the 638 containers incubated and assayed for both seven- and 14-day incubations at 30-35°C. This sample was Gram stained to ascertain its Gram and morphological characteristics. It was determined to be dissimilar to the resin inoculum organism, *B. subtilis.*

Table II — Methodology of *E. coli* derived *limulus* (LAL) challenge to the ALP Bottle Pack Blow/Fill/Seal Aseptic System

Objective: To determine the efficacy of the aseptic filling processes of the Bottle Pack Machine when challenged with an endotoxin-inoculated plastic resin.

Equipment: ALP Bottle Pack Machine No. 301-181 and associated equipment.

Testing Laboratory: Geneva Laboratories Inc., Elkhorn, Wisconsin

Procedure: The systems challenge was divided into three sections:

1 *Preparation of Endotoxin-Inoculated Resin*

1.1 Freeze-dried vial of *E. coli*-derived endotoxin was reconstituted with 5.0mL LAL Reagent Water. The vial contained 125 micrograms lyophilized endotoxin.

1.2 Relative potency of the vial of endotoxin determined by standardizing it against U.S. Reference Standard Endotoxin (EC-5); determined as 625,000 EU (Endotoxin Units) total.

1.3 Three 10-pound portions of plastic resin (Alathon 20) accurately weighed on triple-beam balance.

1.4 The three resin portions were endotoxin inoculated; one at 75,000 EU, one at 150,000 EU, and one at 300,000 EU.

1.5 The resin pyroburden level was verified and calculated for 100-gram samples; portion #1 held 800 EU, portion #2 held 1,600 EU, and portion #3 held 3,200 EU.

2 *Fabrication of Bottles from Inoculated Resin*

2.1 Inoculated resin was transported to the ALP plant in Woodstock, Illinois.

2.2 The lease-potent endotoxin-inoculated resin was poured into the resin extruder hopper.

2.3 The machine then produced bottles filled with purified water (USP sterile water for injection or irrigation), continuing until all resin was used.

2.4 Steps 2.2 and 2.3 were repeated for the remaining two portions of endotoxin-inoculated resin.

2.5 Three cases of bottles, one from each portion of inoculated resin, were shipped to Geneva Laboratories.

3 *LAL Assay and Evaluation*

3.1 The three cases of bottles were thoroughly agitated on an orbiting shaker two hours at room temperature.

3.2 Five bottles from each case were selected at random, and weighed on a pan balance.

3.3 The outer surface of each bottle was scrubbed with an alcohol sponge and air-dried before sampling.

3.4 Each bottle was opened with depyrogenated scissors; samples were withdrawn for LAL testing with a Lysate of 0.25 EU/mL Label Sensitivity.

3.5 Appropriate positive and negative controls were included with the test samples.

3.6 The 15 test samples were covered to prevent gross contamination, and allowed to stand overnight at ambient temperature.

3.7 LAL testing was repeated one month later, but with a 0.06 EU/mL Label Sensitivity LAL, again with appropriate controls.

3.8 The 15 sample containers were emptied and dried. The mass of each bottle (compared to the weight in step 3.2) was used to calculate the endotoxin challenge level.

Test Results: No evidence of endotoxin was noticed in any of the samples tested with 0.25 EU/mL and 0.06 EU/mL *Limulus* Amebocyte Lysate. Verifiable endotoxin reduction was on the order of 300 times.

D. Suspended-matter control

It is essential to avoid the presence of suspended matter in plastic packaging materials. During the extrusion step of the blow/fill/seal system, a homogenous plastic mass is formed upon the melting of the individual grains of plastic granulate. It is here that foreign substances are inseparably trapped by the melt so that cannot migrate from the packaging material and into the liquid pharmaceutical product.

E. Sterile air supply

The packaging cycle begins with plastic granulate which, upon heating to 170°C to 230°C for extrusion, provides a sterile packaging material that is free of loose suspended matter. The natural goal of the remainder of the packaging cycle is to prevent contamination of this now sterile material.

In the process, an endless plastic tube is formed continuously from the plastic melt by extrusion through the parison. The final shaping of the plastic container is with compressed air. This means that to assure continued aseptic processing of sterile packages from start to finish, this forming air must not introduce reinfection. This in turn requires that all lines through which the compressed air passes must be sterile.

The compressed air is supplied by an oil-free compressor, and passes through the four purification stations incorporated in the ALP blow/fill/seal system:

    i.   A liquid separator eliminates high humidity and possible traces of oil.
    ii.   A pre-filter removes suspended matter with particle sizes greater than one micron.
    iii.   An activated charcoal absorber removes typical odor and taste components present in the compressed air.
    iv.   A sterile filter removes particles, microbes and their spores down to a particle size of 0.2 micron absolute.

The lines through which the compressed air must pass are sterilized in situ prior to production. Pyrogen-free clean steam at 30 to 40 psig and 250°F to 270°F is passed through these lines for at least 20 minutes. Condensate is blown out of the lines with sterile air, and the lines are cooled. This procedure prevents reinfections from the compressed air system leading from the four-stage compressed air processing section.

F. Extruded tube sterility

In the ALP blow/fill/seal system, an endless sterile plastic tube, open at the lower end is continuously extruded from the melted granulate (Figure 5). There is a theoretical possibility that microorganisms from surrounding ambient air might intrude into this tube under unfavorable conditions. Such intrusion is prevented, however, by a stream of sterile air that flows continuously downward through the tube while it is still in its open, unexpanded state (See Figure 7). In this case, the sterile air serves solely as support air to prevent the molten tube material from collapsing prior to final shaping.

Figure 7—Sterile air pressure inside the molten plastic tube forms it to conform with the inner dimensions of the container and seal mold.

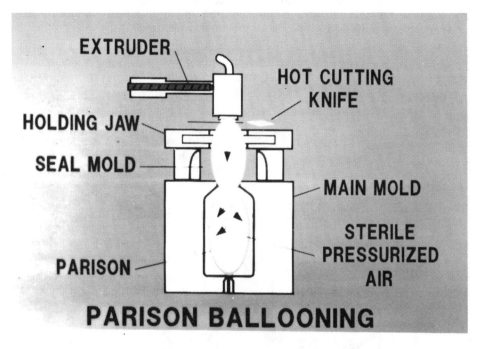

G. Plastic tube separation

As the extruded continuous plastic tube enters the filling cavity of the mold, the portion that is to become the container must be cut free from the upper end of the tube. Before the tube is cut, the pressure of the continuous flow of sterile air through the interior of the tube ensures that the warm plastic is held in firm contact with the vacuum holding jaws.

At this point, the bottom of the blow-mold cavity closes, welding closed what is to be the bottom of the container. This portion of the tube is then cut free by a knife heated to about 300°C to 400°C to ensure a sterile cut.

Once the tube is separated, there is a new problem that must be resolved to maintain sterility. The interior of the section of extruded tube that is in the blow mold is now open at the top where the vacuum holding jaws are located. At this time, since the tube is being extruded continuously, the blow-mold cavity must rotate away from the tube position to allow a repeat of this separation cycle for the next blow-mold cavity. The time required for the mold to move (by hydraulic means) to the container production (or blow-forming) station is about 0.3 to 0.6 seconds (see Figures 8 and 9).

Figure 8—As the mold chamber containing the partially formed container rotates, an outward flow of sterile air prevents contamination.

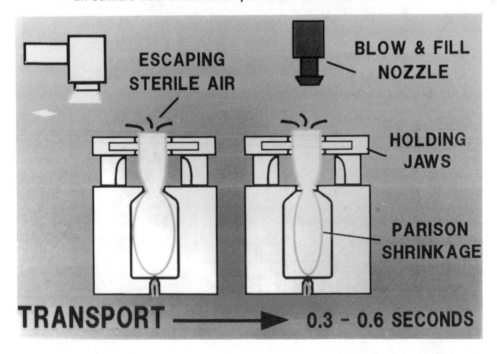

To prevent the plastic tube that is coming from the extruder from landing on top of the next blow-mold cavity, the extruder swings upward. After separation, the hot plastic tube through which cold, sterile air flowed prior to separation, is now merely filled with this sterile air. The tube begins to shrink in the mold as the pressure of the flowing air drops. From this shrinkage in tube volume, sterile air is displaced to the atmosphere, protecting the tube from contamination.

At the same time, the cold sterile air in the tube begins to warm, increasing the volume of air to create a slight excess pressure. This sequence of events makes it impossible for ambient, unsterile air to intrude, and is 100% effective in maintaining the sterility of the inner volume of the tube section while the mold is being moved.

Figure 9 — Mold chamber moves into position below the blow and fill nozzle.

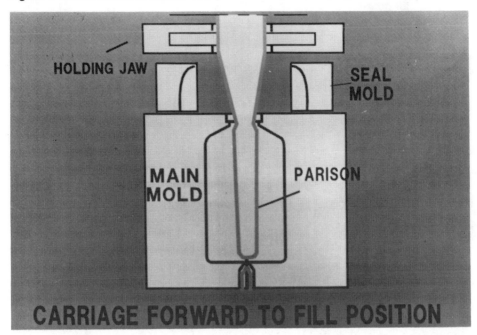

HOLDING JAW

SEAL MOLD

MAIN MOLD

PARISON

CARRIAGE FORWARD TO FILL POSITION

H. Shielding the blowing/filling mandrel

After the mold has been moved away from the tube-extrusion position and into the container-forming position, the combination blowing/filling mandrel is inserted into the upper end of the plastic tube in the body mold. This seals the still unmolded sterile plastic tube. At that time, incoming sterile compressed air inflates the plastic tube and forces it against the mold walls, shaping the container to its final form (see Figure 10).

The blowing/filling mandrel is sterilized in situ at 130°C without disassembly before production. During production, the fill system is bathed with continuous air flow supplied by HEPA filtered air, thus protecting it from contamination. Because of the equipment movement, laminar air flow conditions do not exist. However, the level of microbiological bioburden is maintained at 1 CFU (Colony Forming Unit) per 100 cu. ft., thus reducing or eliminating the risk of intrusion from nonsterile air. With the system, there is continuous purging of the mandrel by sterile air.

There are many methods of liquid sterilization which could interface with the ALP blow/fill/seal system. Each specific liquid product lends itself to the

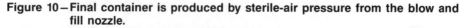

Figure 10—Final container is produced by sterile-air pressure from the blow and fill nozzle.

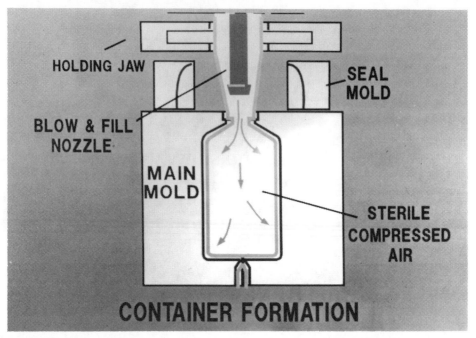

appropriate technique, based on its characteristics. Some examples are: submicron filtration; high-temperature, short-time continuous steam sterilization; and bulk thermal sterilization.

For discussion purposes, we will concentrate on submicron filtration, since it is the method most readily employed with blow/fill/seal technology.

I. Product liquid sterility

A filling system must maintain the product liquid in the sterile state in which it is delivered to the system, and it must provide protection against particulate matter intrusion. In principle, liquid product passes through a hermetically sealed filling system during the process of sterile filling.

After product liquid has passed through the sterile filter, it may not be allowed to come in contact with the atmosphere, not even that of a clean room. All lines downstream from the filter must also be sterilized each time production begins.

A simplified diagram of the solution paths inside an ALP blow/fill/seal aseptic packaging system is shown in Figure 11. It is at this point that the advantages become evident for a system in which the manufacture of the packag-

Figure 11—Simplified diagram of the solution paths inside an ALP blow/fill/seal aseptic packaging system.

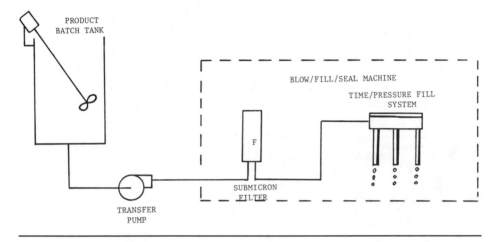

Figure 12—After the container is formed inside the mold, sterile liquid product is introduced into the container.

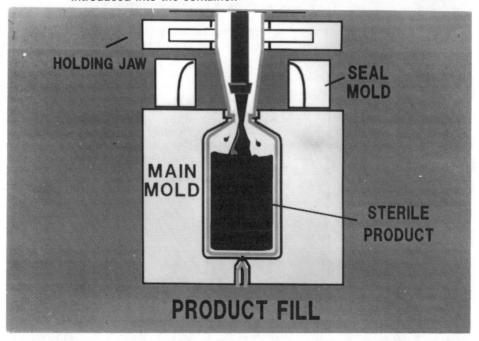

Figure 13—Filled container is sealed in place by the closing of the seal-mold form onto the container top.

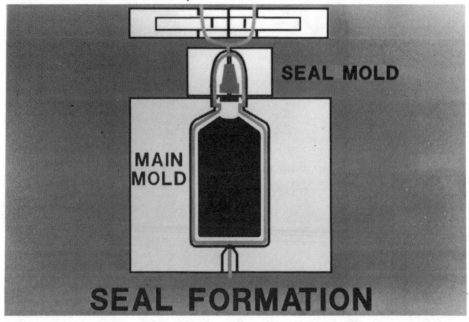

Figure 14—Upon completion of the filling and sealing steps, the mold is separated, producing the sterile filled and sealed container.

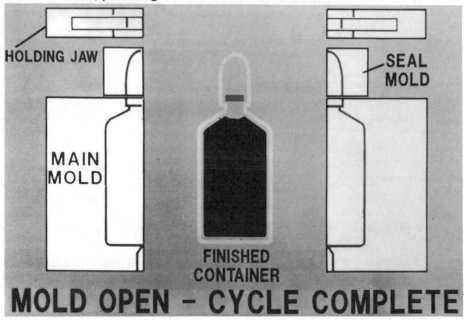

ing container and filling of the container are accomplished in the same location without need to transport an empty sterilzed container to the filling site (see Figures 12, 13, 14).

All of the sterilty-ensuring design measures pertaining to production of the container also apply to the blowing/filling mandrel. Filling lines are designed so that Clean-In-Place (CIP) cleaning is possible, without the need for disassembly at the completion of each batch.

After cleaning-in-place, steam sterilization is carried out for all product (solution) pathways. Before the start of the container filling, all filling lines are blown out with sterile air to avoid mixing of liquid product with residual condensate left in the lines after sterilization.

To ensure that sterility remains in effect throughout the entire production process, HEPA filtered air is supplied to the filling chamber at the blowing/filling station. Despite the fact that in practice there is virtually no chance that suspended matter could be taken up from the filling system, the ALP blow/fill/seal system provides a final filtration step just before the filling step. Sterile filters with retention values of 0.2 to 0.45 microns are installed upstream from the fill tube. These filters are sterilized along with the other components.

This final filtration ensures that particles possibly resulting from abrasion of metal parts in the filling equipment will be eliminated immediately prior to product entering the container.

J. Container-closure sterility

Container closure, as well as container formation and filling, is accomplished in the mold without the need to change the location of the container. The blowing/filling mandrel rises vertically to the upper rest position inside the sterile filling chamber. At that same moment, the mold dies close over the mold body (see Figure 13).

The result of the pressure exerted by the top dies is to weld shut the upper section of the parison. Because the plastic tube has been contact-free in an air cushion during container production and filling, the loss of heat is so slight that thermoplastic deformation and welding are possible without the need for additional heat.

With the lifting of the blowing/filling mandrel, shielding against contamination is again provided by HEPA air filter. In addition, the volume in the upper section of the tube is reduced when the top dies close so that the sterile air above the contents is forced outward. The resulting volume reduction leads to an outflowing bell of sterile air above the upper end of the tube, which lasts until the tube is completely welded shut.

After the top has been sealed, it is molded to the final shape. Because the tube section in the top die is still hot, it can be thermoplastically formed from a vacuum acting at the top die. Thus it is possible not only to squeeze-weld the top, but also to mold a press-on or screw-on top closure of the desired shape and design (see Figure 14).

In conclusion, the maintenance of sterility utilizing the blow/fill/seal method can be represented best through media-fill results obtained by ALP. Media fills have been conducted over the course of eight years under a number of different operating parameters. These operating parameters included:

i.   Normal production startup, moving directly into media-fill validation
ii. Media-fill validation after one full week of production
iii. Media fills without HEPA filtered air
iv. Numerous container designs and sizes.

Statistical evaluation of the results of eight years of media-fill evaluations, shown below, demonstrate that the blow/fill/seal system is successful in meeting and maintaining adequate conditions, as outlined by the FDA for sterile filling:

Total number of media runs 106
Total units filled 398,486
Total units contaminated 16
Percent failure rate 0.004%

7. Looking to the Future

The blow/fill/seal technology for sterile packaging of pharmaceuticals of all kinds, particularly for unit-dose parenterals, ophthalmics, and products, has already proven itself in numerous applications.

Blow/fill/seal technology was first developed in West Germany. More recently, the original patents have expired and ALP has moved to enhance the technology with its own proprietary modifications. Overall, blow/fill/seal technology has found widespread application in both Europe and the United States. Hundreds of such systems are now being used to produce a wide variety of products, ranging from small ophthalmic droppers to various configured solution containers. Early applications in the United States include such sterile products as:

- Nebulizing solutions
- Respiratory therapy products
- Eyewash preparations
- Veterinary injectable packages
- Diagnostic Reagents
- Injectable Diluents

Blow/fill/seal packaging has been proven to be a viable way to achieve highly specialized sterile product delivery goals within reasonable economic boundaries. As health-care costs face further downward pressures from both the public and lawmakers, and as the need for ever more stringent sterile standards develops, the sterile-packaging advantages of blow/fill/seal technology will become more visible for a greater variety of medical-product packaging applications.

10

Isolator Technology for Manufacturing and Quality Control

Patrick Oles with Bernard St. Martin, Jean Teillon,
Didier Meyer, and Claude Picard, la Calhene, Goshen, NY, USA

1. The Role of Isolation Technology for Aseptic Processing

Sophisticated technologies are essential to guarantee the production of pharmaceutical products that have been protected from biological contaminants, particularly in the case of very active products. This is especially true where, in the event of deterioration, these products are capable of causing toxicities. Thus, medical authorities in numerous nations are favoring increasingly rigid controls in the manufacture of pharmaceuticals.

As an alternative to total reliance on final sterility analyses, these controls are becoming the regulations of "good manufacture" that cover the entire production cycle and provide optimum quality guarantees to the product. Therefore, the maintenance of aseptic conditions is a central issue in pharmaceutical production, particularly so in parenterals.

The essential requirements of aseptic processing practice for pharmaceuticals manufacture are set forth in broad terms in "The United States Pharmacopeia", USP XXI, page 1351:

> The requirements for a properly designed, validated and maintained filling or other aseptic processing facility are mainly directed to (i) an air environment free from viable microorganisms, of a proper design to permit effective maintenance of air supply units and (ii) the provision of trained operating personnel who are adequately equipped and gowned...
>
> Certification and validation of the aseptic process and facility is achieved by establishing the efficiency of the filtration systems, by employing microbiological environmental monitoring procedures, and by processing of sterile culture medium as simulated product.

219

USP XXI notes also that there is a substantial class of products, which are not terminally sterilized but are prepared by a series of aseptic steps designed to prevent the introduction of viable microorganisms into components where sterile or once an intermediate process has rendered the bulk product or its components free from viable microorganisms.

Of possibly even greater significance in the next few years, the FDA (Food and Drug Administration), recognizing basic differences between aseptic processing and terminal sterilization, has published proposed new guidelines on aseptic processing. These proposals relate to procedures for preparation of sterile drug products by aseptic processing that constitute acceptable means of complying with certain sections of the current good manufacturing practice (CGMP) regulations for drug products cited in Parts 210 and 211 of Title 21 of the Code of Federal Regulations.

Most of the questions which the FDA hopes to answer with the proposed regulations concern process validation. Employee hygiene, aseptic gowning and cleanroom design are expected to be covered in future revisions. These proposals do not address terminally sterilized drug products. In brief, the proposals add more stringent requirements to cleanroom operation. For example: "The air should also be of high microbial quality. An incidence of no more than one viable organism per 10 cubic feet is considered as attainable and desirable." And in sterility testing, added requirements are proposed for sterility testing under 21 CFR Section 211.167 (Special Testing Requirements).

A. Rationale for isolation enclosure processing

The only known way to ensure that a material or an object is free of bacterial or particulate contamination is to place that material or object into a sterile decontaminated environment, then prohibit recontamination. This is particularly true for the manufacture and packaging of injectable products where even trace amounts of contaminants, not solely biological in nature, may upon injection produce immediate allergic reactions or, over a period of time, produce lesions in vital organs.

Storage or shelf-life is another problem. The presence of trace contaminants in certain alkaloids or lyophilized antibiotics, even though not of themselves biologically harmful, can contribute to chemical deterioration of the active principals when exposed to heat or humidity. Also, during the manufacture of injectable products, personnel must be protected from potential allergic reactions, such as from contact with certain antibiotics or enzymes, as well as from the hazards posed during the production of pathogenic strains or vaccines.

There are problems too when the production process results in fine powders or aerosol mists which may remain suspended in the air for long periods of time, particularly true when particle sizes are smaller than one micron. The unwanted result can be the contamination of those persons adjacent to but not directly involved in the manufacturing process.

The major sources of contamination of so-called clean environments are from the personnel, materials and equipment brought into the processing area. This is the primary drawback of the partial-barrier cleanroom or sterile-bench with laminar-air approach toward sterile conditions. Without an absolute barrier, there will always be some unwanted interchange of contaminants between the protected and the unprotected environments. In contrast, the use of a properly maintained and operated airtight absolute barrier prevents interchange of contaminants between the protected and the unprotected environments. This latter method provides complete protection for both the product and the operator, as well as for nearby personnel.

While the FDA proposals are not the basis for the following material, one cannot ignore the implications, both technological and economical, of increased stringency for sterile conditions, standards already realizable with isolation technology.

B. Evolution of isolation technology

Even before microbes were known to cause diseases, the Bible recognized "miasma" in the air. Evasion and isolation were used to combat infectious diseases. After the discovery of microbes in the 1800s, the methods of germfree research were advanced by plant physiologists who sterilized rearing chambers with heat during their studies of nitrogen fixation. Isolation systems were the simple flasks and bell jars used by early chemists to collect gases.

The first germ-free animal experiments during the 1890s used a modified bell jar as an isolator. From this modest start came the storage box and its more modern version, the metal-walled, autoclavable isolation box with viewing windows and built-in gloves for the sterile handling of materials and animals. By the middle 1950s, it was discovered that inexpensive plastic hoods could be used to create the sterile enclosures required for bacteriological research, reducing the reliance on steel and glass.

In 1913, the steam-tunnel sterile lock, a two-door autoclave, was introduced for the aseptic transfer of materials and equipment between the outside atmosphere and that of the isolation chamber. For heat-senstive materials, there was the so-called Cesearean entry in which a plastic container containing sterilized material was glued to the isolator wall, and an operator on the inside used a hot cautery to cut a hole through the wall and container to remove sterile material from the chamber. A technique for aseptic exiting of sealed containers from isolation chambers, one still in use today, was to pass the containers through a germicidal-liquid bath.

Partial enclosure methods date back to Louis Pasteur. As early as the mid-1800s, he used the nonturbulent (laminar) flow of air to separate a contaminated environment from a test environment, a method still in use. What was perhaps the first "germfree room" (or clean room) was built in the early 1900s. It boasted filtration of incoming and exiting air and entrance through a double-door cubicle. Decontamination was by washing with an antiseptic solution, followed by 48 hours of formaldehyde vapor. Operators wore protective clothing, a technique first used by physicians during the 17th century plagues.

These techniques offered varying degrees of protection from microbial intrusion. Even those approaching absolute protection brought with them their own problems. The autoclave was, and still is, an effective transfer unit, but cannot be used for heat sensitive materials and is of no value for the aseptic transfer of operators into and out of isolation chambers. Mechanical locks were difficult to use, and liquid baths were limited to the exiting of sealed containers.

It was in 1960 that la Calhene developed and patented what is now recognized as an essential key to the efficient aseptic transfer of materials and people into and out of sterile absolute-barrier isolation enclosures, namely the noncontaminating DPTE transfer container, discussed in detail in following sections of this report. The triple-seal design of the DPTE transfer container facilitates rapid and aseptic transfer of materials and objects, limited only by the dimensions of the container and isolation chamber. Although the DPTE transfer container was first developed for the safe transfer of equipment and materials into and out of nuclear environments, the aseptic manufacture of pharmaceuticals is rapidly becoming its a primary use.

C. Freeze drying and sterile conditions

The purpose of freeze-drying is the complete dehydration of the solution without the use of heat, with the consequent improvement of shelf-life over those pharmaceuticals which are packaged as liquids. Then, prior to administration of the pharmaceutical, it can be reconstituted by the addition of sterile liquid.

Where freeze-drying is an integral part of the processing cycle, as in the production of powders from solutions of heat-sensitive materials, the dryers themselves come in a variety of styles and sizes, and are produced by several manufacturers. The important aspects of freeze-drying are that they are sterile enclosures and that it is possible to enter and exit sterile containers aseptically.

An effective way to maintain the integrity of the freeze-dryer's sterile interior is to fill containers (e.g., vials) aseptically in a mobile transfer isolator with a DPTE transfer door (see Section d.). This allows aseptic transfer of the liquid-containing vials from the mobile transfer isolator through the DPTE transfer door mounted on the freeze-dryer. As noted, freeze dryers are produced by several manufacturers. It is possible to retrofit these dryers with DPTE transfer doors.

The alternative to the transfer method just described is to fill the vials within the protected atmosphere of a laminar-airflow bench then move the vials quickly to the freeze-dryer facility in a cleanroom, also under a laminar-airflow unit. Operators would be wearing protective clothing. The obvious problem here is that while the vials are being transferred from bench to dryer, there is an opportunity for bacterial or particulate contamination.

D. Sterility testing

Sterility testing is based on a statistical sample of 20 production units, according to definition in the various pharmacopoeia. (The 20 samples are taken at spaced intervals during a single day of production, i.e., a lot. The requirement of 20 samples per lot is regardless of size for lots with 200 or more units.) Even this requirement as such does not guarantee the sterility of injectable pharmaceuticals. The question arises, therefore, since sterility testing is intended as the official reference point in the event that a dispute arises concerning the sterility status of a lot, how does one obtain reassurance that the test was performed under perfect aseptic conditions.

There is an intrinsic incompatibility between human beings and sterility. This means that there will always be the risk of product contamination from the personnel conducting the sterility testing unless the two are kept absolutely separate. Thus, the answer to the need for reliable product sterility testing by a non-sterile species is to use an enclosed sterile working area, such as an absolute barrier, which provides total environmental separation between the operator environment and the material to be tested. The construction and operation of isolation systems suitable for sterility testing is discussed in detail later.

With the exception of the occasional mention of partial barriers and a comparison to absolute barriers of their relative effectivenesses, the material in this chapter will be concentrated on the design, operation and uses of absolute-barrier technology.

2. Definitions

Absolute barrier: An enclosed volume that allows no interchange between the protected and unprotected environments and usually consists of an airtight enclosure constructed of impervious material (such as transparent PVC plastic) with the processing operations being completed through remotely controlled machinery, or from the outside through arm-length rubber gloves, or from the inside by operators wearing isolation clothing. To prevent contamination from the outside environment, the chamber should be maintained at a slight positive pressure, usually between 1–3mm water.

Enclosed volume: An airtight isolation chamber delimiting the space which is strictly necessary for the production or testing operations. Such a chamber is illustrated in Figure 1. It is the leaktightness of this chamber that isolates the sterile products from the personnel and the surrounding environment, as well as isolates the operator and other personnel from dangerous products.

Partial barrier: Unenclosed processing area, such as a cleanroom or laminar-airflow workbench, which has been decontaminated but not protected to prevent external recontamination.

Figure 1—Typical airtight isolation chamber for aseptic processing of sterile materials.

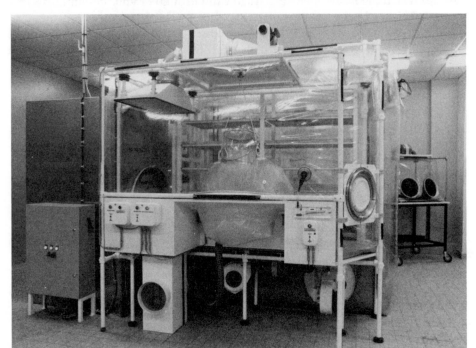

3. Design of Barrier Enclosures

A. The enclosure

Airtight enclosures with volumes as small as 0.5 cu.m. (18 cu.ft.) to as large as 200 cu.m. (7,200 cu.ft.) or greater are commonly made of various materials, flexible or rigid, transparent or opaque. For example, the walls can be of stainless steel, although transparent flexible polyvinyl chloride (PVC) or Plexiglass are preferred.

The advantages of flexible PVC are that it resists scratching and abrasion, and can be formed into contoured fittings. Being pliable, PVC provides superior working reach for outside operators by flexing as the operator moves; being transparent, the PVC allows the operators inside the enclosure to view external surroundings. Conversely, supervisors on the outside can, without special gowns, monitor operations within the enclosure.

Following are some of the factors involved when choosing the type of material for the enclosure walls:

- Flexible walls allow greater reach range and more comfortable handling of isolated materials by operators working with gloves and special suits.

- Transparent walls allow observation and supervision of the operators from vantage points outside of the protected area, and reduce feelings of claustrophobia by operators on the inside.

- Heat generated by machines and equipment inside of the enclosure must be considered and compensated for.

- Compatibilities of the product with the material of the walls (e.g., abrasiveness, corrosivity) can be important.

- Smooth, easy-to-clean inner wall surfaces, such as transparent, flexible PVC, are very desirable when working with fine powders or aerosols.

Another important factor relates to machinery associated with the isolation chamber. It should be separated, where possible, from the working station to allow maintenance in the non-protected outer area. Finally, the isolation chamber should be as small as possible to decrease the cost of air treatment.

B. Handling techniques

There are three basic designs that allow for the aseptic handling of materials inside an absolute barrier enclosure. They are gloves, half suits and total suits (e.g., Scalair). These are illustrated in Figures 2 and 3.

Figure 2 — Use of gloves, half suits and total suits for aseptic handling of sterile materials in isolation chambers.

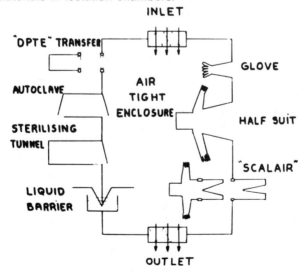

Figure 3—Illustration of full-suit and half-suit operations in airtight isolation chamber.

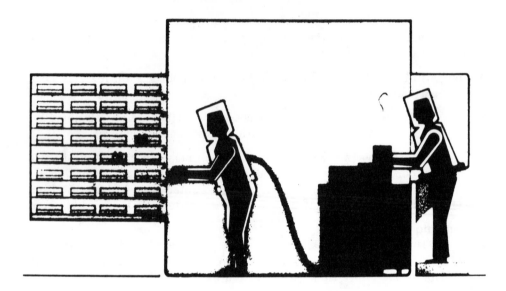

Glove systems herein discussed are improvements over those already well-known. The gloves are attached to sleeves that are in turn fixed with airtight seals to a wall of the enclosure, and permit introduction of hands and forearms of the operator (see Figure 4). Allowing for the length of a sleeve and the typical arm-length of an operator, the range of motion for a glove-and-sleeve method mounted on a flexible PVC enclosure is about two to two and a half feet (see Figure 5). There is provision for aseptic interchange of gloves within the enclosure to accommodate different hand sizes, as well as types (see Figure 6).

Double-walled half suits can protrude through an enclosure wall with an airtight seal. These suits permit aseptic introduction of operator's torso into the working area of the enclosure. Typically, in such a suit, the inner wall next to the operator's body is porous and ventilated for operator comfort and working flexibility. The range of motion for an operator in a half suit is superior to that of a glove system, providing a work radius of some four to five feet with an angular flexibility of 200 degrees (see Figure 5). The same basic technique that is used for aseptic glove interchange (see Figure 6) is used for exchanges when using half suits.

Figure 4—Handling sterile vials in an isolator chamber using an arm-length glove-sleeve facility.

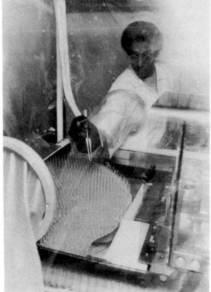

Figure 5—Ranges of motion within airtight isolator enclosure with gloves, a half suit, and a total ["Scalair"] suit.

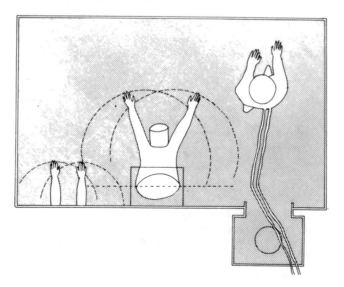

Figure 6—Technique for interchange of sterile gloves within an airtight isolation
         chamber

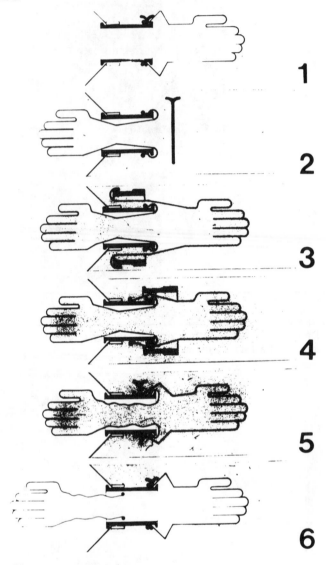

1—Glove is inside of isolator, operator's hand and arm inserted
2—Glove pulled back, i.e., wrongside out
3—With other gloved hand, operator places new glove (sterile, from where it has been stored
    inside the isolator) over the top of the wrist ring holder
4—Replacement glove is being sealed to the wrist ring
5 and 6—Old glove is removed

Total suits (e.g., la Calhene's "Scalair") can be used when it is essential for the operator to aseptically enter and exit a large airtight sterile enclosure. The range of motion for the operator in a total suit is unlimited within the enclosure (see Figure 5). This type of suit first gained popularity in the nuclear industry, and is rapidly gaining acceptance in the pharmaceutical industry where totally sterile conditions are essential (e.g., loading and unloading of freeze dryers and autoclaves, as well as other activities requiring the presence of an operator within a large, enclosed, sterile work area).

Figure 7—Process for sterile entry of total-suited operator into airtight sterile isolation chamber.

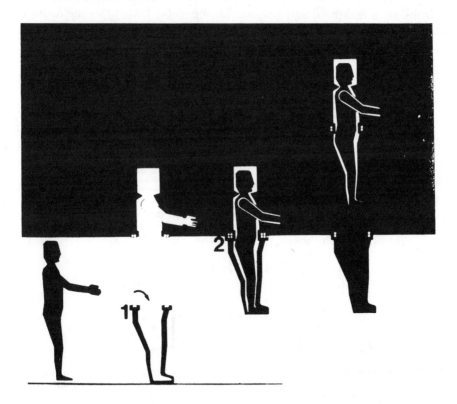

1—Operator steps into the inner of the two-layer trouser portion of total suit
2—Trouser portion is sealed to upper portion of total suit which in turn is sealed to the enclosure wall
3—Total suit is released from enclosure wall, allowing aseptic entry of operator protected by suit with sterile outer surface

The total suit is used mostly when it is necessary to load or unload large volumes of materials before moving them to the peripheries of the enclosure to be within working range of operators equipped with gloves or half suits.

The technology used for physical introduction of the full-suited operator into the enclosure without his being introduced "biologically" is the same as that used for contamination-free introduction of materials and equipment into sterile chambers, the details of which are covered in section 3.d. under "Means of Transfer" in which the mechanism and use of the DPTE transfer container are described.

Referring to Figure 7, it can be seen that the top half of the full suit replaces the door of the enclosure. A double pair of trousers becomes the port and body of a container. When the top half of the suit is locked onto the internal trousers, a leakproof suit results. The operator leaves the enclosure by reversing the procedure. Concentric flexible tubing from an external ventilation station supplies fresh air to the suit, and extracts spent air from it.

C. Sterile air

In the confined volume of an isolation chamber, it is necessary to control the physicochemical characteristics of the specific atmosphere as determined by the requirements of the product being handled. To prevent the introduction of contaminants into the enclosure with entering or exiting air, or into the atmosphere by exiting air, intake and output air pass through entrance and exit absolute HEPA filters (High Efficiency Particulate Air) (see Figure 8).

Figure 8—HEPA filters are located on both the inlet and exit air lines of an isolator chamber to prevent particulate contaminates from entering or exiting the chamber.

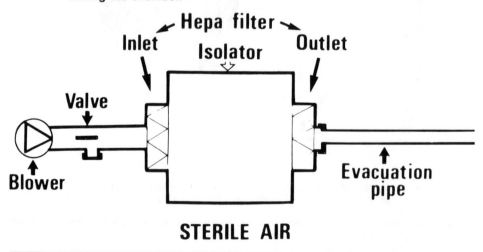

The HEPA filters can remove almost all particulate material, microbial or other, equal to or greater than 0.3 microns diameter. The HEPA inlet filter ensures that only sterile air enters the enclosure. The HEPA outlet filter protects the outer environment from contamination that may escape from the isolation chamber, but also serves to protect the contents of the chamber from outside contaminants should there be a power failure and air from the outside is drawn in as the positive pressure within the enclosure is lost.

It is recommended that a prefilter be installed at the inlet of the air blower to remove larger-sized particulates and to prevent early clogging of the inlet HEPA filter. A manometer is used to indicate and monitor the positive pressure within the enclosure.

D. Sterile transfer technique

Equipment and products must be introduced into the isolation chamber and removed therefrom, or transferred from one isolation chamber to another, without concurrent contamination of the sterile environment. This means that there must be a constantly unbroken seal between the inside of the chamber and the outer atmosphere.

The four known ways to accomplish such non-contaminating transfers are:

i. Pass material or equipment through a liquid barrier filled with a germicide or antiseptic. This is a difficult method to control, and generally used only to exit materials from the enclosure.

ii. Pass material or equipment through a double-door autoclave with an airtight seal to the enclosure wall. The nonsterile item is placed into the rear door of the autoclave, the door closed, the item is autoclaved until sterile, then the front or primary door opened and the sterile item introduced aseptically into the enclosure. While this system is effective, the application of this procedure is limited to items that are not heat-sensitive.

iii. Continuous introduction of items (e.g., vials, stoppers) into the sterile enclosure on a conveyor belt passing through a sterilizing tunnel. Typically, as the belt moves through the tunnel, the items on it will be washed with water and steam, rinsed, then sterilized by exposing the items to high-temperature dry heat.

iv. The DPTE transfer container allows the rapid aseptic transfer of sterile materials into or out of the sterile enclosure without breaking the seal that protects the enclosure from the outside environment.

"The DPTE transfer container" system was developed and patented by la Calhene to facilitate the rapid and safe transfer of hazardous radioactive materials into and out of sealed enclosures. More recently, the technology has been adopted for sterile transfer of materials into and out of absolute barrier enclosures used in the pharmaceutical industry.

Figure 7 shows the three steps in a sterile DPTE transfer. The container is closed by a cover made airtight by a triple seal. On one wall, the isolation chamber has a DPTE cell clamp with airtight door. The container is brought up to and connected to the isolation chamber via a lock on the clamp by rotating it by 60 degrees. At the same time, the door of the container is locked to that of the cell, and then is unlocked from the container.

The double door formed in this manner provides an airtight seal between the two faces which had been in contact with the outer atmosphere. From inside the isolation chamber, the operator can open this double door without breaking the system's seal.

DPTE containers are made in several variations (see Figure 10). The standard model is made of polyethylene. The autoclavable container is of stainless steel with an absolute filter which allows the passage of steam without concurrent passage of particulates. For the transfer of powders in bulk, funnel containers are equipped with mechanical systems to facilitate removal of powders.

Figure 9 — Docking of DPTE transfer container for aseptic transfer of sterile material into an airtight isolator chamber.

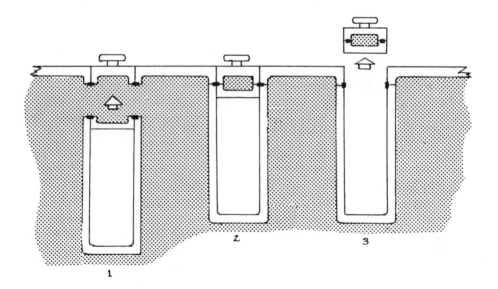

Step 1 — Sealed DPTE container approaches wall-mounted transfer seal
Step 2 — DPTE container engages with transfer seal
Step 3 — Container is opened for aseptic transfer of sterile material into airtight isolation chamber

---

Figure 10—Types of DPTE transfer containers

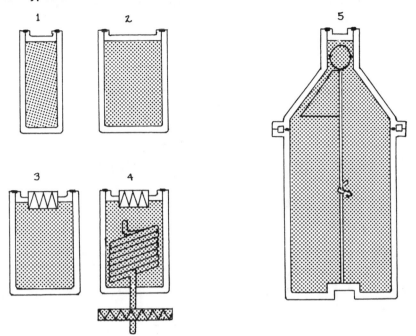

Type 1—105mm diameter polyethylene container
Type 2—270mm diameter polyethylene container
Type 3—Autoclave-sterilizable container with HEPA filter on top
Type 4—Autoclave-sterilizable container with HEPA filter on top and absolute liquid filter at bottom
Type 5—Funnel type container with interior agitator

E. Enclosure sterilization

A partial barrier environment, such as a cleanroom, cannot be completely sterilized. Moreover, it requires periodic decontamination. Walls must be scrubbed, rinsed, and so on. The problem is that the very persons doing the decontamination bring with them a new supply of particulates and biological contaminants. In contrast, the absolute barrier chamber can be sterilized to a sterility assurance level (SAL) of 10^6, and this can be accomplished remotely without need for the presence of operators within the enclosure. Even more important, sterilization of the isolation chamber is needed only when the sterile seal has been broken, a new operation is to be conducted within the chamber, or when validation is required.

Sterilization of the isolation chamber is accomplished by introducing dilute peracetic acid or formaldehyde vapors through the inlet HEPA filters, as shown in Figure 11. While the average sterilization time with peracetic acid is about one-fifth that of formaldehyde, there may exist reasons why peracetic acid cannot be used (e.g., incompatibilities of products and the sterilization material).

Figure 11—Sterilization of the interior of an isolation chamber is accomplished by the introduction of sterilant vapors through the inlet HEPA filter.

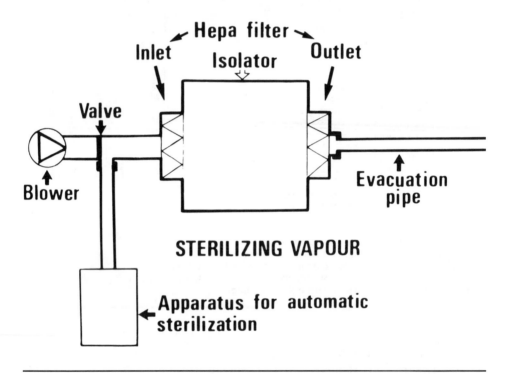

Prior to actual sterilization of an isolation chamber, pre-cleansing is recommended. This is easily accomplished by washing the inner surfaces of the isolation chamber with a 1% solution of peracetic acid in demineralized water, or with full-strength formaldehyde and subsequent rinsing with demineralized water.

The preferred procedure for sterilization of the isolation chamber is as follows:

i. If using formaldehyde or peracetic acid, ambient room temperature (22°–24°C) is adequate.

ii. Compressed air is mixed with the sterilizing agent and heated to force vapors of the sterilizing agent into the chamber until the volume within the chamber is saturated (see Figure 11).

iii. The sterilizing process is continued for a sufficient period of time to ensure complete sterilization. Typical sterilization times are from 45 minutes for a volume of 0.5 cu.m. to 5 hours for a volume of 13 cu.m. Sterilization effectiveness is confirmed by biological indicators containing spores of *"thermophillus" "subtilus niger"*, or *"globigii" at a concentration of 10^6* spores per indicator strip.

iv. The sterilizing agent is purged from the chamber using sterile air that has been passed through the HEPA filter, eliminating sterilizing agent vapors.

Note: Steps (2), (3) and (4) are most easily and effectively accomplished automatically by use of a la Calhene sterilization system.

This procedure sterilizes both the inlet and exit HEPA filters at the same time that the isolation chamber is being sterilized. The procedure, as noted, can be made fully automatic to eliminate the need for constant operator supervision.

E. Validation of enclosure integrity

A number of tests are available to ensure that the isolation chamber is airtight. These include:

- Leaktight test with a detector cloth that reacts to ammonia vapors, or with Freon gas and a sniffer
- DOP test for the HEPA filters
- Checking particulate level per Federal Standard 209B with a particulate counter
- Checking the maintenance of positive pressure within the enclosure via a manometer connected to the chamber through a HEPA filter
- Initial and followup checking of flowrate through the chamber
- Use of biological indicator testing, the same as following sterilization

4. Sterile Production Cycle

The technology for a sterile production cycle is the same when processing either liquid or powder materials within the isolation chamber. The primary differences will be in the type of DPTE transfer container used, the method for packaging product and sealing containers under aseptic conditions, and the precautions needed to prevent excessive loss of powder into the enclosure atmosphere with resultant premature plugging of the outlet HEPA filter. Figure 12 illustrates a sterile production cycle for a powder material. (See also Figs. 13 and 14.) The steps in the cycle are: storage, sampling and quarantine, production, lyophilization (where freeze-drying is a part of the production process), powder work-up, and packaging.

A. Sterile storage

Referring to Figure 12, Stages 1, 2 and 3 relate to pre-process handling of raw materials. While these are not parts of what is conventionally considered the production cycle, they are essential pre-production procedures. They are carried out when the raw materials are received to provide for sterilization of the external faces of the metal delivery containers, and to store them in DPTE transfer containers under sterile conditions.

Figure 12—Sterile production cycle from receipt of materials through final packaging.

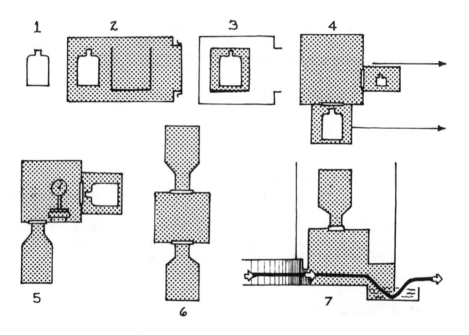

Step 1—Receipt of raw materials
Step 2—Preparation for sterile storage
Step 3—Transfer to sterile container
Step 4—Sample taken and sent to the laboratory, bulk of material to quarantine
Step 5—Weighing
Step 6—Working-up of powder materials
Step 7—Packaging of materials [as shown here, packaging is for liquid materials with vials entering through heat barrier and, when filled and sealed, exiting through a sterilizing liquid barrier

Stage 1: Sterile raw materials arrive in leakproof containers.

Stage 2: The external surfaces of the delivery containers are sterilized in an isolation chamber or sterilization chamber, as are the internal and external surfaces of DPTE containers with doors open. When sterilization is complete, the delivery containers are placed inside of the DPTE containers, the doors of which are closed and sealed.

Stage 3: The sterilization isolation chamber can now be opened. The interiors of the DPTE containers will remain sterile.

B. Sampling and quarantine

Referring to Stage 4 in Figure 12, precautions used in the sampling and quarantine of samples are the same as those used in the conventional processing cycle for production of sterile product.

Samples are taken from the sterile isolation chamber for analysis in the sterile microbiology laboratory, as shown in Figure 10, which is itself an airtight, sterile isolation chamber. The containers in which the sterile samples are taken are initially sterilized. After analysis, the sterile containers are quarantined.

C. Production

Production comprises Stages 5 and 6 as illustrated in Figure 12. They are:

Stage 5: Inside the sterile isolation chamber, the contents of the containers are weighed, then introduced into the DPTE funnel containers. From there, all transfers of powder needed for the production cycle will be carried out in DPTE funnel containers.

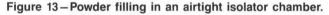

Figure 13—Powder filling in an airtight isolator chamber.

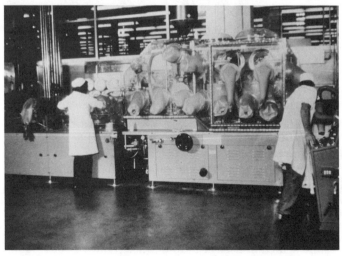

Stage 6: The term "working-up of powders" refers to all of the treatments to which mixtures are subjected to impart the required final physicochemical characteristics.

Figure 14 — Start of cycle for packaging of liquid materials in vials.

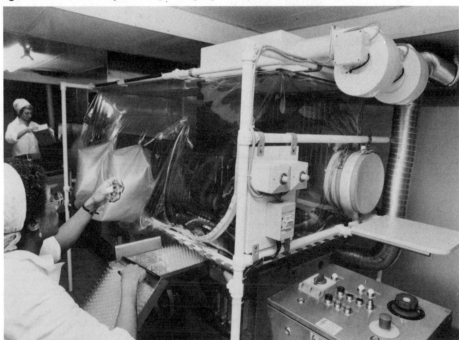

D. Packaging

This portion of the production cycle covers the continuous introduction and removal of the bottles or ampules from the sterile isolation chamber without resultant cross-contamination. In the cycle illustrated in Figure 12, Stage 7 shows the bottles or ampules being introduced through a heat barrier and removed through a liquid barrier.

The heat barrier is a continuous sterilization oven connected in a leak-proof manner to the isolation chamber that protects the packaging machine. When the oven is stopped, or when its temperature falls below a specified level, a leakproof port closes at the inlet of the isolation chamber.

The exiting liquid barrier is located at the outlet of the isolation chamber. The filled and sealed bottles or ampules are removed continuously by passing submerged through the liquid barrier, an asepticizing solution. The barrier

Figure 15—Sterile microbiology laboratory in airtight enclosure.

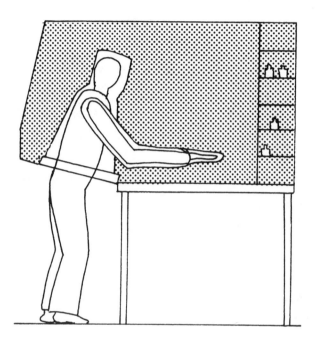

prevents contamination from entering the isolation chamber, and its chemical nature protects personnel from powder that may have been deposited on the exterior surfaces of the bottles during packaging.

E. Lyophilization
Where freeze-drying is involved in the process, there is a lyophilization cycle as shown in Figure 16. The solution to be freeze-dried is introduced into the sterile isolation chamber by passing through an absolute filter for liquids. This filter is mounted on a DPTE container which is sterilized in an autoclave.

After bulk lyophilization, the powder is placed in metal containers which exit the isolation chamber via the DPTE container. Conditions are the same as those used during Stage 4 of the sterile production cycle (see Figure 12).

Finally, after lyophilization in ampules or vials, these containers are stoppered or otherwise sealed, then removed from the isolation chamber via the same autoclave that was used to introduce them into the isolation chamber.

Figure 16—Lyophilization cycle when a process involves freeze-drying.

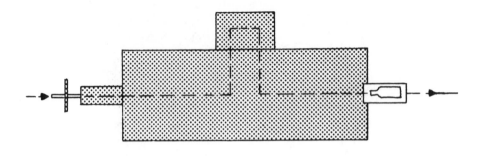

F. Personnel protection

Personnel must be protected during all steps of the procedure. Referring to Figure 17, the operations during which there is particular need to protect personnel include:

   Stage 1: Raw materials arrive in various types of packaging.

   Stage 2: Samples are taken in an airtight isolation chamber, either with sterilized test tubes and transferred by means of a DPTE container, or with presterilized polyethylene bags. Quarantine follows.

   Stage 3: After weighing and mechanical or manual sifting, powders are transferred from their containers into funnel containers in an airtight isolation chamber.

   Stage 4: This stage is similar to Stage 6 of the aseptic production cycle (see Figure 12).

   Stage 5: If there is no need for a specific atmosphere inside the isolation chamber and if it is therefore necessary only to ensure the protection of personnel, the introduction and removal of the bottles or ampules can take place as follows:

> Introduction through a differential pressure barrier: The isolation chamber is ventilated under reduced pressure, avoiding any escape of air concurrently with introduction of the bottles into the enclosure. Also in this case, an airtight door ensures the continuity of the isolation when the production stops, thus avoiding contamination of the external environment.

> Removal through a liquid barrier: The continuous removal of the stoppered or otherwise sealed vials or ampules is accomplished in the same manner as for Stage 7 of the sterile production (see Figure 12).

The maintenance and cleaning of the machines are regulated just as stringently as is the production cycle itself. Powders collected during maintenance and cleaning are chemically destroyed or incinerated. The complete cycle of all production operations—non-sterile, sterile, maintenance—thus form a closed loop with no hazardous contact between products and operators.

Figure 17—Steps during aseptic processing of sterile materials that require special attention for the protection of personnel.

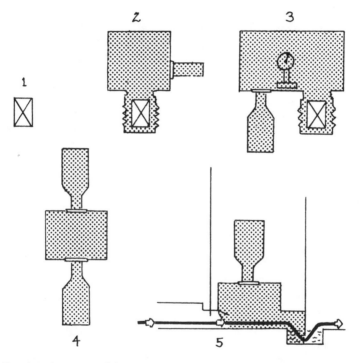

Step 1—Receipt of raw materials
Step 2—Sampling
Step 3—Weighing and sieving
Step 4—Working-up of powder
Step 5—Packaging [shown with product entering through reduced-pressure barrier, exiting through liquid barrier].

---

5. Sterility Testing

As noted earlier, sterility testing must be conducted in a sterile atmosphere to have a maximal statistical validity. Teillon has carried out much work toward development of reliability standards for sterility testing. The method, based on a description by Dr. Teillon, follows.

A. The isolator

As a way of preventing accidental contamination of test samples and resultant false positive readings, Dr. Teillon uses two la Calhene absolute-barrier isolators made of flexible PVC. The isolators are positively pressurized by a slight but constant renewal of sterile air.

Since no human body need penetrate the enclosure, the rate of air renewal is minimized, in turn lessening the load on the HEPA absolute filters. This results in a significant cost savings.

B. Transfers

Transfers into and out of the sterile isolators are made without breaking the sterile seal. This is done with an intermediary airlock, onto which an autoclave or oven can be attached. An alternative method of transfer can be by means of the DPTE container.

C. Manipulations

An operator in a half-suit (described earlier) handles necessary analysis manipulations of the sample without "biologically" entering the isolator. The half-suit is used to provide greater access and flexibility than would be possible with traditional glove-equipped isolators.

D. Sterilization

Sterilization of the isolator's enclosed volume is performed automatically by a device that pumps vapors of peracetic acid into the isolator for a specified period of time. These vapors are obtained by gently heating a 3.5% concentration of commercially available peracetic acid, then circulating the vapors through the isolator via the inlet and exit HEPA filters (see Figure 11). Sterilization is followed by a purge with sterile air.

The commercial peracetic acid used has a 35% concentration of original active ingredients, i.e., a mixture of peracetic acid, acetic acid, hydrogen peroxide, oxygen and water. After three years of using peracetic acid vapors for sterilization of the isolator, Dr. Teillon has found that the abrasiveness of the peracetic acid sterilant has been negligible for PVC plastic as well as for metallic components, such as aluminum and stainless steel.

E. The system and its use

The system used comprised two isolators occupying a total floor area of 6.75 sq.m. The first isolator is the "Sterilization Chamber" and has a volume of 3.35 cu.m. This chamber, equipped with a half-suit, is used to stage material that has been sterilized previously through conventional methods, such as autoclaves and ovens.

Prior to introduction into the Sterilization Chamber, the external surfaces of all glass containers are submerged in a 1% solution of peracetic acid to ensure exterior decontamination.

The second isolator, the "Manipulation Chamber" (the working station), has a volume of 4.74 cu.m., and is equipped with two half-suits. Two airtight plastic portals similar to the introductory portal of the Sterilization Chamber maintain the two isolators as separate, independent enclosures. The transfer of material and samples between the two isolators is through a 490 mm.-diameter transfer airlock. Sterility is maintained between the two isolators by a rubber connection closed with a metallic clamp, covered with flexible shroudings (see Figure 18).

Figure 18 — Interconnection of sterilization isolation chamber to sterile manipulation [working area] isolation chamber for sterile testing of materials.

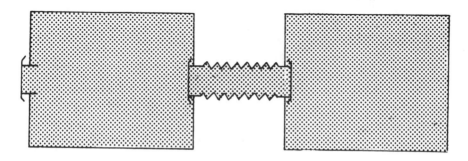

F. Sterility test results

In compliance with the different pharmacopeia, Dr. Teillon performed his sterility tests on injectable pharmaceuticals using the membrane filtration method. To establish a basis of comparison, he tested 2,593 units under partial barrier conditions of a horizontal laminar-flow, Class 100 hood. The test failure result for testing of the 2,593 units was 0.85%. This exceeds FDA standards of acceptability.

Even more significant was the elimination of false positives when using the isolator. Where the testing of 509 units in a sterile room produced 1.18% false positive readings, in contrast the testing of 437 units in the sterile isolator environment produced zero false positive readings.

6. Comparison of Absolute and Partial Barriers

The main differences between aseptic processing in a partial barrier, represented by a laminar air-flow in one protected area, and an absolute barrier are shown in Tables I and II.

Table I—Partial Barrier vs. Absolute Barrier: Comparison of Physical Characteristics

	Partial Barrier in One Protected Area	Absolute Barrier in Sterile Enclosure
Sterilization Requirements	For entire room	For airtight enclosure only
Sterilization Assurance Level	1,000 SAL	1,000,000 SAL
Operator Gowning	According to good manufacturing practice (GMP)	None required
Product Protection	Depends on the operators	Always total
Operator/ Environment Protection	Not absolute; depends on both the operators and design of the laminar airflow facility	Always total
Equipment/ Materials Transfer	Aseptic conditions non-immediate and depend on operators	Leakproof and instantaneous with DPTE system
Transfer/Transport of Dangerous and/or Sterile Products and/or Wastes	Aseptic conditions depend on strict procedures; no absolute warranty	Total protection of both personnel and environment with DPTE transfer system
Glove Leakage	Requires aseptic procedures to change gloves	Glove interchange without breaking sterile seal

Table II—Partial Barrier vs. Absolute Barrier: Comparison of Installation Specifications

	Partial Barrier in One Protected Area	Absolute Barrier in Sterile Enclosure
Room Requirements	Class 1,000 or 10,000 (FS 209b) recommended	No special requirements
Power Requirements	2 Kw	0.1 to 0.2 Kw
Sterilization Requirements	Rooms must be leaktight with exhaust blower; decontamination generally accomplished by rinsing or fuming with formaldehyde	Need compressed air; 110v power source; exhaust from totally enclosed isolator is from isolator to the outside
Power Continuity Requirements	Power failure will break the "air curtain" protection	Sterile isolator protected by inlet and outlet HEPA filters

It can be seen that not only does the absolute barrier reduce the danger of contamination, both internal and external to the working area, but there is a reduction in investment costs. As compared to a clean room, the absolute barrier has no requirement for special corridors and operator changerooms. A smaller area requires treatment of the air, energy requirements are less, and sterile gowns for operators are not required.

7. Summary and Observations

There is no question that the development of the absolute barrier and its capabilities to reduce or eliminate cross-contamination has been and will continue to be a boon to the pharmaceutical industry, especially concerning the manufacture of sterile products.

In addition to the advantages of contamination control during the production and packaging of materials, the same technology has been applied successfully to sterile analyses, resulting in a significant decrease in false positive readings. Also significant, is the greater ease with which the manufacturer can protect both the operators working with or inside of the isolation chamber, and the assurance that deleterious materials will not escape from the chamber to affect those persons in the vicinity of an isolator.

The very near future will see isolation technology applied in the design of dust-free sterile working areas under anaerobic atmospheres in which robots will be conducting all handling operations.

11

Clean-In-Place and Sterilize-In-Place (CIP/SIP)

Dale A. Seiberling
Seiberling Associates, Inc, Roscoe, IL, USA

1. Development of Clean-In-Place Procedures and Equipment

In-place cleaning was first applied in the dairy industry in the late-1940's. From that time until approximately 25 years ago, cleaning of all milk processing equipment involved (a) complete disassembly, (b) manual cleaning by rinsing, brushing with a cleaning solution and rinsing, and (c) reassembly followed by (d) application of sanitizing solutions just prior to processing. The labor required for these procedures frequently constituted as much as 50% of the total labor required to handle all phases of a production operation from receiving through processing, packaging, and distribution.

A review of literature traces the development of Clean-In-Place (CIP) procedures. Though in-place cleaning has been practiced for more than 35 years, the greatest application has occurred since 1965 with respect both to the extent of its use and its effect on the design of processes and equipment. Prior to 1960, piping systems and cleaning operations received little attention until a new plant was placed into operation, whereas the highly automated systems being installed today demand attention to the planning of cleaning and sterilizing operations during the design stages.

Pyrex heat-resistant glass piping was introduced to the dairy industry in 1941 as a suggested means of conserving critical materials for war use (Thom, 1949). Approximately 20 installations of glass piping had been made by 1949, generally for purposes of moving raw milk from a receiving area to raw storage tanks. A bacteriological survey of four milk plants using glass pipe indicated that glass piping installations could be effectively sanitized with savings in both time and labor (Fleischmann, et al, 1950). A report published two years later confirmed these findings and indicated that more than 40 commercial and college dairies were using permanent glass lines at that date (Sheuring and Henderson, 1951).

Both plant operators and equipment manufactures had determined that the fragility of glass piping made it unsuitable for the total piping installation. Attention was given to stainless steel lines of either all welded construction or equipped with special CIP type joints. An early application of welded lines was reported to "explode the common theory that all dairy pipelines must be dismantled for sanitary reasons" (Havighorst, 1951). It was shown "that the permanent system provides fewer sources of bacterial contamination. And consequently, products processed through these lines are of uniform high quality." This initial welded installation utilized crosses with inspection ports at every change of direction. The welding technique involved the use of filler rod followed by subsequent grinding and polishing of the inner surfaces of the weld, using special equipment developed for this purpose.

A 12-month study of Clean-In-Place procedures in a medium-size milk plant revealed labor reductions of as much as 75% as compared with manual take-down cleaning (Parker, et al, 1953). This study gave considerable attention to the factors of temperature, velocity, pressure, and cleaning materials.

Cleaning procedures in milk processing plants were subject to greater lack of uniformity and control than any of the other processing operations, because: (a) they were handled by less skilled and trained personnel; (b) they were accomplished under undesirable working conditions and at night; and (c) less supervision was provided as compared with manufacturing operations. Automation of the CIP procedure minimized some of these deficiencies in an installation in a small milk plant (Seiberling, 1955).

Prior to 1955, most recirculation cleaning was accomplished with existing product pumps by using process tanks or vats or small portable tanks as the solution tank for the recirculating procedure. In 1956 several manufacturers introduced multi-tank CIP systems of packaged design incorporating a rinse water tank, a solution tank, a sanitizing tank, CIP supply pump, heating controls, programming controls, and air blow-down equipment to facilitate recovery of solution.

Early applications of in-place cleaning were restricted to piping systems, generally to only the longer piping systems. Results achieved suggested that even greater benefits could be obtained if similar procedures could be applied to the cleaning of vessels such as transportation tankers, storage tanks, and processing vats. An evaluation of permanently installed spray devices provided bacteriological evidence supporting the ability to satisfactorily spray clean storage tanks and tank trucks (Seiberling and Harper, 1957a). An air-operated CIP cleanable valve was evaluated via radioisotope based procedures later the same year (Seiberling and Harper, 1957b).

Several substantial piping systems cleaned by commercially available CIP equipment were installed in the late 1950's. Automated CIP operations were found to further reduce the labor requirements as compared to manually controlled procedures (Johnson, 1960) and contributed to significant reductions in the amount of effluent and the BOD of the effluent discharged from a dairy.

The first reported major application of automatic cleaning, air-operated valving and welded lines permitted a single operator to control a complex operation in a dairy plant placed in operation in 1960 (Bonem, 1960).

During the decade beginning in 1965, CIP was recognized as the key which would open the doors to many other changes in dairy and food processing technology. The ability to ensure controlled sanitation through mechanical/chemical cleaning led to extensive development of all welded product piping systems, extensive application of air-operated CIP cleanable sanitary valves, appreciable increases in the sizes of processing and storage tanks as compared with vessels that had to be manually cleaned, significant increases in processing flowrates and packaging machinery capacity, and approaches to plant design and arrangement not previously feasible. During this period, Clean-In-Place procedures were applied extensively in many non-dairy food and beverage industries, including brewing, wine processing, meat processing (smokehouses), as well as numerous processes which handled dry or semi-solid products in stainless steel equipment. The author's first work in the pharmaceutical industry involved the application of these techniques developed in dairy and beverage processing to the high volume production of intravenous solutions.

Clean-In-Place and Sterilize-In-Place involve far more than the selection and application of pumps, tanks, sprays, valves and controls. The design of a solutions process requires consideration of materials and methods of construction, equipment layout, specialized cleaning equipment, processing equipment design which must be conducive to CIP cleaning, and finally the design of the process.

2. CIP Systems

As practiced today, in-place cleaning is essentially chemical in nature. Processing equipment and CIP appurtenances are designed to permit solution to be brought into immediate contact with all soiled surfaces and continuously replenished. The results achieved depend upon the combined effects of time, temperature, and concentration, all of which may be placed under automatic control. Since relatively high volumes of solution must be brought into contact with the soiled surface for periods of time ranging from five minutes to one hour, recirculation of the cleaning solution is essential to maintain economic operation.

The term CIP System conveys different meanings in both the literature and the industry, depending upon the background and experience of the reader or user. Some people consider the term to describe the combination of tanks, pumps and valves used to recirculate the flush, wash and rinse solutions. Others consider the term a description for a process which has been designed so as to be CIP cleanable along with the appurtenances and special components required.

For purposes of this chapter, a CIP System is defined to include: (1) the recirculating unit, (2) any required spray devices, (3) the CIP supply/return piping system including valves, pumps and transfer panels, (4) chemical feed equipment, (5) program control equipment and (6) required controls and recording devices.

This chapter is based primarily on work accomplished in the United States. The engineering data is in English units; the metric values which follow the English values throughout the chapter are approximations.

A. Recirculating units

CIP Recirculating Units may exist in many different forms. The design may vary with the application or the method of operation.

i. Re-use recirculating units

The multi-tank re-use system shown in Figure 1 utilizes the same wash solution for many cleaning operations during the production day. This approach requires the use of a cleaning solution at a fixed concentration and temperature for cleaning all connected process lines and vessels regardless of the nature or quantity of soil to be removed. This system further requires the provision of a solution tank of adequate capacity to hold the contents of the largest line circuit to be cleaned. Solution tanks may vary from 250 to more than 1,000 gallons (1000–4000 liters) in capacity. The water supply tank may be of comparable or greater capacity, depending upon the gallons/minute required for the flushing and rinsing operations and the available water supply. Such systems occupy substantial space. Some are commercially available, in packaged form, while others are developed by combining tanks, pumps, and valves to provide the required operating capability.

Chemicals can be supplied to the multi-tank re-use system by venturi feeders, or by air-operated or mechanically-driven pumps which feed the various ingredients in a predetermined ratio under control of a conductivity sensing and control device. Many multi-tank re-use systems are charged by hand with dry powder-type materials. Operating personnel add a pre-determined quantity of chemical after each specified number of programs have been completed.

ii. Single-use recirculating units

The single-use system shown in Figure 2 operates on the basis of making up a small volume of solution automatically, using it once at the lowest possible strength, and discharging spent solution into the sewer at the end of the cleaning cycle. Air-operated piston-type pumps are used to precisely meter the required quantities of four different detergent materials to a controlled volume of water. This operating concept makes it possible to vary concentration and ingredient ratios to suit the specific requirements of each cleaning task and the composition of the water to be used.

The single-use CIP recirculating unit as shown in Figure 2 can handle a line cleaning or vessel cleaning operation with solution volumes only slightly in excess of that required to fill the circuit and supply-return piping connections. For instance, if the supply and return lines from the recirculating unit

Figure 1—Schematic Diagram of 2-Tank Re-Use CIP System

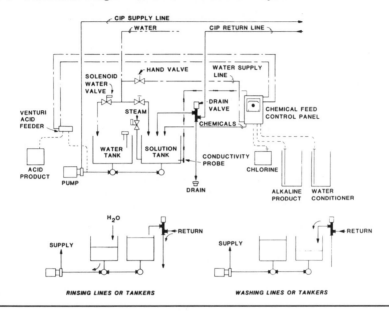

Figure 2—Schematic Diagram of Single-Tank Single-Use CIP System

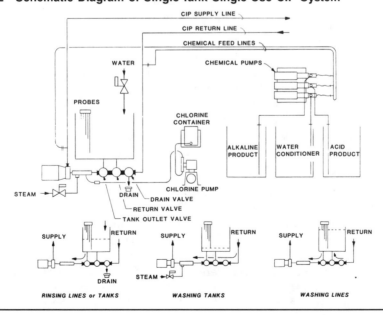

to a particular processing tank hold only 50 gallons (200L) of solution, the tank may be cleaned with not more than 60–65 gallons (225-250 liters) of solution in the system, with the excess being required to provide submergence of the outlet. The unique operation of this system eliminates the problems with synchronization of pumps that exist in the usual application of multi-tank re-use systems in which solution is pumped from the supply tank to the vessel being cleaned and then returned to the supply tank by either pumps or gravity.

Figure 2 includes with the schematic diagram, small flow diagrams which indicate the movement of water when rinsing lines or tanks, washing tanks, and washing lines. During the solution recirculation step of a tank cleaning program, the return pump discharges directly through the return line piping to the suction side of the supply pump. Safety devices in the form of pressure switches and delay-to-temperature circuits are incorporated to provide protection against improper operation on the part of the operator. This system can be programmed to feed chemicals and heat only if (a) a proper circuit is established and (b) the pumps operate properly to first establish recirculation on clear water (cold or perhaps tempered).

The single-use recirculating unit requires a more complex control system than the re-use recirculating unit. More careful engineering is required to properly size the sprays, lines and pumps to assure proper hydraulic balance under all operating conditions, as described by Seiberling (1976). The effectiveness of the single-use system was recognized by several brewers in the late-1960's resulting in the development of a special unit fitted with industrial slide-gate valves, a powered Merco strainer to remove undissolved solids, and instrumentation more typical of that used in the brewing industry at that time (Seiberling, 1970).

iii. Eductor return recirculating units

Both of the above systems require return pumps to be located near the vessel being cleaned. An alternative eductor-type re-use system (Tri-Clover) combines multiple tanks, a high-volume/high-horsepower motive pump, and an eductor to create a negative pressure on the CIP return system, thus drawing the rinse and wash solutions back from the vessel being cleaned. The application of a system of this type for cleaning tanks and parts used in the processing of pharmaceuticals was described by Grimes, et al. (1977).

iv. Eductor assisted single-use systems

Eductor assisted CIP recirculating units (Figure 3) have been applied in the dairy industry to reduce water requirements for CIP cleaning by more than 50% (Hyde, 1983). This is accomplished through recovery of spent wash and rinse solutions and re-use of these solutions for the pre-rinse and wash fill. Systems of this type have been used without the "recovered solution" principle for cleaning parenteral solutions processes with considerable success. The recirculating unit (Electrol) shown in Figure 4 includes a Water For Injection (WFI) buffer tank which is the "break-tank" between the WFI system and the CIP system for normal cleaning programs. This tank holds sufficient WFI to subsequently clean the entire WFI distribution system, as required, on an infrequent basis, following which rinsing is accomplished with fresh WFI direct from the still.

Figure 3—Schematic Diagram of Single-Use Educator Assisted CIP System

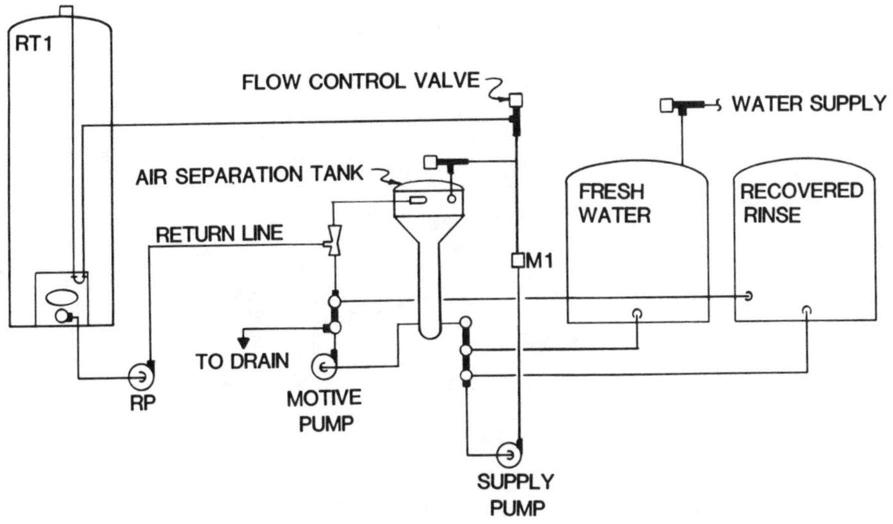

The unique design of the air-separation and recirculation tank used with the eductor-assisted system makes it possible to achieve recirculation of cleaning and sanitizing solutions at flow-rates varying from 50–300Gpm (200–1200Lpm) with as little as 12–25 gallons (50–100L) of solution in the tank. Therefore, when cleaning a piping system, the volume of chemical-treated solution required is only slightly greater than the capacity of the piping. When cleaning tanks, the return system contains an air/water mixture and the tank being cleaned contains no puddle, the volume of solution required is approximately equal to the volume of the CIP supply/return piping, with perhaps a small allowance for the water on the surfaces of a very large tank.

An air-blow at the origin of the CIP system will clear all solution from the CIP supply piping at the end of each cycle step. The eductor-based return system will draw all solution from the CIP return piping, even when return pumps are used to assist in overcoming head loss in the return piping. The design of the recirculating unit permits the motive pump to discharge all but a gallon or two of each solution from the system at the end of each cycle step. Proper design and control virtually eliminates the problem of "rinsing by dilution" which

Figure 4—Single-Use Eductor Assisted CIP Unit with WFI Tank

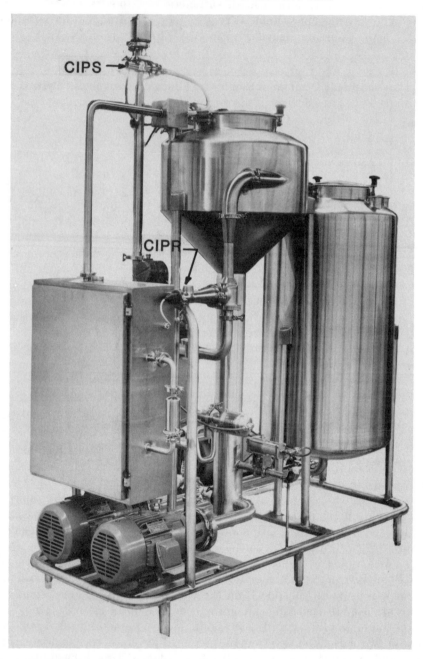

adds substantially to the water requirements for operating re-use systems, whether return pump based or eductor based.

As an example, consider an actual application in a parenteral solution process cleaned by the system shown on Figure 4. The largest circuit in the process included one (1)-3800L tank, two (2)-2800L tanks, one (1)-1500L tank, two (2)-1100L tanks, and more than 400 ft. (120M) of 1½" (38mm) and 2" (50mm) line. This complete circuit was cleaned in a single operation with approximately 80 gallons (300L) of solution in the circuit, and the total program required approximately 1100 gallons (4200L) of WFI. Return flow was via the vacuum produced by the eductor in combination with several process pumps used also as CIP return pumps.

v. The recirculating unit as integral part of the process

It is not always necessary to provide a CIP recirculating unit to accomplish Clean-In-Place operations. Consider, as an example, the High-Temperature Short-Time (HTST) pasteurization system used in the dairy industry (Seiberling, 1985). HTST systems include many combinations of plate or triple-tube heat exchangers, pumps, valves, and interconnecting piping designed to meet the process criteria. The constant-level tank which is a part of every system can be used as the CIP recirculating tank; the process pumps may serve as the CIP recirculating pumps. Heating may be accomplished via proper operation of the heat exchanger already present in the system, under control of the same instrumentation provided for the process. The additional components required include: (1) a 3-port divert valve to control flow of wash and rinse solutions to the sewer or back to the constant-level tank for recirculation and (2) chemical feed equipment.

When considered in this context, the capital cost and space required for a CIP system is already incorporated into that for the processing system. Similar applications have been made throughout the food processing industry for those processes which function for production for a designated period of time, be it a shift, a day, or a week, and then are removed from production and cleaned as an entity.

B. Spray devices

Spray cleaning was first applied to bulk milk tankers used to transport milk from the farm to the dairy processing facility in the early-1950s. The initial efforts involved the application of equipment already in use for cleaning railroad cars and transport tankers used for hauling industrial chemicals. This industrial equipment was designed to emphasize physical action as compared to chemical action and used high-pressure sprays and impact to remove and flush away soil. Such spray devices operated at pressures ranging from 60–200 psi (400–1400 KPa). The design varied from simple rotating spray heads (comparable to a lawn sprinkler) to more complex devices involving simultaneous rotation in two different planes with mechanical indexing to assure proper coverage of every portion of the vessel during a pre-determined number of complete cycles of rotation. Simple rotating spray heads were occasionally permanently installed but the more complex multi-planer devices were moved from one vessel to another, being installed only for the cleaning operation and then removed, requiring access to properly located manways in the upper center portion of each vessel.

When attention was focused on the spray cleaning of in-plant processing and storage tanks via automated systems the mechanical rotating and oscillating spray devices were quickly discarded in favor of fixed-sprays. Intensive evaluation of transport tanker spray devices by a multi-plant dairy processor confirmed previous findings that the permanently installed ball-type spray has the following advantages, as compared to rotating spray devices:

1. There are no moving parts.
2. It can be made completely of stainless steel.
3. Its performance is not affected greatly by minor variations in supply pressure.
4. A properly established installation will continue to provide satisfactory service for extensive periods of time.
5. It sprays all of the surface all of the time, hence reducing the total time required for cleaning a vessel of a given size (Hood, H. P., 1974).

Fixed ball-type sprays (Figure 5) are available with a variety of characteristics in terms of flow-rate, operating pressure, and pattern of coverage (Klenzade). Experience indicates that cylindrical tanks containing almost any complement of agitating equipment and baffles can be adequately cleaned if sprayed at 0.1 to 0.3 gal/min/sq ft (4–12 L/min/M^2) of internal surface, and patterns are arranged to spray the upper one-third of the tank. Sprays must be located and used in sufficient numbers to eliminate any possibility of shadowing. Vertical tanks which are free of agitating equipment, baffles and other internal devices may be cleaned satisfactorily at flow-rates of 2.5 to 3.0 gal/min/lineal ft (30–35 L/min/lineal M) of tank circumference.

Spray cleaning is not limited to processing and storage vessels. Any processing machine which can be fabricated of stainless steel, designed to confine water, and further designed so that all internal surfaces drain to one or more common points, can be effectively cleaned via application of a variety of spray devices and special installation fittings shown in Figure 6 (Electrol). Equipment of this type has been used to clean dryers used for the production of powdered drug products.

To achieve the most effective coverage of the appurtenances such as agitator openings, sight glasses, manhole openings, and inlet nozzles incorporated in most process tank designs, the spray device must be located 18–24" (0.4–0.6M) below the top of the tank. In most instances, this places the spray in the product zone when the tank is filled to operating capacity. For that reason, the spray ball must be fabricated to the same standards as the vessel in which it is installed, and, it must be inspectable. The split-ball sprays fitted with bail clamps shown in Figure 5 fully comply and are self-draining and self-cleaning. Sprays

Figure 5 – Spray Devices for Processing, Transportation and Storage Tanks

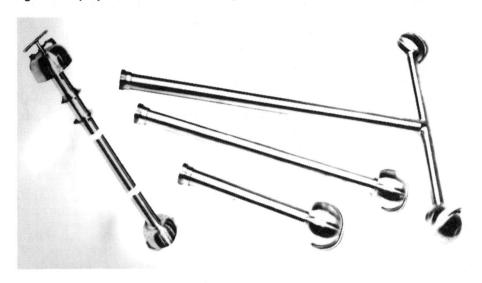

Figure 6 – Spray Devices and Installation Fittings for Various Types of Processing Equipment

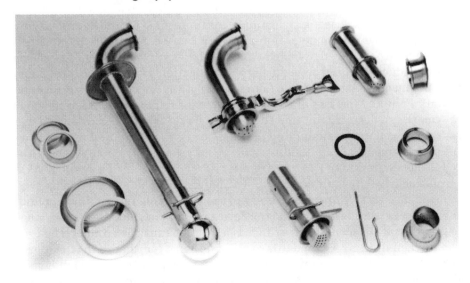

of this type are sometimes placed on elongated supply tubes which extend nearly to the bottom of the vessel for use as an agitating or sparging device, in addition to serving its primary function for CIP cleaning.

The ball-type spray shown in Figure 6 is fitted with a "slip-joint", a specially machined fitting which provides sufficient clearance to assure movement of cleaning solution through the entire joint area, controlling loss through the joint to assure proper performance of the spray device.

Whereas automated Clean-In-Place procedures used in combination with properly selected and installed spray devices make it possible to clean almost any type of processing or storage vessel, the performance and reliability of this procedure can be improved by designing the vessels so as to be more susceptible to mechanical/chemical cleaning. Seiberling (1968) identified design practices then found beneficial in the dairy industry. Subsequent experience in the non-dairy food industry, in brewing and wine processing, and in the pharmaceutical industry has confirmed the validity of these criteria, not only to processing and storage tanks, but to processing machinery in general.

C. CIP supply/return system
The initial application of spray cleaning in the dairy industry was accomplished by use of portable pumps, and later portable recirculating units, via hose connections to sprays installed in the tanks, and to the tank outlet. Whereas effective cleaning could be accomplished without entering the tank, the labor savings were minimal, if any. Portable equipment could not be "automated".

i. CIP solution piping
A permanently installed CIP supply/return piping system was an integral part of the earliest "automated" CIP installations (Bonem, 1960 and Johnson, 1960). In dairy processes and some food processes, it is necessary to clean processing and storage vessels during the production period. A number of those vessels may contain product at a later time during the production day when the process piping is Cleaned-In-Place. The 3-A Accepted Practices for Permanently Installed Sanitary Product Pipelines and Cleaning Systems require that "All connections between the solution circuit and the product circuit shall be constructed as to positively prevent the comingling of the product and solution during processing" (3-A Standards, July 1986).

Compliance with this requirement is best accomplished by the installation of separate CIP supply/return piping. The "make break" connections between the product vessels, the process lines, and the CIP supply/return lines generally consist of movable elbows, U-bends, or "goosenecks" (an elbow on a short length of straight tubing) physically arranged to prevent improper connections.

Whereas the 3-A Standards require the same consideration of materials, gasketing, fabrication technique, and support as applicable to the product piping, these Standards do permit piping used exclusively for cleaning solutions to be fabricated of non-polished tubing, rather than being polished to a #4 finish (120–150 grit) as required for product piping. In most instances, the material used is bright-annealed (non-polished) ID and polished OD to maintain uniformity of appearance in the exposed areas.

Grimes (1977) described a minimal CIP supply/return system installed to clean manufacturing and storage tanks used in a pharmaceutical process. All vessels cleaned by this system were portable and were moved to the wash stations for cleaning. And, the wash stations were located one level above the eductor-type CIP system.

ii. Integrated piping system design for product and CIP solution use

The required "make-break" connections described above are generally manually cleaned and, therefore, represent an opportunity for either improper cleaning or recontamination during assembly for the production run, or both. Considerable attention recently has been given to design concepts which improve the CIP procedure by cleaning a major part of the system as an entity, using the product piping, pumps, and valves to provide and control CIP solution flow (Seiberling, 1979). This concept is applicable to the processing of parenteral solutions. Such process requires the assembly of complete systems or substantial sub-systems prior to initiating the CIP steps. Generally all of the equipment is made available for cleaning, at the same time following completion of the production run.

This non-traditional approach provides several advantages including:

1. Markedly reduced capital cost for CIP supply/return piping.
2. Elimination of labor required for establishing cleaning circuits and then re-establishing processing circuits via make-break connections.
3. Reduction of capital cost and elimination of many areas of potential leakage and/or contamination by elimination of joints associated with those connections.

The solutions process shown in Figures 21–27 in Section 3.C of this chapter maximizes the use of common piping for production, Clean-In-Place and Sterilize-In-Place operations. When using this concept, the process engineer must design and specify inter-connecting piping, valves and pumps in sizes and arrangements which are capable of handling the higher flow-rates required for CIP operations, as compared to those required for production of the parenteral solution.

iii. Return flow motivation

When tanks are cleaned-in-place, the flush, wash and rinse solutions must be returned to the CIP Recirculating unit to establish recirculation for the solution wash or recirculated final rinses. It is desirable to return flush and rinse solutions to this point also, so that one set of valves may control flow for recirculation or discharge to drain, and to facilitate sampling for routine test and validation.

It is much easier to pump water into a tank than to remove it from the tank continuously, at high rates of flow, with a minimum "puddle" in the vessel being cleaned. CIP return pumps are most commonly used for this purpose. A self-priming centrifugal pump would be desirable, but such are not available in sanitary design and construction. Low-speed (1750 rpm) centrifugal pumps are preferred for this application as they are less susceptible to "air-binding" as compared to high speed (3450 rpm) pumps. Air-relief valves are generally required immediately adjacent to the pump inlet; practice has shown that most reliable performance will be achieved if the piping design maintains suction side losses at less than 10 ft. (3M) of head, though a slight negative pressure is required on the pump inlet to close the air relief valve during recirculation. Return line piping must pitch continuously from the outlet of the tank to the inlet of the pump. A single pump will generally support only five to seven tanks due to the suction side head loss limitation. Return pumps are generally required for operation of both the Re-Use and Single-Use recirculating units described in Section 2.A.

The eductor based recirculating unit described in that section uses a high-head motive pump and tank as an integral part of the recirculating unit to replace the return pumps otherwise required at each group of process tanks. The motive pump supplies the eductor, a pumping device which functions on the venturi principle, and the eductor creates a vacuum which pulls the cleaning solution from the vessel being cleaned to the eductor. This concept may reduce the number of pumps required and it eliminates solution loss through air relief valves in the process area, as well as the maintenance problems associated with the installation of those valves. Its performance will not be affected by minimal air-leaks in the return system and it provides puddle-free operation of spray cleaning programs. The primary design limitation is that the eductor can create only sixteen to eighteen inches vacuum. This places a limitation on return system length, requires relatively large diameter return lines, or requires the reduction of recirculating rates as compared to return pump based systems.

Those limitations are overcome in the Eductor-Assisted Single-Use system described under Section 2.A.iv. in which instance a high-speed (3450 rpm) return pump would be used in combination with return lines of only 1½″–2″ (38–50mm) diameter for normal spray cleaning flow rates of 80–120 gpm (300–400 lpm). The high-speed pump provides the head to drive water through the small diameter tubing to the eductor which functions to keep the pump continuously primed.

If the process tanks are pressure-vessels, tank pressurization can be used to achieve return flow under similar distance/line size/flow rate limitations described above for the eductor-based system. This concept is further described in Section 3.C.ii and provides the means of accomplishing CIP cleaning with only one additional particulate generating device (CIP supply pump) in the system, a similar pump already being required to supply WFI.

Gravity return of flush, wash and rinse solutions generally is not feasible as multi-floor construction would be required, with the CIP recirculating equipment installed at a level 20–30 feet (6-9M) below the outlets of the vessels being cleaned.

Substantial experience has demonstrated that operation and maintenance of a CIP system will be simplified if a standardized approach is applied to system design—i.e., select sprays, design the supply/return piping, select and install return pumps, and size tank outlet valves—so that all tanks in a given system are cleaned at approximately the same flow rate and spray supply pressure. Such an approach which permits the use of relatively uniform pre-rinse and post-rinse volumes as well as drain times, reduces the variables in the cleaning program to the time/temperature/solution strength combinations necessary to remove the soil.

4. COP units

In some instances, the "take-down" connections are cleaned in parts washers or COP (Clean-Out-of-Place) systems (Grimes 1977). The author has successfully integrated the COP washer and the automated CIP system in many applications in the dairy industry and in one pharmaceutical facility. Such integration is accomplished by modifying the interconnecting piping on the COP unit so that its self-contained high-volume pump circulates solutions at a high velocity through the manifolds or nozzles located on the tank, while the CIP system provides a lesser flow to this self-contained loop, and receives an equivalent return flow via appropriate level control devices. This concept makes the heating, chemical feed, automatically controlled programs and rinsing capabilities of the permanently installed CIP recirculating unit available to the COP parts washer, which is otherwise manually controlled in most applications.

D. CIP programs

i. An overview of experience in other industries
Cleaning programs for piping systems generally include (a) pre-rinsing with cold or tempered water until the effluent runs nearly clear, (b) recirculation of the cleaning solution for the required time at an elevated temperature ranging from 130–180°F (54–82°C), (c) post-wash rinsing with cold or tempered water, and (d) the application of an acidified recirculated final rinse to aid in removing alkaline films and in controlling water hardness deposits. These steps may occur in one continuous sequence and may be followed by a sanitizing rinse utilizing chlorine or iodophors just prior to placing the equipment back into use.

Spray cleaning programs differ from line cleaning programs in that pre-rinsing and post-rinsing are generally accomplished by a "burst" technique. Water will be discharged through the spray devices in three or more bursts of 15 to 30 seconds duration, and the vessel will be drained completely after each burst. This procedure is more effective in removing sedimented soil and foam than is continuous rinsing and can be accomplished with much less water. Cleaning temperatures may vary from 135–140°F (55-60°C) for storage tanks to as much as 160-180°F (70-80°C) for processing vessels with heat transfer surface.

Chlorinated alkaline cleaners varying in concentration from 1500 to 4500 ppm alkalinity and 50 to 100 ppm chlorine are highly effective in removing all types of fat, protein and carbohydrate based soil. Lightly acidified recirculated post-rinses (pH 5.5–6.0) are effective in removing residual alkaline films and producing a surface which dries free of water spots. Iodophor sanitizers containing sufficient acid to produce a pH of 2.6 to 5.0 at the use concentration are sometimes applied to accomplish the neutralization of the alkaline film and chemical sanitizing in one step. Such programs have been utilized on vessels of stainless steel construction, glass-lined construction and also on mild steel vessels protected by various types of coatings and linings (brewery vessels).

These procedures have been applied in fluid milk plants, ice cream plants, cheese plants, edible soy bean processes, and various types of food processing operations with uniform success. In the brewing industry, they have been applied to clean cookers, mixers, brew kettles, fermentation tanks, storage tanks, and spent grains holding equipment. Extensive piping systems often include centrifugal machines and heat exchangers. Chemical cleaning and sanitizing has produced results substantially superior to those previously achieved through hand-washing and chemical sanitizing or steam sterilization at atmospheric pressure.

It is possible to design and apply equipment and programs which can produce product contact surfaces that are physically clean and nearly free of all bacterial contamination. Standard swab tests from piping and spray cleaned equipment from properly operated single-use CIP system will yield plates showing no growth in 75–80% of all samples and plates showing not more than 3 to 5 colonies on the remaining samples (as compared to an allowable 50 colonies per plate), when sampling is done immediately following cleaning and before sanitizing. If equipment is properly handled, there will be no positive coliform counts on any swab taken from surfaces cleaned by in-place cleaning procedures.

In summary, experience has shown that it is possible to remove any soil, from any smooth, non-corrosive equipment surface, in any water, by use of a chelated alkali, an additive for controlling water hardness and "building" detergency, sodium hypochlorite, and a phosphoric based blended acid. The concentrations, combinations of ingredients, and sequence of application, as well as the application of the detergent solution is best controlled through proper engineering design of the processing system, the CIP system and an integrated control system to assure that all components function in harmony.

ii. An overview of cleaning programs for the pharmaceutical process

The summary statement of the previous section is equally applicable to those segments of the pharmaceutical industry with which the author has had experience. Similar programs, with reference to solutions and sequence of application, have been applied to parenteral solutions systems used for the production of total parenteral nutrition solutions of lipids, amino acids and dextrose water. Other processes effectively cleaned by CIP include human blood plasma fractionation, gamma globulin and serum albumin production, powdered drugs in water solutions, and therapeutic creams and ointments.

Comparable programs have also been applied to cleaning drying equipment used for producing powdered drugs, and with slight modification (depending upon membrane material), for cleaning ultra-filtration systems used for processing pharmaceutical products.

The only significant deviation from these programs is the use of WFI for all functions including the pre-rinse, solution make-up, post-rinse and acidified recirculated final rinse. Additional WFI is used to rinse the acid solution from the process system and supply/return piping. In describing "An Automated System for Cleaning Tanks and Parts Used in the Processing of Pharmaceuticals", Grimes reported the use of a comparable program provided by an eductor-based recirculating unit (1977). This procedure differed primarily in the use of reverse osmosis water as make-up water for the alkaline detergent wash solution and the acidified rinse and a subsequent post-rinse. The final rinse was accomplished with Purified Water, USP or WFI.

iii. Chemicals and chemical feed systems

A major portion of all dairy, food processing and pharmaceutical equipment can be effectively cleaned with a solution (solvent) which is 99½ to 99¾ percent water. The chemicals which make up the remainder of this solution may be supplied in liquid or dry form. The single-use systems require the use of liquid ingredients as these systems lack a solution tank of adequate size in which to make-up the cleaning solution. Therefore, air-operated pumps and/or diaphragm-type chemical feed pumps are generally used to feed the required ingredients in the proper quantities and ratios. Concentration control is accomplished by adding a known quantity of the chemical ingredients to a known quantity of water which is, at that time, recirculating within the circuit being cleaned.

The concentration of cleaning solutions in re-use recirculating units is generally monitored by a conductivity cell. These systems are programmed to "waste" a small part of the solution in the system at the end of each cleaning program, to continuously remove soiled solution from the system. Fresh water is added to bring the solution tank to the operating level, at which point the conductivity-cell based chemical feed system will add more cleaner. The chemical(s) may be provided in liquid form and pumped into the tank (Figure 1) or it (they) may be supplied as dry material(s). In the latter instance, the initial charge is often via manual addition of the cleaner to the solution tank and to a pre-dissolving tank mounted above the solution tank. The conductivity cell signal is then used to add water to the dissolving tank, causing overflow of a solution of high concentration to the CIP unit recirculating tank.

Typical liquid products available from Klenazde for use with either single-use or re-use recirculating units include AC-101™ (heavy-duty alkali), AC-3™ and AC-300™ (heavy-duty acids) and XY-12™ (liquid sodium hypochlorite). Status™ is a water conditioning additive suitable for hard waters (not required when using WFI, or water of comparable quality). These products are typical of those which would be blended under automatic control in widely varying concentrations to remove a variety of soils. Less demanding soils may be handled with Principal™, a blended liquid chlorinated detergent formulated to achieve the results of a mixture of AC-101™, Status™ and XY-12™.

CIP-Pres™ (an alkaline cleaner), Clenesco Chlorinating Liquid™ and Hicid™ (acid) offered by Clenesco may be used in a similar manner, as can Interest® (liquid chlorinated alkali), Sentol® (acid) offered by Diversey Wyandotte. This company also supplies a dry chlorinated alkaline cleaner (Simbol®) suitable for use with the powder-feed systems described above.

Many of the above products are available in both 55-gallon barrels and in bulk, by chemical transport tanker.

iv. Suggested parameters for development of cleaning programs

Reference was made in Section 2.D.i to pre-rinsing piping systems until the effluent runs nearly clear. This application could apply to a piping system which was a single continuous circuit. Some automated processes utilize air-operated valving to control flow through a multiplicity of branch circuits, in which instance it is necessary to assure proper rinsing of each branch until the effluent runs clear. Further, if the air-operated valves are of the compression type, with stem O-rings, it is necessary to move those valves, under pressure and flow conditions, to effectively rinse, wash and again rinse the stem O-ring area. Seiberling and Harper determined that the stem O-rings would clean satisfactorily under experimental conditions if the valves were moved 4–6 times during each step of the cleaning program (1957b). In practice it has been found that the application of valve sequencing programs which move each valve 2–3 times during the pre-rinse, 4–6 times during the solution wash, and 2–3 times during the post-rinse and acidified recirculated rinse produce satisfactory results. This same practice would be applied to the final rinse with Purified Water in a pharmaceutical application.

The volume of water required to rinse a piping circuit is normally found to be 1½ to 2 times the volume contained in the piping. That volume will need to be increased in automated systems if the length of the branches differ substantially unless provisions are made to control the rinsing time for each branch independently. On this basis, the total water requirement for a complete program for a piping system would be in the magnitude of 6 to 8 times the volume of the circuit for a single-use recirculating unit in a dairy application assuming a pre-rinse, solution wash, post-rinse and acidified recirculated rinse. The additional final rinsing required in a pharmaceutical process might increase the total water requirement to 10 to 12 times the volume of the piping system.

This volume would be decreased by 15–20% for a re-use system which utilizes the same wash solution for a number of circuits. The solution tank for the re-use system would need to be large enough to hold the entire volume of the largest circuit cleaned by that system.

v. Cleaning temperature and pressure control and recording

The "3-A Accepted Practice" applied in the dairy industry and often used as guidelines by other users of Clean-In-Place technology states under Item F.(4) "Solution temperature shall be automatically controlled by the use of a temperature regulator with a response range of plus or minus 5°F." This is loosely adherred to in practice, if at all, as there is no requirement for a specific cleaning temperature, for any application.

Item F.(5) of the same Standards requires a "recording thermometer having a scale range of 60–180°F with extension of scale on either side permitted: graduated in time scale divisions of not more than 15 minutes. Between 110–180°F, the chart shall be graduated in temperature divisions of not more than 2°F, spaced not less than $\frac{1}{16}''$ apart, and be accurate within 2°F plus or minus. The sensor shall be protected against damage at 212°F, the sensing element of the recording thermometer shall be located in the return solution line." This requirement is enforced and is given attention on all plant inspections and survey ratings. The intent of this requirement is to provide a chart record of the cleaning time and temperature relationship, in recognition that the effectiveness of this essentially chemical procedure is determined by time, temperature and solution concentration.

This supposition assumes proper hydraulic performance. Richter (1975) evaluated a re-use system and a single-use system to clean transport tankers fitted with permanently installed spray devices, and during this study found it necessary to make many modifications of the re-use system to bring it to the same level of performance as achieved with the single-use system, even though suitable chart records had been previously produced for a long period of time. Cleaning solution may remain stagnant in the return system, at wash temperature, while the return pump is air-bound for prolonged periods of time, and this condition ultimately impacts on the performance of the supply pump, also. Therefore, a temperature recorder alone may suggest a suitable recirculation period, whereas flow (and cleaning) actually occurred for only a portion of that time.

All of the more than 700 single-use and single-use eductor assisted recirculating units installed under the author's supervision during the past 25 years have included a pressure recording pen in the same case with the return line temperature recorder. A special chart with both temperature and pressure graduations is used and the two pens provide a concurrent record of temperature, time and CIP supply pump discharge pressure. The pressure pen produces a record of hydraulic performance during the cleaning program which is an asset in controlling system operation and troubleshooting (Seiberling, 1976b).

Heating during recirculation is mandatory as the total heat required is more closely related to the mass of stainless steel that must be brought to temperature than to the quantity of solution in the system. Until recent years, heating was most commonly accomplished by direct injection of steam, by a mixer in the solution tank in the case of the re-use system, and by a mixer on the suction side of the CIP supply pump in the case of the single-use system. Many current systems are being installed with stainless steel shell and tube heat exchangers in the CIP supply line, permitting high-pressure steam to be used for faster heating, and also provide for recovery of condensate, thereby reducing boiler water treatment requirements.

The single-use eductor assisted system shown in Figure 4, as applied in a pharmaceutical process, uses direct injection of steam produced from WFI via a pure steam generator. The eductor based system reported by Grimes was equipped with a shell and tube heat exchanger (1977).

There are no shell and tube heat exchangers currently available that are fabricated fully in compliance with 3-A Standards, giving consideration to internal gasketing, welding standards, or inlet and outlet connections of sanitary design.

vi. Re-use versus single-use of wash solution

The term "re-use" implies savings in water, heat, and chemicals. Those savings may exist if the equipment being cleaned is so lightly soiled that the major portion of the soil is removed during the pre-rinse to drain. If, however, soil residues remain to be removed by the cleaning solution, then soil build-up must necessarily occur in the wash solution. A chlorinated alkaline detergent loses its effectiveness as the chlorine binds with the soil removed; i.e., the purpose of the chlorine is to enhance soil removal at lower levels of alkalinity. Therefore, re-use systems are generally operated at higher levels of alkalinity than single-use systems when used for removing comparable soil loads.

Soil build-up in a re-use system solution tank is controlled either by extending the pre-rinse to effectively rinse out most of the soil before initiating the wash recirculation, wasting a portion of the solution at the end of each solution wash and replenishing the tank via the addition of clear water and chemical or both.

When reporting a field study of milk transport tank washing systems Richter stated that the re-use system "required more water than the single-use system to achieve (nearly) equivalent results" (1975). The re-use system evaluated in this study included a 500 gallon (2000L) wash solution tank which was dumped only twice weekly, and was used for cleaning 25 tankers and 7 storage tanks per week. This is equivalent to 32 operations per 1000 gallons (4000L) (spray cleaning programs only) for approximately 30 gallons (120L) of solution per vessel cleaned. In addition, the re-use system required between 550 and 800 gallons (2000 and 3000L) of water for the pre-rinse and post-rinse cycles. As suming an average of 600 gallons (2400L) per vessel, this would equate to approximately 19,000 gallons (76,000L) per week or 20,000 gallons (80,000L) total water requirement for 32 spray cleaning cycles. By comparison, the single-use system used 205 gallons (800L) per vessel, or approximately 6500 gallons (26,000L) for 32 vessels, including 45 gallons (180L) of fresh solution for the wash.

Seiberling reported an analysis of the cost of cleaning using liquid chemicals and automatic feeding systems in six dairy facilities which processed comparable volumes of milk, ice cream and cottage cheese on a daily basis (1976d). Seven re-use systems and eight single-use systems were installed in these plants. Whereas it was impossible to make direct comparisons on the basis of loads, equipment cleaned, and the cost of liquid chemicals, the reduction of the data to establish an individual cost for a uniform CIP load suggested that the cost of chemicals was only slightly greater for the single-use system.

A processor conducted study of single-use systems and European-type re-use systems was reported by Olenfalk (1975). This internal report dealt with technical factors, safety problems, sewer problems, steam consumption, space requirements and economic factors. The report was highly favorable to the single-use system and included a comment, "The single-use system has an essential advantage which is not valued monetarily in here. The system requires hardly any supervision, work or adjusting which most of the other recycling re-use systems require, no daily controlling of the concentration and adding of detergent, control of pH or conductivity."

In the early 1970's a solution recovery tank was added to many single-use systems, this tank and associated valving being used to recover spent solution and post-rinse water and re-use that water/solution mixture as part of the pre-rinse for the next cleaning cycle. Internal evaluation of that program by a regional multi-plant processor showed water, chemicals and steam savings estimated at approximately $4,000/yr. when cleaning 200 tanks/week (Seiberling, 1976a).

During the past decade, the cost of water and its disposal has been one of the most greatly accelerated costs related to Clean-In-Place procedures. In the pharmaceutical application, this water must be further processed through conversion to WFI or equivalent before use in a CIP system, at further capital and operating costs. Giving consideration to the risk of cross contamination which accompanies the application of a re-use system, it would appear that the processor of parenteral solutions should carefully review both types of systems before reaching a decision based on economic factors heavily weighted with regard to the cost of the required cleaning materials. Reliability, performance and control should receive primary consideration.

3. CIP Application to Solutions Processes

As noted previously, Clean-In-Place procedures were initially developed for dairy processes which necessitate continuous receiving, temporary storage, process ing and packaging on a 24-hour basis in the larger plants. Regulations require that each processing tank and the complete piping system (or any portion thereof) be cleaned following each period of use. This makes it necessary to install the traditional (extensive and expensive) CIP supply/return piping system previously described in Section 2.C. However, product flow may be controlled via air-operated valves under either manual or automatic control. These valves may be installed individually on tank inlets and outlets, individually for shut-off purposes or for flow-rate or pressure control within transfer lines, or in large valve manifolds for controlling flows from multiple sources to multiple destinations in a very flexible manner. In this latter instance, a single air-operated valve is frequently the only separation of one product stream from another and failure to achieve proper closure would result in inter-mixing of two product streams.

The production of parenteral solution requires, by comparison, the ability to establish and maintain the integrity of the product through every step of the process, an objective best accomplished by eliminating all valves between various product streams.

A. U-bend transfer panel design and application

i. Description and derivation

U-bend transfer panels have been combined with highly-automated "sub-systems" in developing designs, installing, and placing into operation several successful parenteral solution systems. This approach provides the maximum flexibility for the production function, yet makes it possible to assure controlled sanitation through mechanical/chemical cleaning and further guarantee the integrity of all individual product and cleaning and/or sterilizing flow-paths. The U-bend transfer panels (Electrol) are the result of continued modification and application of the component commonly referred to as a "flow-verter" or "cleaning hook-up station" used in the past primarily to control CIP solution distribution.

ii. Application

Figure 7 is a schematic drawing of a panel and interconnecting piping between four process tanks and four processing systems. The number of tanks could be increased by lengthening the panel and adding additional rows of ports identical to those shown on either side of the breakline. Additional processes would require design modifications including the provision of more horizontal headers.

With reference to Figure 7, the pairs of lines numbered 1–4 and identified as Lines To and From Processes might, for example, connect each of those tanks to (1) a CIP system, (2) a drug mixing system, (3) a filtration system enroute to one filler and (4) a filtration system enroute to a second filler. The options are limited only by the requirements and are determined by the need for simultaneous, but totally isolated, operations. This concept has been converted to practice (Figures 8, 9 and 10) in an operating installation which makes it possible to use any of 8 tanks, individually or simultaneously, in the following manner:

Figure 7—Schematic Diagram of U-bend Transfer Panel Application

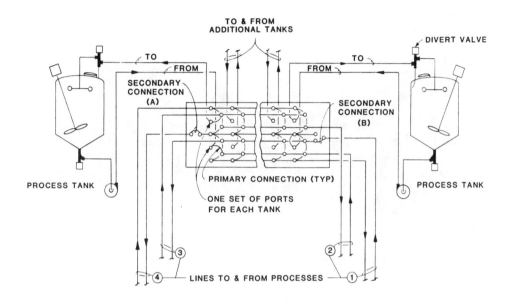

1. Rinse a tank or transfer path with WFI to drain.
2. Fill a tank with WFI for solution make-up.
3. Recirculate WFI from the source tank through a mixing tank for incorporation of the drug ingredients.
4. Pre-coat a pre-filter with a filter aid prepared in a pre-coat tank.
5. Establish flow from any one of eight tanks through any one of three pre-filter lines, each providing access to either of two available pre-filter housings, and continue flow from the selected pre-filter to a packaging line through final filters at that location.
6. Steam sterilize any tank or transfer line individually.
7. Steam sterilize the total system including all eight tanks, all pumps, all pre-filter housings, all piping, and all of the headers and piping associated with the U-bend transfer panel in a single operation at completion of day's production.

Figure 8—Shop Fabricated Flow Control System (Front)

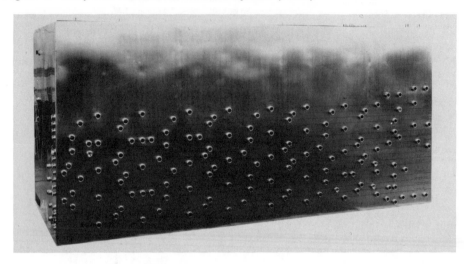

Figure 9—Shop Fabricated Flow Control System (Rear)

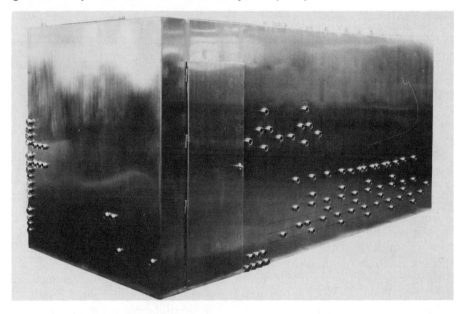

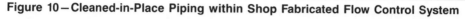

Figure 10—Cleaned-in-Place Piping within Shop Fabricated Flow Control System

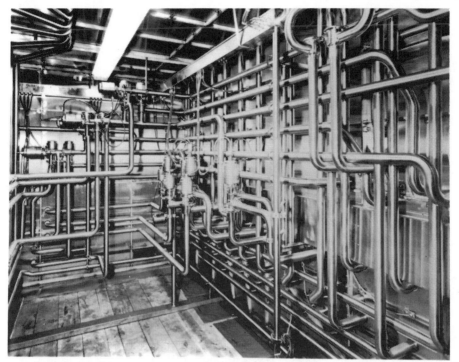

The through-the-wall transfer panel illustrated in Figure 11 was developed to permit installation of tankage in a warehouse area, with all of the connections from that tankage terminating on the clean room side of the panel. The components provided for product/CIP flow-control automation include air-operated CIP cleanable valves, air-blow control valves, and filters for the sterile air or gas blow-down system. A smaller free-standing transfer panel equipped with WFI and steam shut-off and leak-protection valves is shown in Figure 12. This is typical of a panel designed to permit installation of final filters in a filler supply line as well as providing the means of rinsing and steaming those filters and completing integrity tests prior to placing the system into operation.

iii. Elimination of dead-ends

The utilization of headers in transfer panels as described above requires special emphasis on the elimination of any dead-ends. A branch of a tee (for example, the port from the header to the skin of the transfer panel) must be limited to approximately 1½ pipe diameters to allow recirculation cleaning at normal velocities. Figure 13 shows two methods of keeping a header "live" from one end

Figure 11—Transfer Panel with Valves and Filters

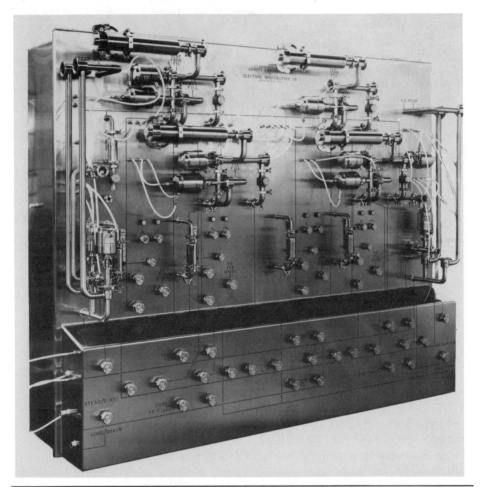

to the other, even though flow may be to the header and from the header at intermediate points. The double-tube arrangement is the least space consuming but requires access to one or both ends to install the internal tube, or remove it for inspection. The loop-type header functions equally well hydraulically, but requires more installation space in the enclosure. Figure 14 shows typical components utilized to convert the double-tube header concept to practice. Figure 15 more clearly illustrates the installation of the internal tube in a short header on a small transfer panel and shows one set of spacers (spider) used to center and support the internal tube. In dairy applications this concept has been used

Figure 12—Filter Transfer Panel

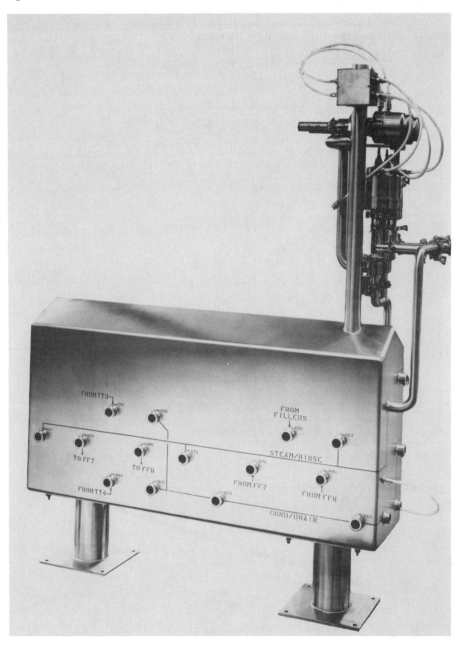

to construct 4″ (100mm) headers with 2½″ (65mm) internal tubes in excess of 120 feet (36M) total length to operate at flow-rates up to 600 Gpm (2400 Lpm).

Figure 13—Double-Tube and Loop-Type Headers

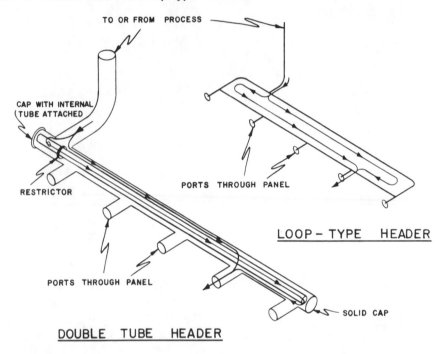

TO OR FROM PROCESS

CAP WITH INTERNAL TUBE ATTACHED

RESTRICTOR

PORTS THROUGH PANEL

LOOP-TYPE HEADER

PORTS THROUGH PANEL

SOLID CAP

DOUBLE TUBE HEADER

Figure 14—Internal Parts of Double-Tube Headers

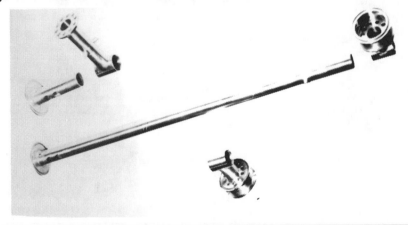

Figure 15—Transfer Panel with Double-Tube Header

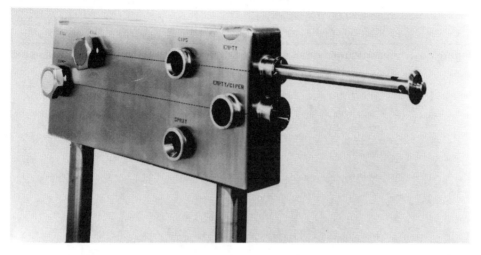

iv. Proximity sensors

The use of manually positioned U-bends for establishing processing, Clean-In-Place, and Steam-In-Place connections in a highly automated system requires some means of verifying the integrity of the required flow paths. This has been accomplished in practice by installing permanent magnets in stainless steel enclosures welded to the center of the U-bend connections (Figure 16). Proximity switches located behind the skin of the panel (Figure 17) may then be used to detect the presence or absence of a U-bend between any selected pair of ports. The computer or progammable controller data base is developed to include the "allowed" or "required" connection for every established flow path necessary for processing, cleaning, or sterilizing procedures. The use of this data may be as simple as not allowing a process to start until proper connections have been established or, in a more sophisticated system, providing operator prompting for removal and reinstallation of U-bends. These systems have proven highly reliable and effective; the associated control logic can be used for both interlock (preventing improper starts) or inhibits (providing automatic shut-down and alarm) purposes.

The transfer panels shown in Figure 16 were designed to incorporate small filter housings at precise points within the piping system. The identification names and numbers on these stainless steel panels are Lectroetch® on the surface of the stainless steel and are quite durable, requiring physical grinding and/or polishing with a harsh abrasive to remove the mark. Brief and concise nomenclature on the panels is easily referenced in operating manuals. With only a general understanding of the process, an operator can determine most of the connections for a given operation from the legends on the various ports.

Figure 16—Transfer Panels used as Filter Supports, with U-Bend Position Sensors

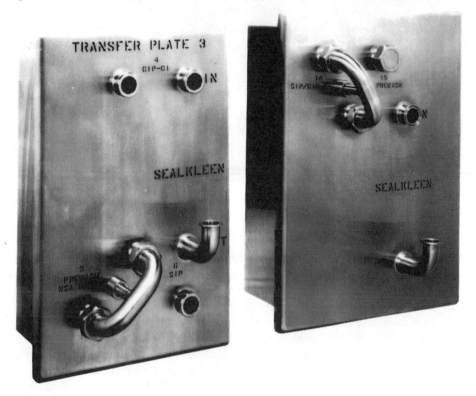

B. Air-operated valves

Both diaphragm-type and compression-type valves have been used satisfactorily for parenteral solutions processing systems (Tri-Clover). A sterile system requires either a diaphragm valve (Figure 18) or a compression valve of aseptic design (Figure 19). Conventional compression valves are widely used in systems which are steam sterilized but which are not operated aseptically, the general criteria being a piping system design which places all valves and connections in the clean room area.

The effective recirculating cleaning of a complex piping system requires valve sequencing programs to operate the valves in proper combinations throughout the cleaning program to cause water and/or cleaning solutions to first pass through the piping system in one direction, then another, in as many as six or eight different manners so that every port of every valve will be effectively cleaned, and so that valve stem O-rings on compression-type valves are properly cleaned (Section 2.D.iv). All portions of every valve and every part of the piping system must be exposed to equivalent mechanical/chemical treatment.

Prior to late 1985, the pharmaceutical process engineer was unable to select air-operated valves, tubing or fittings of sanitary construction, in sizes of less that 1″ (25mm) O.D. tube diameter. Fractional size fittings and valves fabricated to 3-A Standards are now available. Typical valves are shown in Figure 20.

Figure 17—Proximity Switch Installation behind Transfer Panel Face

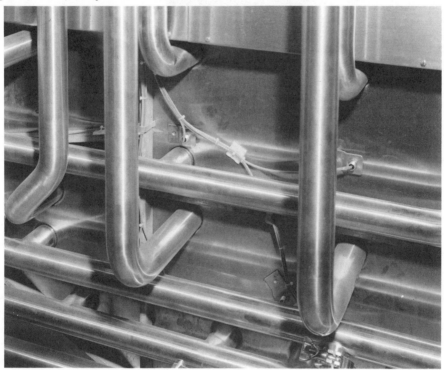

C. Overview of solution manufacturing process

Figure 21 is a Schematic Diagram of a composite system which embodies many of the concepts used in actual practice. This system includes the following:

Figure 18—Air-Operated Diaphragm-Type Valve with Bevel Seat Thread Connections

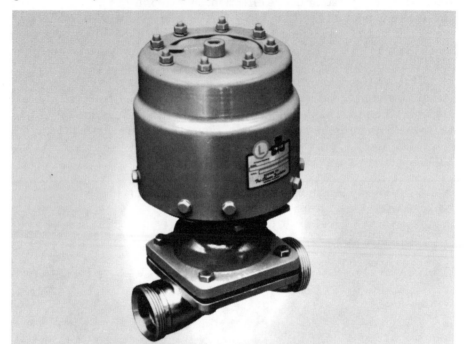

1. A WFI bump tank with breather filter, pump and WFI recirculation/supply loop which provides the means of separating the WFI supply to this system from the remainder of the processing facility. This system could include a heater or cooler, as required.
2. A mechanically agitated mix tank for dissolving drugs in WFI.
3. A filtering system consisting of a pre-filter (F1) and two final filters (F2-3) between the mix tank and a hold tank.
4. Vent filters and the required complement of vent, gas and steam valves for the pre-filter, final filters and hold tank, permitting these items to be operated as a sterile system.
5. A cleaning hook-up station CHS-1 which makes it possible to physically connect the CIP recirculating unit into the WFI loop so as to utilize the WFI piping as the CIP supply line, and simultaneously clean the WFI bump tank and pump.
6. A product hook-up station PHS-1 to provide a manual disconnect of this portion of the process from the continuation so that these tanks, filters, and interconnecting piping can be cleaned as a unit while product remains in the downstream portion of the system.

Figure 19—Air-Operated Compression Valve for Aseptic Processes

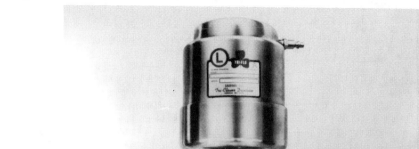

This schematic drawing identifies the major lines and components and identifies all valves by number, the valve nomenclature including an alphabetical character which defines control of water, CIP solution, sterile gas, steam, product or drain flows. Note also the identification of traps, level transmitters and level sensors. In practice, this schematic diagram would also include and identify all RTD's, proximity sensors, pressure sensors and all other required instrumentation. This nomenclature is necessary for the development of process system descriptions, control program sequences, operating manuals, and validation documentation.

Although it is a common engineering practice to develop schematic diagrams showing a process from left-to-right with the utilities at the top and the drains at the bottom, for CIP/SIP (Clean-In-Place and Sterilize-In-Place) purposes it is beneficial to prepare the schematic diagram to conform with the geo-

Figure 20 — Air-Operated and Hand-Operated Compression Valves of Various Types in Fractional Sizes

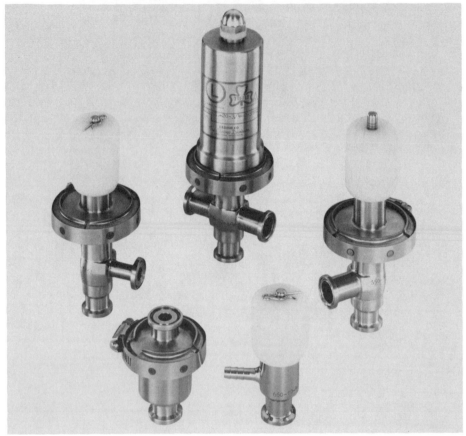

graphical arrangement of the equipment in the processing facility. This approach enables better understanding of the product flows, pitch directions, and drain points, all essential to the completion of the detail design of the cleaning and sterilizing piping and control systems.

Assuming that the system has been cleaned, assembled in the process configuration, sterilized, and is ready for production, the operation of the system shown in Figure 21 for processing, cleaning and sterilizing would be as follows:

Figure 21—Schematic Diagram of Solutions Process with CIP System

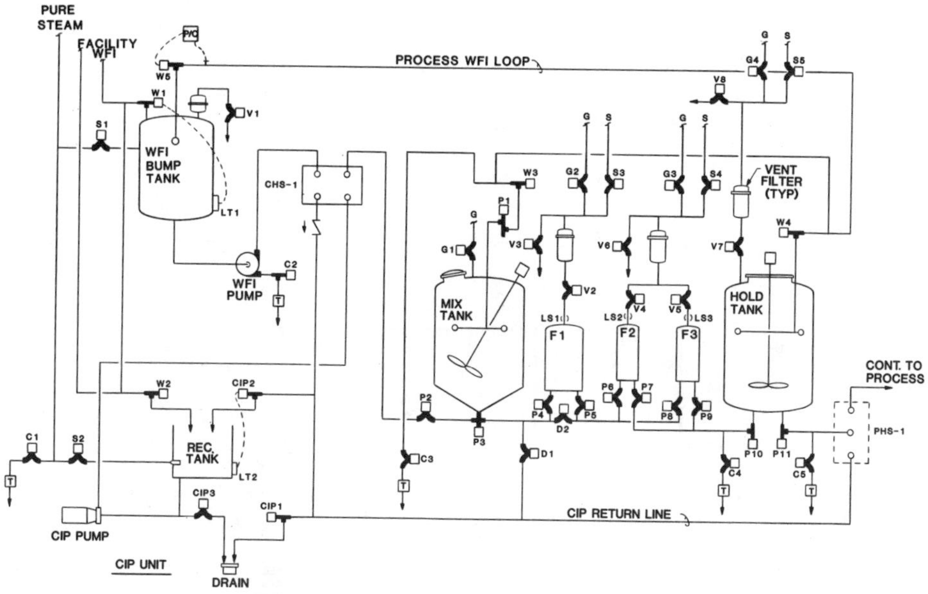

i. Processing

The operation of the WFI supply loop is shown as a heavy-line on Figure 22. The arrowheads identified WFI indicate the direction of WFI flow. Water from the facility's supply loop would be admitted to the WFI bump tank via valve W1 under control of LT1. The WFI pump would provide recirculation through the process system WFI loop, back pressure valve W5 being used to maintain a fixed pressure on this loop at all times. WFI would be supplied to the mix tank via valve W3 following which other ingredients of the solution would be added through the manhole, or through alternative support systems which might discharge to this point. The mix tank could be load-cell mounted, if required.

Following agitation, sampling for any required analysis, and approval of the mix formulation, the product would be discharged through pre-filter F1 and one of the final filters F2-3 in accordance with the heavy-line flow path identified with the "P" arrowheads. A typical sequence to accomplish automatic filling of the filters would include (a) open valve P9, P4, V2 and V3 and pressurize the mix tank via valve G1 to fill F1, and when liquid reaches level sensor LS1,

(b) close V2 and V3 and open P5, P6, V4 and V6 to continue flow to F2. Then, when liquid reaches LS2 (c) close V4 and V6 and open P7 and P10 to establish flow to the hold tank, opening V7 and V8 at that time to vent the tank through the breather filter.

Figure 22 — Tank-to-Tank Transfer through Filters

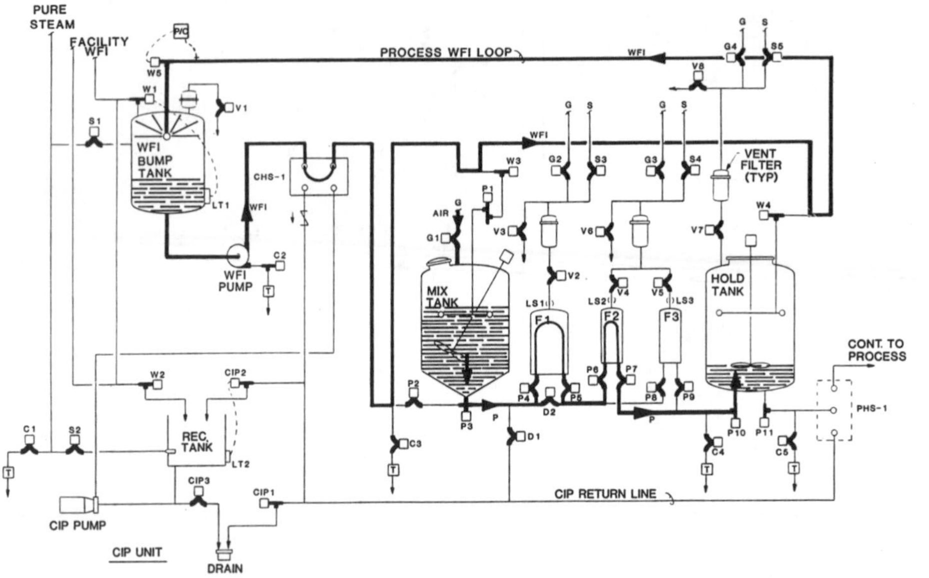

When the mix tank empties, the gas supply valves would be utilized to clear the final product from F1 and F2-3 and the continuing piping to the hold tank. At the end of the required hold period in the sterile tank, that tank would be pressurized via the gas supply line, vent filter and valves G4 and V7 as P11 was opened to provide flow through the product hook-up station to the continuation of the process.

A WFI rinse of the product solution to the continuation of the process is available under automatic control as shown on Figure 23. As the hold tank empties, valve W4 would be opened to spray the vessel with WFI, the quantity being determined by timed flow at a constant pressure or by weight if the tank were mounted on load-cells. This quantity could be established and controlled on the basis of that necessary to fill the pipe to the next process vessel.

Figure 23—WFI Rinse from Hold Tank to Remainder of Process

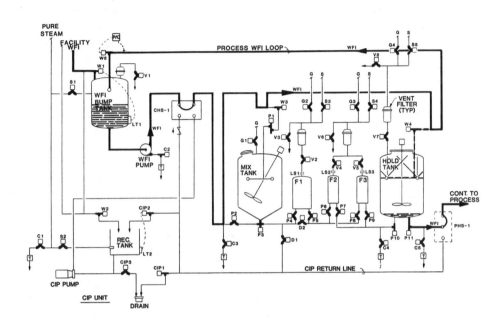

ii. Recirculation cleaning of process tanks and piping

Following completion of the use of this portion of the system, preparation for cleaning would include:

1. Removal of filter elements from F1-3 and the vent filters and reassembly of the filters for the Clean-In-Place operation.
2. Reposition U-bends on CHS-1 to place the CIP system into the WFI recirculation loop.
3. Reposition the U-bend on PHS-1 to connect the discharge line from valve P11 to the CIP return line.
4. Manually clean the manhole gasket and manhole rim on the mix tank, and then close the tank for the Clean-In-Place process.

The CIP circuits for cleaning the mix tank, hold tank, transfer piping and filters are shown on Figures 24 and 25. The initial step of the cleaning procedure would be to pressurize the tanks with gas or sterile air via the available supply header to the gas valves. The pressure required would be equal to the pressure drop through the return system at the cleaning solution flow rate, plus 2-3 psi (14-20 KPa) additional to achieve proper throttling control of valve CIP2, based on level in the CIP unit recirculation tank. To make this return flow concept function, the CIP program would be developed to start the solution wash with sufficient water in the recirculating tank to fill the supply/return piping, provide the desired operating level in the recirculating tank, plus 5 to 10 gallons (20–40L) to form the puddle in the vessel being cleaned. When the tanks are load-cell mounted, an alternative approach found workable in practice uses tank weight to control the puddle volume by operating the outlet valves.

Figure 24 – CIP Circuit for Cleaning Mix Tank and/or Hold Tank

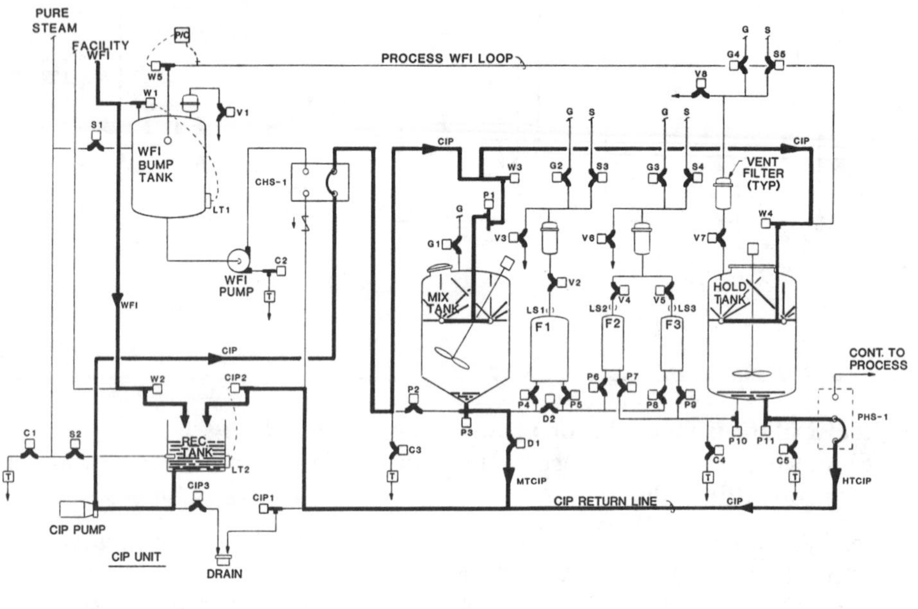

Following tank pressurization, WFI would be supplied to the CIP unit from the main facility system via valve W2 and the CIP pump would start, producing flow through the WFI loop and the tanks in a sequence of 4 steps:

1. The first sub-circuit would treat the filters and lines in accordance with the CIP circuit shown on Figure 24. The CIP pump would discharge through valve P2 and the downstream valves in an appropriate sequence to pressure wash F1-3 inclusive, with discharge from the filters continuing through valve P10 to the hold tank, thence through valve P11 to the CIP return line.

Figure 25 – CIP Circuit for Cleaning Filters and Transfer Piping with Hold Tank

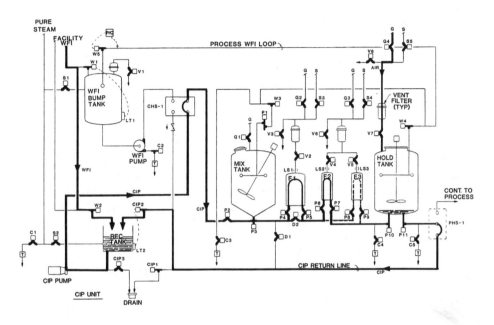

2. Water and/or solution would be supplied to the mix tank spray via valves W3 and P1, with valve P1 being pulsed to provide intermittent flow through the tank fill connection. The tank outlet valve P3 and drain valve D1 would be open, providing return flow from the tank to the CIP unit via tank pressurization. This flow path is shown on Figure 25 by the arrowhead identified "MTCIP".

3. Open valve W4 to supply the hold tank spray and open P11 to provide return flow via PHS-2 to establish flow via the arrowhead HTCIP on Figure 25.

4. During the above steps, return flow would be via CIP1 to the drain for the pre-rinse and post-rinse. For the solution wash return flow would be via valve CIP2 to the solution tank, this valve being operated under instrument control on the basis of a signal derived from the solution tank level transmitter LT2, thus maintaining a fixed volume of solution in the recirculation tank to eliminate "blow-down" of the tank being spray cleaned, hence loss of top pressure.

During the solution wash recirculation, pure steam produced from WFI would be introduced directly to the recirculation tank via valve F2 to heat the solution to the required temperature and chemicals would be added either manually or automatically, depending upon the type of system provided. At completion of the CIP program, drain valve CIP1 would be open as would all of the process valves and gas or sterile air admitted to the tanks and to the top of the filters would clear the final rinse solution from all of the piping.

The flow paths described above would be established in a repetitive sequence as previously described to assure proper pre-rinsing, solution washing and post-rinsing of all portions of the system.

iii. Recirculation cleaning of WFI loop

Following completion of use of the complete system supported by the WFI recirculation loop, the WFI piping, bump tank and pump would be cleaned in accordance with Figure 26. WFI would be supplied to the CIP unit from the main facility system via valve W2 and the CIP pump would start, providing flow through the WFI loop to valve W5 which would supply the spray in the WFI bump tank. Valve W5 would be opened under instrument control on the basis of a signal derived from the bump tank level transmitter LT1, thus maintaining a fixed volume of solution in the bump tank to prevent cavitation of the WFI pump due to vortex development at the tank outlet. The WFI pump would provide return flow to the recirculating unit, and valve CIP2 would be fully open for this program. As for the process tanks and lines, the cleaning program would include a pre-rinse to drain, a solution wash, and a post-rinse to drain.

iv. Sterilize-In-Place procedure

Following completion of the Clean-In-Place programs for both the process tanks and piping and the WFI loop, manual preparation for steam sterilization and subsequent production would include the following:
1. Filter elements would be reinstalled in the filter housings.
2. The U-bends on CHS-1 and PHS-1 would be restored to the process configuration.

The automatically controlled sequence would be initiated to provide Steam-In-Place sterilization of the complete system including the process system WFI recirculation loop, the process tanks and piping and the filter housings with the filter elements installed. This automatically controlled sequence would include three major steps:

1. Condensate drain valves C1-5 would be opened to permit condensate discharge through the traps to the drain or an appropriate collection system.
2. Vent valve V1 on the WFI bump tank would be opened to vent that tank and back pressure valve W5 would be opened following which pure steam from WFI would be admitted to the WFI bump tank. Following venting of the bump tank and closure of V1, the WFI recirculation loop

Figure 26—CIP Circuit for Cleaning WFI System

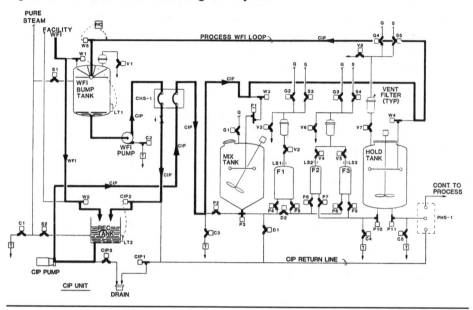

Figure 27—Steam-in-Place Circuit including WFI System

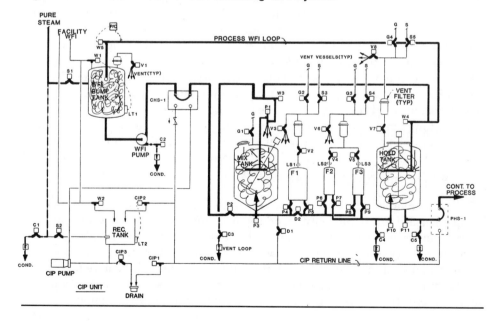

would be used to supply steam to the mix tank and hold tank. The outlet valves and drain valves associated with these tanks and the filters would all be opened and steam would be admitted to the two vessels and the three filters in an appropriate sequence, automatically controlling the vent valves to first vent the vessels, and then closing these valves and adding additional steam via steam valves S3-5 inclusive.

3. Following sufficient time at the required temperature and pressure, as determined by properly located RTD's, the steam supply would be turned "Off" and the gas valves G1-4 would be utilized to pressurize the system with sterile gas during the cool-down period, blowing the final condensate through the traps. The Steam-In-Place circuit is shown on Figure 27.

A system designed and installed per the above example may be expanded to incorporate other items of equipment such as homogenizers, heat exchangers, and filling machines if this equipment is designed and installed so as to be compatible with the Clean-In-Place/Steam-In-Place procedures.

It should be noted that the capital investment for Clean-In-Place equipment in the above example is minimal, being limited to the CIP recirculating unit, two U-bend transfer panels, two spray devices, and several additional flow control valves. The remainder of the equipment and interconnecting piping would be necessary to meet the normal operating requirements for any process of like capability, the major difference being the replacement of hand-actuated valves with air-operated automatically controlled valves.

Whereas the above described system demonstrates the use of a very simple recirculating unit consisting primarily of a tank, pump, steam injection mixer, temperature and level controls, and five valves for controlling WFI and solution flow, the same general procedure would apply to alternative CIP systems described in Section 2.A. If pressure vessels were not required, thus providing the innovative use of tank pressurization to achieve return flow, a return pump could be located at the end of the CIP return line to pump through valves CIP1 and CIP2 to single-use or re-use systems. Alternatively, an eductor-based system could connect directly to the return system and draw water from the mix tanks and hold tanks. In either instance, these tanks (if not pressure-vacuum vessels) would require proper venting to prevent collapse due to the development of negative pressures, via the return pump or eductor, or due to rapid cooling of the air when following a solution wash with a lower temperature post-rinse medium.

The requirement for continuous monitoring of pressures, levels, flows and temperatures from many points, and the need for precise sequential control of valves, pumps and associated components would make it impractical to attempt to operate a system as described above under manual control. Automation of production operations, clean-in-place procedures and sterilize-in-place procedures is essential. For the remainder of this chapter, the phrase CIP/SIP solutions system will refer to a processing system designed to incorporate automatic control of production sequences and provide for automatically controlled Clean-In-Place and Steam-In-Place procedures.

4. Instrumentation for CIP/SIP Solution Systems

Automation of the Clean-In-Place and Steam-In-Place procedures for a solutions processing system requires the control of process variables including temperature, pressure, level, flow and possibly weight. There has been little instrumentation developed specifically for the parenteral solutions process. The process engineer must choose from available components used in dairy and food processing, and in other industries. The sensing devices described below, while not necessarily the ultimate, have provided satisfactory results in past installations, for a period of up to 10 years.

A. Temperature
An RTD (Resistance Temperature Device) may be easily interfaced to a programmable controller or computer via the appropriate input devices and provides an acceptable method of measuring temperature for processing, cleaning and sterilizing functions. Two different devices are shown on Figure 28. The strap-on RTD is non-intrusive and inexpensive (Degussa Corp.). However, process applications requires physical protection (and insulation) of the device and protection of the required wiring connections. Elaborate (and expensive) fittings have been developed to install strap-on RTD's on piping, and on the exterior skin of tanks. The simple method shown at the top of Figure 28 has provided equally acceptable performance with greater flexibility of application and at a lower cost.

A direct immersion RTD is available with sanitary clamp-type connections (Pyromation, Inc.) and may be used through tank sidewalls and in piping systems. This component provides complete protection of the sensing device and the wiring connections and will withstand substantial flow, pressure and physical abuse. When used in piping systems, the branch of the tee must be in a horizontal plane to assure proper cleaning. Installation in the sidewall of a processing tank requires use of a conical nozzle to assure effective cleaning by CIP procedures.

B. Pressure
Several different pressure sensors are available in sanitary construction. Figure 29 shows the typical application of a strain-gauge based sensor which can be clamped to an opening in the piping system or in a processing vessel (Viatron Corp.). Similar devices which use air as an intermediate measurement transmitting medium work equally well via installation of an I/P (current-to-pressure) transducer in the control loop.

C. Level
The measurement and control of level is both more diverse and more difficult than temperature or pressure. Liquid level in a process vessel may be determined

Figure 28—Temperature Sensing Devices

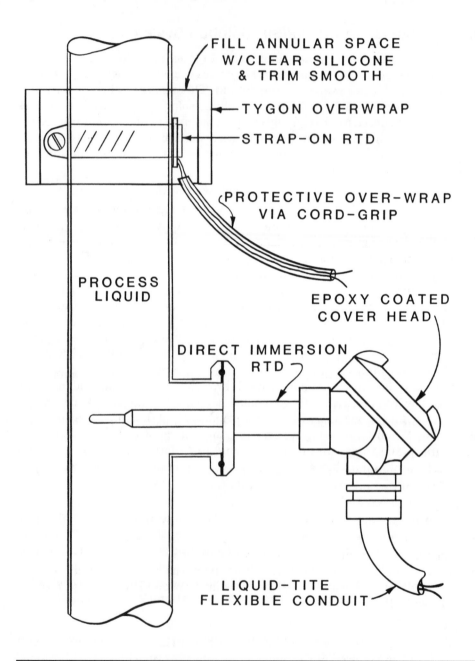

FILL ANNULAR SPACE
W/CLEAR SILICONE
& TRIM SMOOTH

TYGON OVERWRAP

STRAP-ON RTD

PROTECTIVE OVER-WRAP
VIA CORD-GRIP

PROCESS
LIQUID

EPOXY COATED
COVER HEAD

DIRECT IMMERSION
RTD

LIQUID-TITE
FLEXIBLE CONDUIT

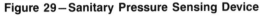

Figure 29—Sanitary Pressure Sensing Device

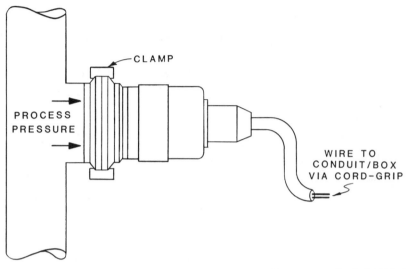

by using the diaphragm-type pressure sensor described above via an appropriate pressure/level algorithm in the control system. Since the pressure sensor must be located in the sidewall of the vessel to be susceptible to CIP cleaning, it is not possible to determine the level when the tank is approaching an "empty" condition.

A capacitance or RF probe with the appropriate amplifier (Endress & Hauser, Inc.) may be installed in a piping system to sense an air/liquid interface as shown in Figure 30. Probes of this type are generally impervious to foam or product build-up on the probe. They work best in liquids with a low dielectric constant (high conductance). Liquids having a low conductance; i.e., oils, may require substantially longer probe surface or may not work at all.

Probes are most generally used for sensing the interface at a specific point such as a high-level, low-level, or lack of solution at a pump inlet as a result of an empty tank. However, the analog output of a continuous capacitance probe has been successfully applied in some dairy processes to measure and control level in tanks ranging from 2 feet (0.6M) to 5 feet (1.5M) in total depth.

The ultrasonic clamp-on level sensor (Figure 30) is especially useful for sensing an air/liquid interface in a vertical pipe, and is the method used for controlling the automatic venting and filling of filters and described under Section III.C. These devices must be carefully installed, using an epoxy or silicone grease between the sensor and line to assure proper sonic attenuation (National Sonics).

D. Flow
The eductor-assisted CIP system (Figures 3 and 4) requires measurement of flow rate and volume to control the program sequence. The flow rate input is processed

Figure 30—Level Sensing Devices

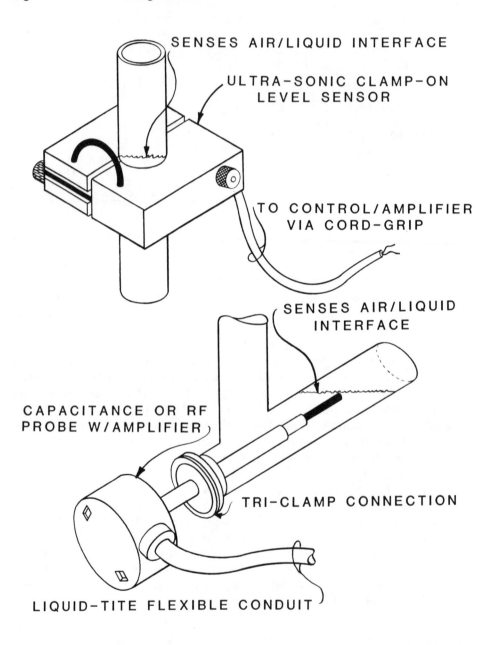

SENSES AIR/LIQUID INTERFACE

ULTRA-SONIC CLAMP-ON
LEVEL SENSOR

TO CONTROL/AMPLIFIER
VIA CORD-GRIP

SENSES AIR/LIQUID
INTERFACE

CAPACITANCE OR RF
PROBE W/AMPLIFIER

TRI-CLAMP CONNECTION

LIQUID-TITE FLEXIBLE CONDUIT

by the associated controller to regulate a throttling valve in the CIP supply line, assuring proper pressures on all sprays and proper velocities in all piping circuits and sub-circuits, under software control. The flow rate output is scaled and converted to pulses equivalent to gallons and all rinsing and wash recirculation is programmed on the basis of the quantity pumped through the system, rather than by time. This is a more precise and reliable approach then the conventional time-based system as the end result of the CIP program is based on a controlled quantity of solution having passed through the piping at a controlled rate of flow.

Sanitary vortex meters (The Foxboro Co.) have worked effectively for control of the CIP solution flows and have also been used for measuring the quantity of WFI delivered for automated preparation of buffer solutions.

E. Weight

Section 3.C. made reference to a load-cell mounted mix tank and suggested that the weighing system output would be utilized for control of both processing and CIP functions. The process vessel in Figure 32 is shown installed on load-cells of recent design more appropriately described as load beams (BLH Electronics). These devices require minimal deflection for weighing and the vessel can be rigidly connected to a properly supported welded piping system designed for CIP/SIP procedures. Practice has shown that the provision of as little as 3–4 feet (0.9–1.2M) of tubing between an outlet valve and a rigidly mounted pump, or between an inlet fitting and the interconnecting supply line will prevent the piping from affecting the accuracy of the weighing system. This is contradictory to the recommendations of the load-cell manufacturers who generally suggest the incorporation of flexible connections between the rigid piping and the load-cell mounted process tank. Those connections create substantial problems with respect to CIP/SIP.

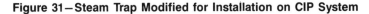

Figure 31 — Steam Trap Modified for Installation on CIP System

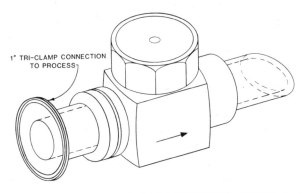

1" TRI-CLAMP CONNECTION TO PROCESS

5. Installation of Piping, Valves and Control System Components

To enjoy the maximum advantage of CIP/SIP procedures, the total solution processing system must be designed, engineered, and installed giving as much attention to the cleaning and sterilizing procedures as to the basic process requirement. The functional parts of the system to be considered in this respect include:

1. Product transfer piping, filters, valves, and pumps
2. U-bend transfer panels, if any
3. Process and CIP/SIP control system sensing devices and electrical and pneumatic connections

The design process must also give consideration to building arrangement, the installation and maintenance of the HVAC system, lighting, materials of construction for floors, walls and ceilings, and movement of people and material within the functional areas.

A. CIP/SIP piping system design

i. Material and finish

A product transfer system designed and installed for CIP/SIP procedures will be of stainless steel material, permanently installed. The tubing, fittings, valves, filter housings, pump heads and impellers and all other metal product contact components will be Type 304 stainless steel, or better. The pharmaceutical industry preference is generally for Type 304L or Type 316L, for welding considerations. Bigelow and DiVasto suggest that the exclusive choice for WFI systems is ANSI Grade 316L (low carbon) ASTM A270 stainless steel (1986). The ASTM A270 standard requires that the tube weld be rolled or hammered to a thickness matching the parent metal, with inside surfaces smooth and without severe scratches. The tubing will then be mechanically polished via a multi-grit process with the final grit varying from 150 to 320 depending on the individual user's specifications. The mechanical polishing process may be followed by electropolishing which further smooths the surface and contributes to the formation of a passive oxide film which adds to the corrosion resistance of the stainless steel. The final tubing should be free of weld bead, weld splatter, pits, folds, cracks and crevices, and weld porosity.

Highly finished stainless steel surfaces are considered to be more easily cleaned. Villafranca and Zambrano conclude, "The traditional stainless steel sanitary finish consists of a misleading and altered surface, having poor cleanability and poor corosion resistance (1985). On the other hand, the electro-polished finish provides the greatest cleaning feasibilities, reveals any flaws and can be used to produce a truly sound and smooth surface with a far greater durability than a conventional sanitary finish because of its corrosion resistance." Scanning electron microscopy techniques were applied by Zoltai, et. al to evaluate milk-contact surfaces as sites for possible microbial attachment (1981). However, this study did not evaluate the surfaces following attempted removal of the microorganisms by physical or mechanical/chemical cleaning procedures. The relative cleanability of Type 302 stainless steel panels having a No. 2B, 3, 4, and 7 finish respectively under identical conditions of soiling and spray cleaning was evaluated by Kaufmann, et. al using the Direct Surface Agar Plate procedure (1960). These investigators concluded that no significant difference in bacterial cleanability was observed when the experimental cleaning treatment approached the recommended practices of washing and sanitizing, even though only in a minimum manner. "The high rate of compliance for all finishes after a complete cleaning cycle, as contasted with the low rate of compliance for all surfaces after only a poor rinsing, indicates the desirability and need for adherence to the recommended cycle to insure the desired end point." This study was completed prior to the wide spread application of automatic control to the clean-in-place procedure. Subsequent experience in practice has demonstrated the validity of this conclusion.

High surface finishes may be essential to longevity of the processing system, but practice suggests that a poor weld is better than the best gasket, and that surfaces of any type are more easily cleaned by rigidly controlled mechanical/chemical procedures as compared to manual brushing, spraying or foaming.

ii. Fittings for welded CIP/SIP piping

A specification for stainless steel tubing and fittings should further require that all components should exhibit true roundness and uniform wall thickness. In practice, suppliers have been found capable of meeting criteria which include:

1. The outside diameter of finished tubing and fittings shall be plus or minus 0.010' (0.25mm) in sizes ¾" (19mm) through 2½" (65mm) and plus or minus 0.016' (0.4mm) in the 3" (75mm) size.
2. The maximum variation in ovality shall be less than 0.020' (0.5mm) in sizes ¾" (19mm) through 2½" (65mm) and 0.032' (0.8mm) for 3" (75mm) material.
3. Elbows and tees must be true right angles. Some users specify the angle and planer tolerance.
4. Elbows should be fabricated on a tube bender with a mandrel. Lead is an unacceptable mandrel material.
5. Tees should be fabricated with a pull-out ball. The use of tee-drills should not be permitted.
6. Port spacing tolerance on U-bend transfer panels shall be within plus or minus 0.015' of the specified U-bend center-to-center dimension and all ports for a designated U-bend shall project through the face of the panel to within plus or minus 0.020' of the specified dimension.

Certain components are not available with sanitary connections of the weld, clamp, or threaded type. The industrial steam trap shown in Figure 31 is typical of other devices which may be required to complete a specific installation. It is desirable to eliminate threads and the requirement for the use of pipe wrenches in the maintenance of sanitary systems of welded tubing. Hundreds of steam traps similar to that shown in Figure 31 have been modified for use in both dairy and pharmaceutical systems by boring-out the threads on each end and welding on pipe or tubing extensions which are in turn welded to clamp-type connections.

iii. Design criteria for CIP/SIP piping

Some general recommendations regarding piping system design and installation include:

1. All parts of the piping system must be pitched 1/16' to ⅛" per ft (5mm to 10mm/M) to drain points such as removable elbows, valves, or special openings provided for draining purposes.
2. The support system should be of rigid construction to maintain pitch and alignment and should be designed so as to preclude electrolytic action between the support(s) and the pipeline(s). Supports shall be close enough to each other, generally not more than 10 feet (3M) apart, so that piping will not sag or settle and will be so aligned that there is freedom to expand and contract with thermal changes without distortion or strain on the hanging system, piping or equipment.
3. A complete processing system may be cleaned in a single circuit, but normally the product transfer piping should be developed into two or more circuits compatible with start-up and shut-down of the production operation.
4. Where possible, the spray cleaning of vessels and pressure washing of piping should be combined in a single circuit to minimize the need for make-break connections and the requirement for extensive separate CIP supply/return piping.
5. The generally accepted minimum velocity for CIP cleaning of lines if 5 ft/second (1.5M/second). However, satisfactory results have been achieved at velocities as low as 2 ft/second (0.6M/second), and in excess of 10 ft/second (3M/second). Total circuit length and line size must be controlled so as to achieve these velocities with the available pump and/or other motive sources such as vessel top-pressure or eductor-based CIP return systems.
6. Dead-ends such as capped tees should be located in a horizontal position and must be limited in length to not more than 1½ pipe diameters. Vertical dead-ends are undesirable because entrapped air prevents cleaning solution from reaching the upper portion of the fitting for those positioned vertically upwards, and undissolved solids are likely to accumulate in those which are positioned vertically downwards.
7. The piping system design should provide for inclusion of the maximum amount of piping and equipment in the CIP circuit(s). It is preferable to install several small CIP jumpers or tie lines than to remove and manually clean an equivalent amount of the system in the form of short

lengths of tubing and fittings. Mechanical/chemical cleaning is much more rigorous and subject to better control than manual cleaning.

B. CIP/SIP piping system installation

Three different types of connections are generally utilized for CIP/SIP systems:

1. Tungsten Inert Gas (TIG) welded joints for permanent connections

2. Clamp-type joints of CIP design for semi-permanent connections

3. Threaded joints with hexagon nuts and CIP gaskets for those connections opened daily for processing and cleaning procedures.

Welds are required even for clamp-type and threaded joints to join the ferrule to fittings and tubing.

i. Welding Procedures

Automatic welding is preferred and should be utilized whenever possible. All stainless steel welding must be conducted in a manner which minimizes carbide precipitation and stress. This requires that welds on 16-gauge tubing be made in the following times or less:

Tube OD		Maximum Weld Time
Inches	Millimeters	(Seconds)
1	25	42
1½	38	50
2	50	58
2½	65	67
3	75	75
4	100	120

All welds should be shielded with welding grade argon, supplied at a controlled rate through a flow meter. In addition to shielding the external weld area, the inside of the pipe should be purged with argon to prevent oxidation of the inner surface. Initial purging to displace the air in the pipes should be accomplished at a rate of approximately 20 cu. ft. (0.6M³) per hour until a volume of argon equal to about 6 times the volume of the system has been used, introducing the gas through a sealed connection at one end of the pipe and bleeding off the displaced air through a small hole at the other end. Gas plugs may be used to reduce the required volume of argon. After the initial purge is complete, the argon flow rate may be reduced to between 2-5 cu. ft./hr (1000–2300 cc/min or 0.06–0.14 M³/hr) during the welding operation. Enough gas should be used to keep a slightly positive pressure inside the tubing. Two separate argon cylinders are preferred, one for purging the inside of the pipe and the other for shielding the electrodes. When welding in drafty areas, the welding operation must be protected so that the shielding gas is effective.

If valves which contain heat-sensitive parts, such as plastic or rubber are being welded into the system, these parts must removed during welding to prevent heat damage. Heat sinks must be used for welding valves where recommended by the valve manufacturer, and in the manner the manufacturer prescribes. Ends of valves or other accessories, such as instrumentation fittings or industrial (non-sanitary) design steam traps (Figure 13), are to be machined to match the pipe and/or fitting wall thickness and diameter.

The application of the above described criteria and procedures has resulted in the installation of many dairy and food processing industry CIP systems that have provided highly acceptable performance for more than 25 years.

The most important step in managing the welding process is the qualification of the fitter and welder. Each welder working on a stainless steel solution system installation should be prequalified to the Owner's satisfaction. This is accomplished by requiring the production of sample welds using the various sizes, thicknesses and conditions represented on the job, including welds on both horizontal and vertical pipes, by both manual and automatic methods. Owner representatives must participate in this qualification process. If new welders are added during the job, this same procedure must be followed for each individual who joins the installation team.

ii. Weld inspection and documentation

Weld inspection is generally via visual methods. The completed weld must be smooth and even, with as little build-up or under-cut as possible. The weld must be free of pits, crevices and cracks. Full penetration must be achieved. An optic fiber boroscope may be used to inspect internal welds up to approximately 20 feet (6M) from the end of a piping system. Cameras may be used in combination with boroscopes for production of permanent records of the condition of a weld. Documentation of the weld is generally in accordance with the criteria established by the user. Bigelow and DiVasto suggest several alternative methods of documentation including video cassette records of photographs, print-outs produced by welding machines, and reports (1986). They note "Such documentation does not assure that variables like alignment and surface preparation have been carried out correctly" and emphasis must once again be placed on the proper qualification of the welder.

iii. Passivation of the completed installation

The corrosion resistance of stainless steel is the result of the development of an invisible protective "passive" film on the surface. This film develops naturally when clean metal is exposed to oxygen in the air. Stainless steel components which have been electro-polished and thoroughly washed in hot water and components which have been finished by polishing and buffing generally require no further treatment to establish this protective film. Welding, however, destroys this passive film in the weld area.

A solution of dilute nitric acid may be used to passivate a completed piping system. This treatment is considered especially beneficial in removing particles of steel from cutting tools, iron bearing dust and dirt which contacts the surface during fabricating operations, and oxide scale residues from the welding operation. One procedure which has been found effective:

1. Clean the system via recirculation of a NaOH solution at 0.5%–1.0% for approximately 30 minutes at a temperature of 140°F (60°C).
2. Rinse thoroughly with fresh water and inspect for freedom of all grease and oil. Check final rinse for removal of NaOH.
3. Recirculation clean with citric acid at 2.5%–3.5% by weight for 30 minutes at 90°–110°F (45–50°C).
4. Rinse thoroughly with fresh or distilled water again testing the final rinse for complete removal of the citric acid.
5. Recirculate a nitric acid solution at 15%–20% concentration by weight for 60 minutes at 110°–125°F.
6. Rinse thoroughly with fresh or distilled water, testing the final rinse for removal of all nitric acid.

Stainless steel surfaces can be evaluated for passivity by applying a few drops of 1 Molar copper sulfate to the surface with a swab. Surfaces not in a passive state will cause the copper to plate out.

C. Comparison of dairy and pharmaceutical piping practices

When the installation of welded systems began in the dairy industry in the late-1950s and early-1960s, many Health Departments required boroscope inspection of every weld. Local regulations frequently required the installation of "inspection elbows" thus providing a means for boroscope inspection of welds both following completion of the installation and following some period of use of the piping system. These elaborate requirements have, for the most part, given way to proper qualification of the welding personnel.

The author has been responsible for the design and installation of more than 150 welded piping systems for dairy, food and beverage processes since 1960. The contract documents for the installation of most of these systems required that a boroscope be available for use by regulatory personnel as desired. It was understood, and sometimes part of a contract document, that either the owner or regulatory personnel had the prerogative of requesting any weld to be removed from the system by cutting it out for visual examination or any other means of evaluation. It was understood that if the weld were defective, that the affected portion of the system would be replaced at the installer's expense; if the weld were satisfactory it would be replaced at the owner's expense.

None of the above systems received a nitric acid passivation treatment. However, special attention was made to assure that tools used for fabricating stainless steel, including hole saws, cut-off saws, drills and grinding and polishing equipment were used for stainless steel exclusively. This was the beginning of the use of all-stainless-steel support systems, as it proved impossible to allow a single crew to build support structures of mild steel and also fabricate stainless steel piping without causing some transfer of mild steel contamination to stainless component surfaces through use of the available tools.

These systems ranged in magnitude from several thousand feet of tubing to up to four miles of tubing in sizes varying from 1½" to 3" (25–75mm). At least twenty systems contained in excess of 18,000 feet (5500M) of type 304 stainless steel tubing, thousands of fittings, and hundreds of valves. The CIP supply/return piping in these installations was generally fabricated of No. 5 material (picked or bright-annealed ID, polished OD) and would represent 25–35% of the total tubing installed. Hand-welding was used almost exclusively between 1960 and 1965, and in combination with machine welding during the subsequent decade. Final "in-position" welds were always made by hand.

There has been no recorded evidence of failure due to corrosion of any component in any of these systems. Whereas there were occasional problems with the quality of the product processed through these systems due to poor sanitation, the cause of the trouble was always found to be improper operation and/or maintenance of the CIP system. More importantly, the fouled (or soiled) systems were restored to 100% performance via application of intensive CIP treatment, and following restoration to use, were again properly maintained in a satisfactory condition by normal cleaning procedures. All of these systems were capable of producing results as described under Section 2.D.1 at any period in their life cycle, and many are still in full-time use on a twenty-four hour per day, seven day per week basis. Many of these systems have been modified for renovation or expansion purposes and when cut-up to accomplish that work, both No. 5 and No. 7 tubing were found to be in excellent condition and was, in most cases, reused during the modification work.

Several very large parenteral solution systems were designed and installed to similar standards in the mid-seventies, the only difference being the substitution of type 316L tubing and fittings for the type 304 material used in the dairy application. These systems have met all performance requirements for the first ten years of their productive life.

D. Installation of CIP/SIP systems in the clean room

Complex, automated, large volume parenteral solutions processes substantially increase the amount of equipment and piping in the clean room as compared to previous laboratory or pilot-plant scale processes. The installation of this equipment, and the necessary control and power wiring and air piping to interface it to the Process/CIP/SIP controller, mandates the development of new approaches to the design of the clean room and associated support areas. Typical installation problems which must be addressed include, but are not limited to:

1. The design and installation of a piping support system which meets clean room and process criteria
2. The mounting and connection of load-cell equipped tanks to a welded piping system
3. The installation of instrumentation, control and power wiring to meet generally established clean room criteria and provide accessibility for maintenance
4. The provision and control of process utilities including sterile gases and heating and cooling fluids.

Some of the above problems require attention within the clean room whereas others will impact on the intersticial space above, beneath or to one or more sides of that specialized enclosure.

The first objective should be to minimize penetrations through the walls, ceiling and floor separating the clean room from the remainder of the structure. Consideration should be given to reducing the intrusion of equipment, and people required to maintain that equipment, in the clean room area. This may be accomplished by locating tanks outside of the perimeter wall and using a connecting alcove to provide access to the valves, manway, and vent connections. Certain types of machinery can be specially constructed so as to be bulkheaded through the perimeter wall; i.e., a homogenizer may have the drive in the intersticial area with only the head and homogenizing valve exposed on the clean room side. A plate heat exchanger could be arranged to be similarly installed with the fixed head sealed to the perimeter wall so that all utility connections are external to the clean room area. These suggestions are to stimulate the innovative engineer. The opportunities are unlimited.

Figure 32 is a cross-section view of an arrangement of processing system components and a structure which illustrates problems encountered in practice, and their solutions. These are not represented as the only or best solutions, but rather as typical approaches which have provided satisfactory performance for nearly a decade in pharmaceutical applications.

With reference to this figure, the process vessel (1) is represented as a dome-top, CIP cleanable tank, with a jacket for heating and/or cooling. It is fitted with a top inlet, a spray device for CIP cleaning, a top-mounted sweep-type agitator, a temperature sensor and a level sensor. This tank is mounted on load-beams (2) and is equipped with a fill/CIP selector valve (3) which provides for use of a common line to fill the vessel and conduct CIP solutions through the fill nozzle and to the spray device. The outlet valve is connected via welded line to the inlet port of a centrifugal pump. A single pair of lines from the heating/cooling jacket protrude through the ceiling to the equipment mezzanine where all control valves for selecting and regulating flow of heating and cooling mediums would be located.

The electrical connections to the tank mounted RTD (4) are via a length of stainless steel tubing used as conduit with an appropriate fitting for a cord-grip at the lower end. An air junction box (5) of gasketed stainless steel construction installed in that conduit run near the fill/CIP selector valve (3) provides for the transition from internal polyflo tubing through a bulkhead fitting to a vinyl hose and quick-disconnect for the final connection to the valve. The stainless tubing used as conduit is welded to a stainless steel wire chase mounted flush with the ceiling (11). Other wire chases of similar construction provide for the power connection to the agitator motor, and air piping and instrumentation wiring to an additional air junction box (AJB) located near the tank outlet valve and pump discharge line. From that point, flex cable and cord grips are provided for the pneumatically operated level sensor and a strain-gauge based pressure transducer installed in the pump discharge line, and final air connections to the actuators on the tank outlet valve and pump casing drain valve are via quick-disconnects and vinyl tubing.

Figure 32 — Installation of Clean-in-Place and Sterilize-in-Place System in Clean Room

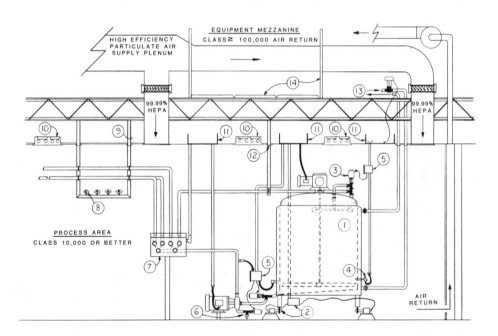

Note that the piping design, equipment layout, and instrumentation requirements must all be coordinated to make maximum use of a single length of stainless steel conduit (tubing) and a junction box for these final connections. The third stainless steel wire chase would provide for the power supply to the pump motor and wiring to the proximity switches in the small U-bend transfer panel (7) fitted with a sloped-top to minimize partical accumulation and be easily cleaned.

The stainless steel product/CIP piping would be supported from schedule 40 pipe (9) welded to the bar-joists which support the equipment mezzanine, with sealed stainless steel escutcheons at all penetrations. The piping would be supported in rubber-bushed hanger clamps welded to the support structure, the design providing for the required pitch to be established at the time of the installation and maintained forever after.

The general procedure for installing this type of support system through a "hung-ceiling" is to weld stubs of sufficient length to penetrate the ceiling to the bar joists prior to installation of the ceiling. Before proceeding with installation of the welded process/CIP piping, all equipment would be placed on the mezzanine to establish the final deflection of the bar joist. Pre-fabricated hanger supports with all hanger clamps installed would be welded to the projecting stubs, a transit being used to establish the height of each support with reference to a selected datum. The hanger supports would be trimmed as appropriate to establish that height before final welding.

The flush-mounted light fixtures (10) shown in the ceiling would be designed and installed as outlined by Kaul (1985). The air inlets from the HEPA filters would be strategically located through the ceiling as required, the filters being accessible from the equipment mezzanine. A catwalk arrangement above the bar joists, with hand rails, would permit ready access to all of the interconnecting power and instrumentation wiring, air tubing, and HVAC equipment, as well as the utility valves, pumps, and heat exchangers which might be located in this area.

Not all systems are installed in new structures. When it is necessary to install a new system in an existing structure, the overhead equipment mezzanine may not be available. An alternative approach to supporting a pair of similarly equipped tanks is shown in Figure 33. This stainless steel enclosure contained the necessary utility valves for controlling heating and cooling mediums to multiple-zone jackets on the processing tanks. The solenoids for the air-operated valves, air piping and wiring instrumentation, and power wiring all entered this enclosure via the retangular stainless steel duct which was sealed to the ceiling above which a minimal intersticial space provided only main headers with branches to each of these utility enclosures. Troubleshooting and maintenance required opening the utility enclosures at which point differential air pressure assured air movement from the clean room to the intersticial space.

The installation of a highly automated processing system in a clean room affects many disciplines and requires a common understanding and coordination of work by the architect, mechanical and electrical engineers, the process engineer, and production and quality assurance personnel.

Figure 33—Shop Fabricated Utility Valve Enclosure for Installation in Clean Room

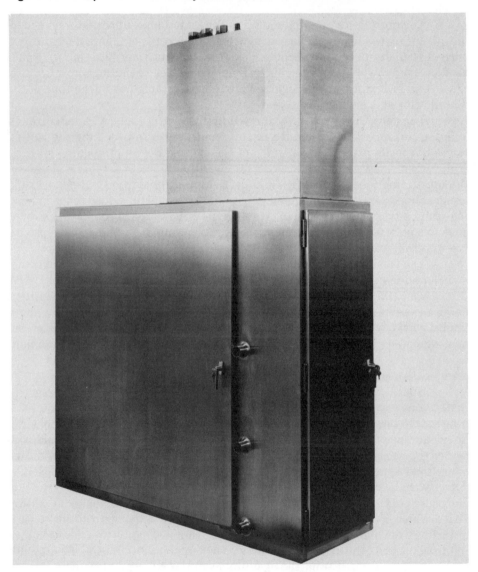

6. Validation of the Automated CIP/SIP System

The design and installation of an automated solutions process system which can be cleaned-in-place and sterilized-in-place provides the pharmaceutical process engineer both new opportunities and new challenges. Harder has observed, "One phase of the overall process of pharmaceutical manufacturer that has not always received the close scrutiny it deserves is the cleaning of the processing equipment" (1984). He subsequently defined a validated cleaning procedure and listed those elements considered essential to the development of such a procedure. Harder emphasized the need for "a good protocol – one that is clearly written and has been reviewed and approved by scientifically and technically competent individuals." Wash efficiency tests were suggested by Grimes as the means of establishing a general wash program that would handle all troublesome products (1977). He reported, "It was found only necessary to adjust the concentration of the alkaline detergent and duration of rinse cycles to achieve no detectable levels of detergents or products after washing tanks soiled with all products processed."

Validation of a CIP/SIP solutions system will generally be handled in combination with the validation of an entire facility or portion thereof including a HVAC system, and WFI system. Blackmer suggested a Validation Protocol Outline applicable to a complete Sterile Operations Facility (1984). The validation of cleaning procedures has been reviewed by Harder in substantial detail (1984).

Validation criteria for a CIP/SIP system must include consideration of the following:

1. The cleaning program, in terms of time/temperature/concentration relationships must be demonstrated to be capable of removing the selected test soil reliably, and repeatedly, under all anticipated variable operating conditions. A residue which has dried on the surface may prove more tenacious than one which has remained moist. A heat transfer surface which is not fully covered during the production operation may cause the development of a heavy deposit at the liquid/air interface near the top of the processing vessel.
2. In addition to demonstrating the effectiveness of the chemical part of the cleaning program, the validation procedure must also be designed to prove that all surfaces are effectively contacted by the cleaning solution. This is especially important for spray cleaning procedures with respect to appurtenances including agitator shafts, steady-bearings, baffles, and heating coils.

The performance of an automated solutions system is significantly affected by variables including design, installation and operation. The validation process must give full consideration to each of these activities. This requires attention to documentation of the design, confirmation that the installation is in accordance with the design, and a rigorous review of the operation of the system for production, cleaning and sterilizing on a trial-run or test-shot basis, preferably with a product which is expected to create the maximum cleaning problem.

A. Documentation

When reporting on field problems with High Purity Water systems, Avallone suggested that the first requirement for validation is a print, preferably an isometric drawing which identifies slopes, drops, and dead legs (1986). The documentation for an automated solutions process must be far more extensive.

i. Drawings

The schematic flow diagrams and working drawings prepared for the installation of the system, if properly done, are an important part of the system documentation. These drawings should be updated to an "as installed' version using the Installation Check-Out procedure to be described below. A complete set of drawings would include: (a) the process schematic flow diagram; (b) prints produced from sepia reproducibles of the schematic flow diagram on which the various product flow paths, CIP circuits and steaming circuits are established; (c) isometric, plan and elevation drawings of the piping (working drawings) to establish all connections, pitch directions, and drain points; and (d) shop drawings of the major components incorporated in the system including tanks, filters, U-bend transfer panels, and CIP recirculating units.

These drawings should establish all equipment nomenclature as well as a numbering scheme for pumps, valves, tanks and instrumentation. The schematic flow diagrams should include line sizes and flow rates as appropriate on the product flow path/CIP circuit versions. The drawings should include pump schedules, valve schedules and instrumentation schedules.

ii. Specification

A written detailed specification should accompany and include references to the above drawings. This specification should establish all requirements for system installation with respect to standards for fit, pitch, support, welding and other required work. This specification may further define the required fittings, valves, and pumps, and specify materials of construction for components such as rotary seals, valve plugs, valve diaphragms and piping system gaskets.

iii. Installation records

Records of weld production and inspection should be included in the system documentation. Chemical passivation procedures or electro-polishing of welded sub-assemblies should also be recorded.

iv. Process description

People from many different disciplines including management, engineering, production, quality control and maintenance from within the company, in addition to regulatory personnel, may be concerned with many aspects of the automated system. A concise, but complete description of the proposed system, its components, its arrangement within the allocated space and its use during operation, cleaning and sterilizing will prove beneficial. This document may be a part of the intitial proposed design. It should be updated and expanded during the subsequent detail design. Further, it should refer to the appropriate building and equipment arrangement drawings to facilitate orientation and to the schematic flow diagrams as an aid to understanding system operation.

A format which has been found suitable includes:

1. Building and Equipment Arrangement: a description by functional area, including references to the major processing equipment and control system components in that area.
2. Control System Design: a narrative description of the interface between the control system and the operator (panels, keyboards, displays) and the interface between the control system and the process (enclosures containing solenoid valves, I/O devices, amplifiers and similar devices). This section should also include a brief description of the general operation of the system giving attention to operator actions, system responses, proposed interlocks and inhibits, system alarms, messages displayed and reports.
3. Process Operations: a narrative review, by function, of each specific production operation, identifying the physical preparation, control system input, and the sequential operation of the process system components to accomplish the desired results.
4. CIP Operations: a narrative description of the CIP circuits, in the sequence in which they would normally be cleaned. This will include the manual preparation, the handling of the controls, and a description of the movement of flush, wash, and rinse solutions through the complete circuit. The approximate cleaning program should be defined in terms of time, detergent type and concentration and temperature required. Error messages, alarms and reports must be defined for all automated cleaning procedures.
5. Sterilize-In-Place Operations: a similar narrative description for the sterilization procedures, in terms of either individual components or the complete system. This shall include reference to manual preparation, movement of air and steam for venting and heating to sterilization temperature, condensate drain points, temperature monitoring and recording, and the method for cooling system for subsequent production use.
6. Maintenance: a brief outline of the anticipated operated problems, their detection and correction, and including a prescribed preventive maintenance program for valves, pump seals, and other components requiring occasional replacement.

Following completion of the validation procedure, the Process Description should be modified to include any changes determined during the validation process. Similar attention should be given to the "as installed" drawings of the piping system.

More importantly, the need for every requirement of the SOP will have been established in the previously listed documentation and is easily supported if challenged.

B. Installation check-out

At completion of the installation of the processing equipment, the interconnecting piping and the control system, it is necessary to check all of the hardware to confirm compliance with the working drawings and specifications, and to assure the availability of complete installation records. An effective approach to control this procedurè, demonstrated by practice, is to again use a special version of the schematic flow diagram, with line numbers, as described under Section 6.A.i. This drawing makes it possible to identify every removable connection, permanently installed welded connection, pump, valve, filter, tank and all instrumentation devices on a line-by-line basis, within a functional area of the process. The drawing can be used to develop a check list after which the check list and the drawing may be used as the documentation for completing the installation check-out. Those items requiring attention include, but are not limited to:

1. Confirm tank design and installation is in accordance with the drawings.
2. Verify line pitch and drain points to assure conformance with the installation drawings.
3. Check surface finish of all materials accessible for visual examination.
4. Confirm that all instrumentation and sensing devices are in accordance with specifications and are properly installed.
5. Review utility connections (electrical, water, compressed air, steam and sterile gases) to assure conformance to the drawings and specifications.
6. Check all control system components, including panels, sub-panels, and all enclosures containing solenoid valves and other components which interface the control system to the process. It is essential that these be properly installed and fully connected to both the process and the control system prior to beginning the operational check-out.

The appropriate documents must be signed and dated by the party or parties responsible for qualification of the system hardware and its installation.

C. Operational check-out

In most instances, this part of the validation process requires the coordinated efforts of the project or process engineer and installation vendors. The facility maintenance personnel should be involved in this procedure, also, as it provides an initial opportunity to become familiar with how the system is expected to operate and thereby become better qualified to handle future troubleshooting and maintenance assignments.

The operational check-out is best handled as a multi-step program including but not limited to:

1. Power-up the control system and evaluate the performance of the operator interface, checking all keyboards, push-buttons, thumbwheel input devices, and machine tool switch components for proper function.
2. Manually enable every control system output "On" and confirm the operation of every valve, pump, agitator motor, or other similar component. Air-operated valves should be checked for movement in the proper direction. Pump rotation should be checked and corrected as required.
3. Calibrate all level, temperatures, flow, pressure and load-cell devices, and other instrumentation as applied.
4. Then, place the system into operation under automatic control, by evaluating and adjusting the CIP programs first. This procedure is beneficial in locating all leaks, missing gaskets and improperly tightened connections and maximizes the number of components placed under evaluation and scrutiny from a single operator input. The control logic for the CIP program and any valve sequencing program required should incorporate "hold" and "manual advance" capability to facilitate the check-out and adjustment of the total system.

   The CIP check-out procedure should include the evaluation of all temperature control systems, chemical feed systems, spray supply pressures and flow-rates through the system. The CIP pressure/temperature recorder instrumentation should be made operative, as should the logic which produces CIP error messages and CIP reports.
5. Following evaluation and adjustment of all CIP circuits, proceed with the check-out of the steam-in-place program(s). This will include an analysis of operation of all temperature sensing and recording devices, confirmation of proper venting and proper operation of all condensate traps, and may require a re-check and re-calibration of temperature sensing devices.
6. After having established proper functioning of the operator/control system interface, the control system/process interface, and having confirmed the ability to clean and sterilize the system, proceed with the evaluation of the system's production capability, using WFI initially, and then combining water with other ingredients as desired. Every functional operation must be checked for proper response to the control system outputs in accordance with the above described Sequence of Events. The calibration of all instrumentation required for controlling and/or recording variables must be fine-tuned. And, the system must be reviewed for proper response to any system errors or operator initiated stops. A well developed program for operational check-out will maximize the use of the available data logging and reporting logic, both as an aid to the evaluation of the process, and as the means of confirming the development of proper error messages and reports.

   Again, the necessary documentation for the operational check-out must be completed, signed and dated by the responsible party or parties.

D. CIP/SIP system components as validation tools
The well engineered CIP/SIP solutions system may, as the result of its unique design requirements, facilitate the development and application of the required validation procedures, and assure greater confidence in the end results than is possible with the systems and practices of the past.

i. U-bend transfer panel impact on validation process
Properly designed multi-port transfer panels may be beneficial in that they provide access to various portions of the interconnecting piping and tankage via temporary connections to special equipment used for the validation process. For example, a portable tank containing a product to be used as a test soil may be connected to a transfer panel port and then pressurized to introduce the test solution. Similar connections may be made elsewhere in the system to recover the test solution, for re-use or disposal. Following cleaning and sterilizing, similar procedures might be followed to move a batch of WFI through the system, collecting it at the discharge end for assay.

The joints and gaskets on U-bend transfer panels conversely represent a potential problem in accomplishing system validation. Operating personnel must understand that the internal headers, interconnecting piping and interior surfaces of the U-bends may be subjected to the rigorous CIP/SIP processes. However, the joints and gaskets are not CIP cleanable and must receive proper manual attention when connections are being made to establish the desired CIP circuit.

ii. The eductor-assisted CIP system as a validation tool
This unique recirculating unit, if fabricated with the appropriate surface finishes, can be constructed to meet the same criteria as the remainder of the process, with respect to CIP/SIP susceptibility. That is, the CIP recirculating unit can itself be cleaned and sterilized to the same standards as the remainder of the process. Since its function requires proper connections to a WFI supply, it provides the innovative pharmaceutical engineer the opportunity to use modifications of CIP programs for validation purposes. Specifically, the provision of one additional valve on the supply side of the CIP pump would provide the means of introducing test solutions which could then be pumped through the entire processing system, including CIP supply and return lines, and via the spray devices to all surfaces which would subsequently be contacted by flushing, cleaning and rinsing solutions. Following the cleaning and sterilizing processes, this system would provide a highly effective means of recirculating WFI through the entire system for sampling purposes. It provides the capability of contacting extremely large areas of processing equipment surface with a relatively small volume of water, thus effectively concentrating the traces of residual soil and/or cleaning chemicals remaining in the system. An essentially standard eductor-assisted CIP unit would be suitable for use with inorganic or organic soils of non-biological nature. If it is considered necessary to use a biological soil in a

system which is otherwise totally enclosed, a retention tank can be installed downstream of the recirculating unit to receive the discharge from the CIP unit drain valve and from the vent on the air-separation tank. The effluent collected in that retention tank may then be filtered enroute to sewer or disposed of in any other acceptable manner.

E. Suggested test areas

A well planned method of rinsing the equipment by recirculation of WFI as described above would provide a sample of the entire system, including areas not accessible for swabbing. However, pump or spray recirculation may not be considered an adequately rigorous procedure for removing tenacious soils. Swabs may be used to extract the soil in a manner similar to that outlined by Grimes (1977). Surfaces selected for evaluation by this technique must be easily reached, and should represent those areas considered most difficult to wash and rinse. Suggested areas would include, but are not limited to:

1. Openings (nozzles) in the head or sidewalls of tanks which are spray cleaned
2. Baffle surfaces and support arms
3. The upper area of any bottom-located side outlet
4. Gaskets associated with inspection covers, manhole covers, and filter housings, and the grooves in which they are installed
5. The stem O-ring area of air-operated compression type valves
6. Slip-joints of essentially metal-to-metal construction associated with certain types of spray devices
7. Tees or branches in headers or transfer lines, especially if located vertically upward.

7. Summary

Mechanical cleaning utilizing spray or pressure recirculation of cleaning solutions under controlled conditions of time, temperature, and detergency has gained wide acceptance in the dairy and food processing industries. Experience has shown that solutions of strong alkali, moderately strong acids, and sodium hypochlorites are highly effective in removing organic and mineral soils of almost any nature when these solutions are utilized in the proper combination and/or sequence.

Parenteral solution processes are adaptable to the incorporation clean-in-place technology. The processing equipment must be designed to permit cleaning solutions to be brought into contact with all product contact surfaces. The equipment and system must confine these solutions to eliminate loss and to prevent damage to personnel or other equipment in the immediate area as a result of splashing, spilling, or leakage. Cleaning procedures must be given as much consideration during system design as the requirements of the process itself.

A system designed for CIP is readily adaptable to SIP. It is necessary only to properly incorporate the additional hardware to accomplish and control the steam sterilization cycle; i.e., steam traps, vent valves and resistance temperature device (RTD's).

8. References

Avallone, H. L. (1986). "High Purity Water", Pharmaceutical Engineering Vol. 6, No. 1, pp. 29-33.

Blackmer, R. A. (1984). "Sterile Operations Facility", Journal of Parenteral Science and Technology, 38, No. 5, pp. 183-189.

Bonem, F. L. (1960). "Single Operator Controls Complex Operation," Food Processing, Vol. 2, July, pp. 36-38.

Fleischman, F. F., Jr., White, J. C. and Holland, R. F. (1950). "Glass Lines: Do A-1 Job; No Take-Down to Clean," Food Industries 22, No. 10, pp. 1686-1690, 1821, 1823.

Grimes, T. L., Fonner, D. E., Griffin, J. C., Pauli, W. A. and Schadewald, F. H. (1977). "An Automated System for Cleaning Tanks and Parts used in the Processing of Pharmaceuticals," Bulletin of the Paternal Drug Association, 31, No. 4, pp. 179-186.

Harder, S. W. (1984). "The Validation of Cleaning Procedures," Pharmaceutical Technology, 8, May, pp. 29-34.

Havighorst, C. R. (1951). "Revolutionary Advance in Dairy Engineering: Permanent Welded Pipelines," Food Engineering 23, No. 9, pp. 74-79.

Hood, H. P. (Staff), Inc. (1974). "Ten-Years Success Story on Automated CIP Cleaning of Milk Tankers," Milk Hauler and Food Transporter, 14, No. 8, pp. 4-5.

Hyde, J. M. (1983). "State-of-the-Art CIP/Sanitation Systems," Dairy Record, 84, No. 7, pp. 101-107.

International Association of Milk, Food and Environmental Sanitarians, "3-A Accepted Practices for Permanently Installed Sanitary Product Pipelines and Cleaning Systems," Int. Assoc. Milk Food Env. San., P. O. Box 701, Ames, Iowa 50010, (No. 605-02 Continually revised; July, 1986)

Johnson, C. R. (1960). "Automated CIP Improves Quality of Product," Food Processing, 1, June, pp. 36.

Kaufmann, O. W., Hedrick, T. I., Pflug, I. J., Pheil, C. G., and Keppeler, R. A. (1960). "Relative Cleanability of Various Stainless Steel Finishes After Soiling with Inoculated Milk Solids," Journal of Dairy Science, Vol. XLIII, No. 1, pp. 28-41.

Kaul, M. (1985). "Electrical Design in Clean Rooms," Pharmaceutical Technology, 9, December, pp. 40, 42-43, 46.

Kuzel, N. R. (1985). "Fundamentals of Computer System Validation and Documentation in the Pharmaceutical Industry," Pharmaceutical Technology, 9, September, pp. 60, 62, 66, 68, 72, 76.

Olenfalk, L.O. (1975). Personal Correspondence Regarding Internal Report.

Olenfalk, L. O. (1975). "Detailed Economical and Technical Study of Various Cleaning Systems," Mjolkcentralen Internal Report, (via personal correspondence).

Parker, R. B., Elliker, P. R., Nelson, G. T., Richardson, G. A., Wilster, G. H. (1953). "Cleaning Pipelines In-Place," Food Engineering 25, January, pp. 82-86, 176-178.

Richter, R. L., Bailey, J. and Frye, D. D. (1975). "A Field Study of Bulk Milk Transport Washing Systems," Journal of Milk and Food Technology, Vol. 38, No. 9, pp. 527-531.

Seiberling, D. A. (1955). "An Ohio Plant Applies Automation to the Cleaning-In-Place Operation," American Milk Review, 17, February, pp. 32-34.

Seiberling, D. A. (1968). "Equipment and Process Design Related to Mechanical/Chemical Cleaning Procedures", Proc. Chem. Eng. Progr. Symp. Ser. 64, No. 68, pp. 94-104.

Seiberling, D. A. (1970). "Automated Cleaning of Brewing Vessels and Lines", Master Brewers Association of America Technical Quarterly, Vol. 7, No. 1, pp. 73-80.

Seiberling, D. A. (1976). "Typical Variations in Automated CIP System Design, Control and Application," New Zealand Journal of Science and Technology, Vol. 11, No. 3, September, 1976 and Vol. 11, No. 4, December, 1976.

Seiberling D. A. (1976). "Fluid Flow Processes" in "Dairy Technology and Engineering," (Harper, W. J. and Hall, C. W., eds.), pp 403. AVI Publishing Company, Westport, CT.

Seiberling, D. A. (1979). "Process/CIP Engineering for Shelf-Life Improvement," American Dairy Review, Vol. 41 No. 10, pp. 14-22, 64-67.

Seiberling, D. A. (1985). "Recirculation Cleaning of HTST Systems," Milk Pasteurization Controls and Tests, 2nd Edition, 159.

Seiberling, D. A. and Harper, W. J. (1957). "Ball Spray Cleaning of Storage Tanks and Pick-Up Tankers," Milk Dealer, 46, No. 4, pp. 40-41, 48.

Seiberling, D. A. and Harper, W. J. (1957). "Automatic Sanitary Valves for Dairy Plants," American Milk Review, 19, No. 1, pp. 30-31, 34.

Sheuring, J. J. and Henderson, H. B.,(1951). Southern Dairy Products Journal, pp. 49, 52-53, 64-65.

Thom, E. (1949). "Glass Sanitary Piping in Dairy Plants," The Milk Dealer, Vol. 39, No. 1, pp. 42-43, 134-138.

Villafranca, J. and Zambrano, E. M. (1985). "Optimization of Cleanability," Pharmaceutical Engineering, Vol. 5, No. 6, pp. 28-30.

Zoltai, P. T., Zottola, E. A. and McKay, L. L. (1981). "Scanning Electron Microscopy of Microbial Attachment to Milk Contact Surfaces," Journal of Food Protection, Vol. 44, No. 3, pp. 204-208.

12

Sterility Testing

Wayne P. Olson
Hyland Therapeutics, Los Angeles, CA, USA

1. Introduction

An enteral drug is intended to pass through the stomach. Topical drugs pass through the skin. Drugs administered by other routes (intracutaneous, subcutaneous, intramuscular, intravenous ophthalmic) are referred to as parenteral drugs or, more simply, parenterals. All parenterals must be sterile (Riggs, 1979). Although there is little evidence of major complications arising as a result of the microbial or particulate contamination of small-volume parenterals (SVPs), the consequences of the administration of contaminated large-volume parenterals (LVPs) are well documented (Felts et al., 1972). LVPs, e.g., 5% dextrose in water, are sterilized by steam autoclave when the product is in the final container. When the autoclave process is verified by suitable physical and biological measurements to be consistent and reliable in the killing of heat-resistant bacterial spores (validation of sterilization), the probability of any given final container being non-sterile is less than one in a million. Some antibiotics, allergenic extracts and all therapeutic proteins and peptides are not autoclave sterilized in the final container because they are heat labile. A possible way around heat lability is radiation sterilization which has been done with corticosteroids in solution in the final container (Bussey et al., 1983). Usually, the SVP manufacturer relies on filtration methods to sterilize the product and to remove particles. Sterilization by filtration is highly effective in practice (Olson, 1979; Olson, 1983), but laboratory experiments with an unusual organism have shown that sterility failures are possible when microporous membrane filters are used (Wallhausser, 1979). Serious questions have been raised about the need for sterility testing on terminally-sterilized LVPs (Mascoli, 1981) and SVPs (Odlaug et al., 1984) but sterility testing of SVPs is a matter of regulation in the United States, 21CFR211.167(a).

This chapter is about sterility testing, and other tests that relate to the quality of make-up water, the product, and the manufacturing environment. Because SVPs and all therapeutic proteins (albumin, immune serum globulins,

315

clotting factors) are sterilized by filtration, the sterilization process also removes particles. Robotics systems for sterility test applications are still in an experimental stage, and as such are not discussed in depth. Dupe and Peters (1984) have described a system for performing sterile culture operations in an incubator, but the unit is described as an engineering exercise and not a system in use.

The sterility of parenteral drugs is an absolute requirement by law, but the only way that the sterility of a lot can be verified is by testing all final containers, leaving none for use. Some statistically sound means of sampling for sterility that does not exhaust the supply of product is needed. Such a sampling method, wherein most of the product is available for use rather than tested, gives rise to problems of test sensitivity. For example, if one percent of 5,000 final containers were contaminated with viable microbes, and the sterility test system was perfect, 300 final containers would have to be sampled for there to be a 95% probability of selecting (randomly) and testing the contaminated containers (Table I). That is to say, if 50 final containers in a lot of 5,000 were contaminated with bacteria, one would have to test 300 final containers to show that any of the containers were contaminated. Six percent of the product is a considerable amount to sacrifice, and is considered uneconomic by most manufacturers. By way of contrast, the more realistic scenario is one in which a sterile product in a sterile receiving tank is fed to a filling machine and 0.1% of the final containers are contaminated with microbes. By inspection of Table 1, it is apparent that even if 500 final containers, 10% of the hypothetical lot, were tested, the probability of detecting any nonsterile containers (using the perfect hypothetical sterility test system) would be .39, less than 40%! So the sterility test is not capable of detecting a small number of final containers contaminated with bacteria or fungi out of the total number of final containers in a product lot. This has been recognized for many years. Bowman (1969), the editor of the Pharmaceutical Journal (1977), Murray Cooper (1982) and many others have concluded that sterility testing is useful as an adjunct to fully validated process, the steps of which ensure the production of a sterile product. Key steps in performing such validation activities are detailed in the tests outlined in this chapter, and in other segments of the text.

2. History and Development of Sterility Testing

Beloian's (1983) chapter on sterility testing is a useful account of the development of the sterility test but better historical overviews are to be found in Alegnani (1979), Borick and Borick (1972), and Bowman (1969).

A. Direct inoculation

Among official compendia, the British Pharmacopoeia (1932) was the first to incorporate a sterility test. Tests for the sterility of liquids are mentioned in USP XI (1936) and are primitive by modern standards. A beef broth was prepared by grinding 500 g beefsteak (freed of fat, tendons and bone) and mixing

Table I—Probability of lot rejection, based on the extent of contamination and the sample size for sterility test

N	% Contamination											
	0.1	0.3	0.5	1	2	3	4	5	10	15	20	30
10	.01	.02	.04	.09	.18	.26	.33	.60	.66	.81	.90	.98
20	.02	.06	.10	.18	.33	.46	.56	.65	.89	.96		
50	.05	.14	.22	.39	.64	.78	.87	.92	.99			
100	.09	.26	.39	.63	.87	.95						
200	.18	.45	.64	.87	.95							
300	.26	.59	.78	.95								
400	.33	.70	.87									
500	.39	.78	.92									

well with 1 liter distilled water. The mixture was left in a refrigerator for 18–24 hours and then heated in "streaming steam" for one hour, followed by 30 psig (approximately 2 bar) steam for half an hour, and so forth. At least 25mL of the beef broth was placed in each of a number of test tubes ("Smith fermentation tubes") and re-sterilized in 15 psig steam for half hour. Presumably, the tubes were plugged with cotton, still a common practice in many microbiological laboratories, but this was not stated in the monograph. To each tube was added 1mL of 1% dextrose for each 25mL of beef broth and the autoclave procedure was repeated. The tubes were to be incubated for at least 24 hours at 37°C, to ensure sterility. To some of the tubes (number not specified), 5 drops (approximately 0.25mL) of the product under test was added, and to the other half of the tubes, 20 drops (approximately 1mL) was added. Test materials were to be incubated at 37°C for 7 days, and material from the turbid tubes was to be transferred to fresh medium and incubated an additional 7 days to verify the presence of microbial contaminants. Three percent of the final containers were to be tested, but the number need not exceed 10. For retest, twice the initial number of containers was required. Sterility testing of bulks required the testing of 10mL from each container of more than 1 liter product, and 3mL from each container of less than 1 liter.

There were no notes on gowning, gloving, or any paraphernalia accepted today as necessary to perform sterility tests with minimal levels of false positives.

At this point, it is useful to consider the statistical "realities" of sampling for sterility. Let V = volume sampled from a bulk (or from a final container), X = a random variable representing the number of organisms per unit volume, λ = contamination level (average number of organisms per unit volume), r = probability that a captured organism will reproduce in the medium presented to it, and p = probability that at least 1 organism will be present in sample volume V. Then, as X follows a Poisson distribution, it can be shown that

$$\ln (1 - p) = -\lambda v$$
$$\text{or } (1/\lambda)\ln(1/(1-p)) = V$$
$$\text{or } V = (1/(r\lambda)\ln(1/(1-p))$$

(Gee et al., 1985) on the assumption that r = 1, i.e., that any organism would grow in the medium presented to it. That is not realistic; some organisms are unlikely to grow in a particular single medium. If, for example, a bulk contains 1 organism/L and the mixing of the bulk is superb (such good mixing seldom occurs in bulks that are alleged to be sterile) so that r = 0.99, and the organisms contaminating the sample will be exposed to a medium in which the bacteria have a 0.95 probability of growth, then the required sample volume is 4.85 liters of product from the bulk tank. There are additional assumptions: no adventitious contaminants, and no inhibitors to growth of contaminants in the product, i.e., the product is not bacteriostatic.

Hence, there are two problems that have plagued sterility testing since its inception in Britain around 1925; the test is insensitive to small numbers of contaminated final containers in a filled bulk, and all possible microbial contaminants are unlikely to grow in a given sterility test media (Alegnani, 1979; Bowman, 1969). For the effective testing of bulks, very large volumes must be sampled for the evaluation to be meaningful statistically (Gee et al., 1985). The basic testing by direct inoculation of samples into growth media test has undergone a number of iterations, relating primarily to the choice of media, the volumes to be sampled from final containers or bulk solution, and the numbers of final containers to be sampled for the initial test or for retests. For example, USP XIV (1950) included Sabouraud Liquid Medium and Fluid Thioglycollate Medium. Sabouraud's was intended primarily for yeasts and molds and as a general aerobic medium. Fluid thioglycollate was primarily intended for anaerobes and facultative anaerobes such as the various clostridia, even though sodium thioglycollate is somewhat toxic to these organisms (Mossel and Beerens, 1968). Today, two media, soybean-casein digest and fluid thioglycollate, are used for USP sterility tests (USP XXI, 1985). Although thioglycollate inhibits the growth of some clostridia (Hibbert & Spencer, 1970), no suitable substitute for the simple, routine culturing of anaerobes and facultative anaerobes has been proven in widespread use. Fortunately, glucose at 5.5 g per liter reduces the inhibitory effect, and this is reflected in the medium composition given in USP XXI.

Direct inoculation testing does not require sampling of the entire contents of a final container. For example, from the 20 final containers currently specified for sterility testing of the final product, one need take only 20mL from each; ten mL for each of the media (soybean-casein, fluid thioglycollate) from each of the containers. The tested product is lost; recovery from either of the growth media poses significant problems, even if there are no bacterial contaminants. We are, of course, ignoring the sampling problems posed by the adsorption of organisms to surfaces such as the wall of the final container or the exposed surface of the elastomeric closure, events that are likely in view of the tendency of microbes to be retained on many types of surfaces (Bitton & Marshall, 1980).

Before any testing is done, the media must be shown to support the growth of inocula of 10 to 100 of the organisms indicated in Table II. Note that all of the organisms are available from the American Type Culture Collection, Rockville, MD 20852. If the organisms produce a turbidity when incubated at the temperatures indicated in Table 2 for 7 days or less (usually, turbidity will form in several days), the media are deemed suitable. However, when product is inoculated directly into the growth media, the thioglycollate must be incubated at 30°C to 35°C and the soybean-casein must be incubated at 20°C to 25°C for 14 days, so as to accommodate any slow-growing organisms, or very small numbers of organisms.

Table II—Standard USP organisms used in the validation of sterility test methods

Organism	ATCC No.	Gram Stain
Listed in USP XXI:		
Bacillus subtilis	6633	Positive
Candida albicans	10231	Not applicable
Bacteroides vulgatus	8482	Positive
Clostridium sporogenes	11437	Positive
Micrococcus luteus	9341	Positive
Not listed in USP XXI:		
Pseudomonas aeruginosa	9027	Negative
Pseudomonas cepacia	17765	Negative
Serratia marcescens	13880	Negative

Just as there has been an evolution in the particulars of the sterility test, there also has been an evolution in the means of interdicting adventitious organisms. Sterile gowning and gloving became standard practice, together with the use of high efficiency particle air (HEPA) filtration (Bowman, 1968). However, despite the best techniques available for direct inoculation, inadvertent contamination of sterile liquids, likely during pipetting and transfer (i.e., false positives), persisted at rates of about 0.2 to 0.5% higher than could be attributed to contamination during the filling operation. For a process requiring a large number of manipulations, each under aseptic conditions, such as in sterility testing, it is necessary to carry several blanks, i.e., sterile water or sterile saline, through the process so that manipulative problems will surface, and will not be confused with an inappropriately high level of contamination among the final containers.

An alternative type of direct inoculation has been proposed wherein medium is added to some of the sterile containers to be filled (Rycroft & Moon, 1975). It was a clever idea, and obviated the problems of sample transfer. However, the method also eliminated the possibility of random selection of samples for test, and included no means of eliminating microbial growth inhibitors.

B. Membrane method

The membrane method is preferred over direct inoculation (USP XXI, 1985) because it is more sensitive (Christianson & Koski, 1983), less expensive (needing less media), and results in a faster reporting of test results. The membrane test is performed over a seven day period, whereas direct inoculation tested product requires 14 days incubation. Since product is in quarantine during the period of the sterility test, the faster turn-around time can be significant.

The membrane method of sterility testing was an outgrowth of public health procedures for the testing of potable water supplies. The original process of Zsigmondy (1922) became the basis for microporous membrane production at Membran-Filtergesellschaft, Germany, now known as SartoriusWerke. Production commenced in 1929 or 1930 and German public health personnel developed rapid and sensitive membrane methods of testing potable water for fecal coliform (sewage) organisms, indicating contamination of potable water lines with sewage. The same methods, with embellishments, are in use today (Standard Methods, 1981) and involve passing a known volume of water through a presterilized 0.45 micron -rated pore diameter (RPD) membrane filter (membrane filter) that then is placed atop an appropriate bacteriological medium (see this chapter's section on microbiological assessment of water quality for particulars of the method). The medium could be provided either by placing the membrane, downstream side downward, on a Petri dish of the appropriate agar-medium, or by applying 1 or 2mL of liquid medium to a fiberglass depth filter placed beneath the membrane filter; the liquid medium wicks upward into the membrane filter, providing nutrients to the organisms on the surface of the membrane filter. The obvious advantages of the technology were that large volumes of low particle burden liquids could be passed through a single small membrane, concentrating organisms on the filter surface, and growth inhibitors could be rinsed through the filter and away from the organisms, improving conditions for the replication of viable microbes. The membrane filter technology was brought to the U.S. from Germany by Al Goetz (CalTech, Pasadena), more or less as spoils of war, Additional work on the casting of membrane filters was carried out at CalTech by Goetz. Jack Busch, of the Lowell Corp. in Massachusetts, bid for the technology and, on the strength of the work in Göttingen and subsequent improvements by Goetz, founded the Millipore Filter Corp. The initial products were directed to the public health sector, but Charles Shaufus and others at Millipore worked closely with Frances Bowman, Mack White and others at the USFDA Sterility Test Branch (since disbanded) to develop the membrane filter method for sterility testing. The method was first applied to antibiotics (Holdowsky, 1957).

It seemed the simplest and most effective way to remove microbial growth inhibitors with minimal sample manipulation. Simple sterile solutions were (and are now) required for rinsing drugs from the filters. Preferably, such sterile rinse solutions would also promote growth. The various fluid rinse solutions are, themselves, nutrient broths of a sort as discussed later in the chapter. A six-place membrane sterility test manifold is standard equipment for sterility testing. A vacuum is applied to the pipe connecting the individual filter units and the vacuum draws liquids through the filters. Individual filter units are turned on or off with the valves. The liquid drawn through the filters and into the central vacuum pipe is drawn into a vacuum trap established only for that purpose.

All work is performed in a room fed with filtered air, at a slight overpressure, and in a HEPA bench. Since most false-positives are bacteria of human origin (e.g., Staphylococcus aureus), operators are masked, hooded, gloved and gowned in sterile clothing, as is done in the aseptic filling rooms. The workspace, especially the HEPA bench, is wiped down with a lint-free cloth dampened with a bactericidal solution such as Betadine. Note: Recent work indicates that povidone-iodine, as received from the manufacturer, can itself be contaminated with *Pseudomonas aeruginosa* (Anderson et al., 1984; Berkelman et al., 1984) and that 2% chlorhexidine can be contaminated with *Serratia marcescens* (Marrie and Costerton, 1981). Benzalkonium chloride, which is used widely as a preservative and for the disinfection of skin, also can be contaminated with S. marcescens (Sautter et al., 1984). Therefore, there is cause for caution; a screening of such solutions, prior to routine use, is indicated. If the manufacturer(s) do not membrane filter the decontaminating solutions of local choice, it might be best to do so with 0.2 to 0.45 micron RPD membrane filter. This is a clear instance in which the solutions should be checked for contamination by means of the membrane filter technique. Commercially prepared solutions that may not require filtration include Sporicidin™, which contains 7.5% phenol and 2.0% glutaraldehyde, and Alcide™, which is an organic acid-stabilized form of chlorine dioxide. When product in the final container is introduced to the sterility test room, the containers usually are contaminated on the surface as exceptional care is not taken to maintain the sterility of the exterior of the final container after it has been filled, stoppered, and sealed. Consequently, some disinfectant should be applied to the outside of the final containers before they are sampled for sterility. Two percent glutaraldehyde or 3% hydrogen peroxide commonly are used in this step (Eskenazi et al., 1982). Clearly, care is required to avoid contaminating the sample or the sterility test system with the sanitizing agent.

In the earliest membrane sterility test systems, the outside of the final container was disinfected, then the container was opened, e.g., with sterile pliers. The sterility test unit(s) were opened and the liquid under test poured into the membrane sterility test unit(s). This step was a likely source of adventitious microbial contaminants. Consequently, the next step was the use of manifolded feed lines from final containers to the membrane sterility test units. Such arrangements obviated the need for pouring a sterile liquid from one container to another. The pouring of liquids causes disturbances in air flow in the recipient container and in the source container, consequently, any means of obviating the movement of nonsterile air into either container during the transfer process potentially may reduce the level of false positives. False positives mean retest and quarantine of the product until the retest results indicate the absence of microbial contaminants. Persistent false positive results will result in the destruction of what is, in fact, an acceptable product. A high level of false positive sterility test results could, in theory, put an otherwise satisfactory pharmaceutical manufacturer out of business. The older membrane methods, outlined in Millipore Application Manual AM201 (1971), sometimes have shown false-positive levels of 0.1%, but more commonly somewhat lower. With the Steritest™ (Millipore) system (Bush and Lomonier, 1977), which is current (1987) state-of-the-art, false positives are reduced by almost an order of magnitude.

3. Curent Methods of Sterility Testing

A. Non-antibiotics and non-preserved aqueous products

The standard membranes for sterility testing have a pore size rating of 0.45 micrometers. As a practical matter, the membranes should have a porosity of about 75% or more. Most commonly, the material of composition is mixed esters of cellulose (about 85% nitrocellulose and 15% cellulose acetate). However, cellulose diacetate and cellulose triacetate, as well as other polymers are suitable. What is required is that the membrane be capable of retaining virtually all of the commonly occurring microbial contaminants and that, when the organisms are on the surface of the membrane and are supplied with nutrients, the organisms are not inhibited from growth by the filter or the topology of the membrane filter system. Consequently, before proceeding with actual tests of product, we first establish that the USP organisms, deposited onto the membrane filter, are fully retained and, when the filter is placed in fluid thioglycollate or soybean-casein digest medium, will grow to a discernible turbidity, usually within 3 to 4 days.

Although emulsion particles are highly deformable, they are capable of clogging a 0.45 micron RPD membrane filter unless it is operated under positive pressure. Pressure differentials of up to 2 bar (about 30 psig) are required to drive emulsions through such a membrane filter. However, when a conventional membrane sterility test unit is operated in the conventional way, i.e., negative pressure, with a vacuum applied to the downstream side of the filter, the maximum pressure that can be applied to the filter is 1 atmosphere. This pressure differential is insufficient to cause emulsion particles to deform, and the filter clogs almost immediately. However, a surfactant may be added to disperse the particles. A 10% solution of Tween 80 is more than adequate for this purpose, but 10% or less of Triton X-100 would be equally as effective. The surfactant must, of course, break the emulsion to render it filterable without affecting the viability of microbes. The Tween, Triton X-100 or other surfactant can be added to the system in several ways. The surfactant cannot be added to the solution immediately above the membrane; assuming the volume above the membrane to be about 30mL, the surfactant concentration would be depleted rapidly as additional test solution is added. It can be shown that over 90% of the surfactant would be eluted through the membrane filter, and unavailable to solubilize additional droplets, with the addition of 60mL or more. This means that the surfactant concentrate must be added directly to the final container, or must be pumped at constant rate into the feedstream to the sterility test filter system. The simplest way to sterilize the surfactant solution concentrate is by membrane filtration through a 0.2 micron RPD membrane filter that has been validated for this particular purpose. The validation should be with Bacillus pumilis spores, which definitely will be resistant to the surfactant, and with Pseudomonas diminuta, which may or may not be resistant to the effect of the surfactant.

B. Antibiotic and preserved aqueous products
Preservatives are added to final containers that are entered more than once. Gamma globulin is a good example. A final container of gamma-globulin solution may be entered with a sterile needle many times, therefore thimerosal (ethylmercurithiosalicylate), phenylmercuric acetate, or another preservative usually is added to the product to inactivate adventitious bacteria from the air-filled syringe (emptied into the container so as to provide an overpressure, which expels the liquid into the now-empty syringe). Consequently, it is important that the product in the final container initially is sterile. The numbers of organisms that might be introduced on an 18 gauge needle or from a syringe filled with air is very modest, and likely would be inactivated by a preservative such as thimerosal. But no such preservatives are added to antibiotics as they are bactericides. The only real concern here is the removal of the antibiotic from any possible contaminating microbes, so that microbial contaminants might grow and produce a detectable turbidity.

It is for antibiotics that the membrane filter sterility test originally was introduced (Holdowsky, 1957). The antibiotic solution is filtered through a 0.45 micron RPD membrane filter and organisms are retained on the filter. If the antibiotic has a high affinity for the membrane filter, e.g., mixed esters of cellulose, the antibiotic sorbed to the filter may inhibit the growth of microbes trapped on the filter surface. Residual antibiotic may be rinsed from the filter with Fluid A (1% peptic digest of animal tissues that is clarified by filtration, pH-adjusted to 7.1, and autoclaved) or Fluid D (1mL Polysorbate 80 added per 100mL Fluid A prior to autoclaving). Fluid D rinses should be warmed to 30°C to improve antibiotic solubility. Should a Fluid D rinse prove inadequate, one might consider the availability of microbial enzymes that inactivate the antimicrobial, e.g., the aminoglycoside-modifying enzymes that inactivate gentamycin (Blank, 1983).

C. Products containing penicillins

The development of penicillins was paralleled by the discovery and use of penicillinases, which are beta-lactamases produced by organisms other than Penicillium spp. Consequently, the United States Pharmacopeas has, since the XIII edition published in 1947, indicated the use of microbial penicillinases in the sterility testing of penicillins. This was critical at the time, as the membrane method was then in use only in Germany, and only for the coliform testing of potable water. The amount of penicillinase to be added was determined by experiment, based on the penicillin concentration estimated in Levy units. The enzyme solution currently is filter-sterilized through a sterile 0.2 or 0.45 micron-RPD membrane filter; many suitable units are available commercially, e.g., the Millex (Millipore Corp., Bedford, MA 01730). Equivalent products can be purchased from Schleicher & Schull, Gelman, and other laboratory filter manufacturers.

Penicillins pose special problems of containment. Just as a penicillin-manufacturing facility should be self-contained and incapable of contaminating other products, so must the sterility test facility be dedicated so that other products, perhaps contaminated with pencillin-susceptible organisms, cannot become contaminated with penicillin particles, leading to false-negative results. This also means that the sterility test HEPA hood must be kept scrupulously clean, and wiped down with a cloth wetted in a suitable solvent, e.g., ethanol or methanol. Other enzymic and nonenzymic additions, to inactivate antibiotics or to facilitate filtration during sterility testing, are now commonplace (see Clotting Factor VIII and Insulin in this section).

D. Ointments and oils

At first consideration, ointments seem unfilterable and untestable for sterility. The filterability problem is one of viscosity. If the viscosity of the ointment can be reduced significantly, at least slow filtration through a sterility test membrane filter can be done. The primary methods for reducing viscosity are gentle heating to 30–35°C, or dilution with an aqueous solution of a surface-active compound such as Tween 80 at 10%. Tween-diluted ointments are readily filtered through the 0.45 micron RPD membrane filter closed canister sterility test filters such as Steritest™ (Millipore) and Sterisart™ (Sartorius) (Gee et al., 1985). Prior art involved the addition of isopropyl myristate (Bowman, 1966; Bowman et al., 1967; Tsuji et al., 1970). A similar diluting fluid, Fluid K, is listed in the current USP (USP XXI, 1985). The composition of Fluid K is:

Peptic digest of animal tissue . . . . .5 gram
Beef extract . . . . .3 gram
Polysorbate 80 . . . . .10 gram
Water, to . . . . .1 L

Steam autoclave, Post-autoclave pH, 6.9 ± 0.2

An alternative method that has worked with fat emulsions is the aseptic addition of sterile dimethyl sulfoxide (DMSO) to about 10% by volume (Placencia et al., 1982).

The physical manipulations pose some problems. For example, under HEPA laminar flow in the hood, the outside of the ointment container (e.g., a plastic tube) must be decontaminated with very high intensity UV or with a solution such as Alcide™. If the port through which the ointment is expressed is a male Luer, then the cap can be removed and a sterile needle attached. The tube contents then are squeezed through the needle into a sterile evacuated transfer vessel with an elastomeric closure. Sufficient 10% Tween solution is then added to ensure solubilization of the ointment. Total solubilization may not be necessary. For example, intravenous emulsions can be intruded through the canister systems with 2 bar (approximately 30 psig) positive pressure, which can be generated with the peristaltic pumps of the canister systems or with the intermittent positive pressure system of Gee et al. (1985) (see Figure 2). Note that intrusion of the membrane is not immediate. There is a lag time, during which no filtrate is observed on the downstream side of the membrane filter. However, after a minute or so at pressure, the lipid droplets (which initially clog the filter) deform, coalesce, and continuous flow through the membrane filter is observed. If the system shown in Figure 2 is used, the suspension is pulled from the final container or transfer vessel (FC) into the feed lines by the peristaltic pump (PP) until the canisters are full. The pump then is shut off, and compressed nitrogen is applied to the liquid-loaded canisters via the two-way gang valve (2GV) and the canister vent filters (CVF). The process is repeated until all of the solubilized ointment has been filtered through the two canisters. The downstream sterile tubing (DST) and sterile evacuated vessel (SEV) are not needed when ointments or oils are under test. If the canister system is used as-is and the pump generates all pressure, the canister vent filters must be capped and the caps clamped in place.

The same basic methods can be used with oils, but warming of the oil and the filtration system is simpler and obviates the need of a positive-pressure system like the Steritest or Sterisart units. Heat tapes can be wrapped around the filter holder to warm it, and the final container can be heated in the same way. Sterile shrouds of Tyvek™ can be prepared for the heat tapes. It is best not to add any water to warmed oils.

Figure 1—Steritest™ system. *Photo courtesy of Millipore Corp.*

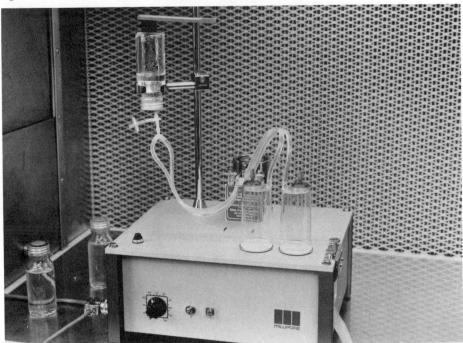

E. Albumins

Five percent human serum albumin (HSA) is a viscous product and filters slowly. The viscosity is reduced somewhat by heating, but the improvement in filterability is insufficient to make filtration times practical. Twenty-five percent HSA is, for practical purposes, unfilterable through conventional sterility test membrane filters under negative pressure, but can be filtered well under positive pressure. The preferred system is that shown in Figure 2, operated under intermittent positive pressure as described under Ointments and Oils (above). With proteins such as HSA, it is critical that intermittent positive pressure is used, wherein the gas pressure is applied only when the peristaltic pump is off. If that is not done, foams form in the canister effectively blocking the membrane filter, making filtration through the membrane filter impossible. Consequently, continuous pump pressure, one of the alternatives under Ointments and Oils, cannot be done with proteins as foams form under these conditions. Routine filtration of 5 liters or more of 5% HSA, or 2 liters of 25% HSA, can be done through a set of canisters. The canisters are fitted aseptically with sterile downstream tubing to the downstream ports of the canisters. The tubing terminates

Figure 2 — The Gee modification (Gee et al., 1985) of the canister sterility test system

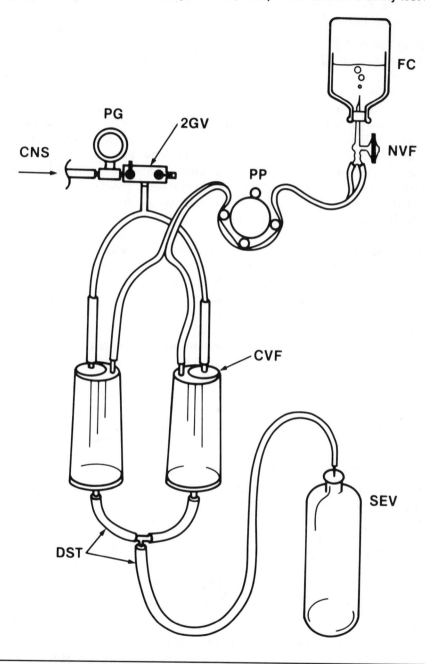

in a sterile evacuated vessel (Figure 2). Because the system has been validated for process as well as for sterility testing, product can be recovered for subsequent addition to later lots (Gee et al., 1985).

F. Clotting Factor VIII

Albumin has a relatively low molecular weight (69 kDaltons) and is stabilized by many intramolecular disulfide bridges; it is a compact, globular molecule and filters more readily than some of the asymmetric proteins of high molecular weight. Human clotting factor VIII, also called antihemophilic factor or AHF, is a freeze-dried preparation (to promote shelf stability) containing fibrinogen (a very asymmetric molecule of 340 kDaltons), gamma 2-macroglobulin (800 kDaltons), fibronectin, and other large proteins. The reconstituted product is quite viscous. Prior to drying, the AHF concentrates are sterile-filtered through 0.3 micron RPD membrane filter cartridge filters (Olson, 1983) but are extremely difficult to filter through 0.2 micron RPD membrane filter operated in the dead-end mode. Why product that filters well through 0.3 micron-rated cartridge filters is all but impossible to filter through a 0.45 micron-rated 47mm diameter disc filter, even if the viscosity is equivalent to that of 25% HSA. Why AHF and HSA preparations filter so differently is not obvious, and deserves attention.

Because the membrane filter sterility test can be completed within 7 days, compared to the 14 days required with direct inoculation, and because the membrane method is more sensitive and requires less medium (hence is less expensive), some means of making Factor VIII concentrates more filterable is desirable. Gee and Olson (1986) found that reconstitution of freeze-dried concentrates with 0.9% sterile porcine trypsin for 0.5 to 1 hour at 20–21°C dramatically reduced the viscosity of the reconstituted material, which then became readily filterable. Incubation with trypsin had no statistically significant effect on colony-forming units of *Bacillus subtilis* or *Candida albicans* or *Clostridium sporogenes* for periods up to 6 hours. Over longer periods (up to 24 hours), there was a significant decline in colony-forming units; however, bacterial or fungal counts were always higher in the samples to which trypsin was added. We concluded that trypsin at 0.9–1.0 mg%, the concentration at which trypsin is used to disperse mammalian cells during tissue culture manipulations, does not impair fungal or bacterial growth and improves the survival of microbes in Factor VIII concentrates by digesting a bacteriostatic protein. Considering the general lack of effect of trypsin on mammalian cells (Seeds et al., 1977; Stanley et al., 1975), and the durability of bacteria and fungi, the results with trypsin are not surprising. However, one should routinely use sterile Millex™ (Millipore) or equivalent disposable 0.2 micron RPD filters to ensure that the trypsin solution injected into the final container is, indeed, sterile.

G. Insulin

Insulin zinc forms precipitates in soybean-casein digest and fluid thioglycollate broth. The precipitates are indistinguishable from microbial growth. Ascorbic acid at 1% in 0.1% peptone (w/v) dissolves protamine zinc insulin and insulin zinc in no more than 1 minute without harming organisms (Calhoun et al., 1970). Conventional sterility test media can be used.

H. Validation

All test methods used in the characterization of product must be written down (21CFR211.80a). Details of analytical methods validation must be recorded unless a compendial or other recognized standard reference method (such as Association of Official Analytical Chemists Book of Methods); in which instance, citation of the method source is adequate (21CFR211.194(a)(2)). However, even when a USP method is used, the method must be validated for the specific product or process. Validation is performed by taking a putatively sterile product and introducing to it none or fewer than 100 CFU per milliliter of standard organisms: *Bacillus subtilis* ATCC 6633 (Gram-positive, aerobic, spore-forming bacterial rod), *Bacteroides vulgatus* ATCC 8482 (Gram-negative, anaerobic bacterial rod), and *Candida albicans* ATCC 10231 (yeast). Alternative organisms are *Clostridium sporogenes* ATCC 11437 as an anaerobe in place of *B. vulgatus,* and *Micrococus luteus* ATCC 9341 (formerly designated *Sarcina*) as a substitute for the *B. subtilis*. These are mentioned in USP XXI. One may use *M. luteus* in place of *B. subtilis,* or *B. vulgatus* in place of *C. sporogenes,* but that is unlikely. The spore-formers are far more convenient to use.

4. Microbiological Assessment of Water

A. Introduction

Water is ubiquitous in the manufacture of pharmaceuticals. For parenteral drugs, make-up water invariably is Water For Injection (WFI) which must be nonpyrogenic in rabbits and contain less than 100 colony-forming units (CFU) of total counts per 100mL and no coliforms (fecal organisms). Organisms from the atmosphere can be introduced to a distilled water loop when a valve is opened; small numbers of retrograde *Pseudomonas* can multiply, even in distilled water, to levels of 10^5 to 10^6 per milliliter in warm standing WFI (Carson et al., 1973; Favero et al., 1971). In a WFI system, usually a distilled water loop, warm standing water can occur in dead-legs which are defined as dead-ends more than 5 to 6 pipe widths in length, and which extend downward, either straight or at an angle, from the loop. The problem with such dead-legs is that the standing water that accumulates in them provides a thermal and a chemical buffer. If the loop is drained and steamed at 1 bar (approximately 15 psig), the dead-legs with their standing water will never achieve the temperature of the steam. Similarly, if hypochlorite or bleach is circulated in the loop, the concentration in a dead-leg is unlikely to reach that of the main circulating loop. There is a distinct possibility of microbial survival under such circumstances.

Even with dead-legs no longer than 1 or 2 pipe widths, e.g., at outlet valves, some levels of microbial counts are inevitable in WFI. Some organisms

Table III — Rapid identification, by colony color, of *Pseudomonas aeruginosa* on agar media

	Agar type		
	Cetrimide	Pyocyanin	Pseudomonas Agar F
Color in white light	Green	Green	Colorless to yellow
Color in ultraviolet light	Green	Blue	Yellow

will be present on and in the manufacturing equipment, in the air, and on the skin and clothing of personnel, hence microbial contamination of make-up water and product is inevitable, even using state-of-the-art operating procedures. However, the contamination of WFI and liquid product must be minimized. The microbial quality of the make-up water, the liquid product prior to sterilizing filtration, and the air in the filling environment must be monitored. In this section, methods of water monitoring will be developed.

The primary microbial contaminants of water systems are Gram-negative organisms, e.g., *Pseudomonas cepacia* (Winstead, 1967; Pickett, 1982). The best methods of test, whether of WFI or cooling water for autoclaves or other high-purity water, are for total microbial bioburden and not for the lipopolysaccharides (LPS) (also known as endotoxin) (further detailed discussion of Pyrogens and Depyrogenation is provided in another chapter of this book). The preferred method is the luciferin-luciferase technique for ATP quantitation, which is discussed later.

The powerful advantage of the luciferin-luciferase method is that it provides almost real-time information, whereas most other methods require incubation of samples in or on culture medium for at least 24 to 48 hours. Consequently, current methods provide information that is largely of historical interest.

B. Sampling

The first consideration in sampling water from a WFI loop is care in avoiding microbial contaminants other than those in the water system. The commonest method is sampling from a valve into a sterile screw-top container. Open the valve to be sampled and let the water run freely for 2 to 3 minutes so as to purge the valve of accumulated organisms. Fill the screw-top container (usually 100mL volume), leaving a small head-space to facilitate mixing by inversion. Re-cap. It is best that the container neck and shoulder is covered with a hood that also is replaced directly after the sample has been taken and the cap replaced. Sample processing should be immediate. If that is not possible, then samples should be refrigerated at about 5°C for no more than 4 hours prior to processing. Up to 6 hours transit time plus 2 hours processing time, all unrefrigerated, are permitted by Standard Methods (1981). This is an excessive allowance in a pharmaceutical plant or hospital pharmacy, where such testing should be possible under the best conditions and where the most accurate results are needed.

The preferable method is sampling the loop from a valve specifically designed for that purpose, such as the sampling and venting valve from Valex (catalogue no. V2025 or V2050, with one of various suffixes depending on the configuration) (Figure 3). This valve has a replaceable PTFE valve stem tip that extends proximal to the inlet connection. The stem of the valve occupies most of the valve body, reducing dramatically the liquid holdup volume. Because the outlet connection can be as small as 0.635cm (0.25 inch) in diameter, the pressure of water from the loop should create sufficient viscous drag to ensure a thorough flush of the valve when the stem is retracted. The valve and stem are 316L stainless steel, and the fittings are Tri-Clamp (TC).

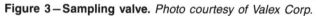

Figure 3 — Sampling valve. *Photo courtesy of Valex Corp.*

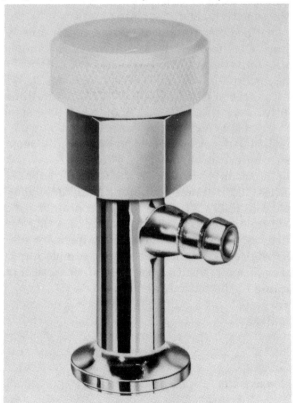

Alternatively, one may use the Millipore sterile sampling port. The unit has a replaceable self-sealing diaphragm behind a covered chamber holding an alcohol-saturated cotton wad. A sampling probe (sterile needle) is used to recover the sample into a bottle or through a membrane filter.

The larger the volume that is sampled in the estimation of total counts for low bioburden water, the more accurate the results are likely to be.

A note on practice: Valves not in use should be blanked off with a TC blank. The intent is reduce as much as possible the contamination of valves with dust and organisms when the valves are not in use.

C. Standard plate counts

What we refer to as standard plate counts are described (Standard Methods, 1981) as an empirical measurement because bacteria and fungi occur singly, in pairs, chains, clusters and packets, each of which may account for a colony-forming unit; and because no single growth medium or set of conditions can satisfy the physiological requirements of all microbes.

Because the sensitivity of direct plate counts is quite poor for low levels of bioburden, this method is suitable only for detecting grossly contaminated systems. An optimistic estimate of the sensitivity of the standard plate count is 10 colony-forming units per milliliter, which is two orders of magnitude less sensitive than the maximal allowable level of organisms in WFI or autoclave cooling water. Best precision is with 30 to 300 CFU per milliliter. Because the method is inherently insensitive, a 100mL sampling bottle is satisfactory. Rather than monitoring microbiological quality of the make-up water, standard plate counts are best applied to the evaluation of product quality during process steps upstream of sterilizing filtration.

Standard plate counts are done in the following manner: Preparations consist of petri dishes (100 × 15mm) containing plate count agar and four screw top 100mL sample containers. The first sample container is empty and is intended for the neat (undiluted) sample. To each of the other containers, 99mL of saline or distilled water are added and the containers are autoclaved at 1 bar (approximately 15 psig) for 30 minutes. Sterile, disposable 1 and 0.1mL pipettes are put to hand. For the petri dishes, about 600mL or more of plate count agar is prepared according to the formula:

Tryptone . . . . .5.0 gram
Yeast extract . . . . .2.5 gram
Glucose . . . . .1.0 gram
Agar . . . . .15.0 gram
Distilled water to . . . . .1.0 Liter

Post-sterilization pH: 6.8 to 7.0

Commercial plate count agar also is acceptable. At least 10 to 12mL of medium, at 44 to 46°C, is poured into each petri dish; the cover is replaced but propped open to allow moisture to escape. The dishes must be on an approximately level surface. The agar hardens within 10 to 15 minutes at 20 to 25 °C. Incubate the inverted plates for 3 days at ambient temperature and for 2 days at 30 to 35°C. Examine and discard any that show growth.

From the neat sample, plate 1 and 0.1mL samples, spreading the samples uniformly over the agar surface with a sterile, L-shaped glass "hockey stick." Replace the dish covers and tape them in place with 2 or 3 small pieces of cellophane tape. Mark the sample designations on the dishes and incubate them, inverted (so that condensate will not drop onto the agar surface) and at 30 to 35°C. Also from the neat sample, pipette 1mL into a sterile 99mL diluent container and mix by inversion and 25 up-and-down arm movements in no more than 10 seconds. From this, 1 and 0.1mL samples are plated as above. These plates should show (in triplicate) CFU per milliliter at neat, 10^{-1}, 10^{-2}, 10^{-3}, and 10^{-4} dilutions. Additional dilutions and plates are prepared to a final dilution of 10^{-7} if the bioburden of the sample is unknown. Plates are examined at 24, 48 and 72 hours and total counts recorded.

In the examination of the microflora of product, one of the advantages of this method is that individual colonies can be recovered, streaked, and identified tentatively so as to establish an overview of the microflora found in in-process material. At the higher dilutions, the most populous organism(s) will predominate and a rough ranking by prevalence can be done.

D. Membrane methods

Because standard plate counts are too insensitive by two orders of magnitude for the evaluation of WFI, some other means is needed to concentrate the organisms in large volumes of water. Because WFI is a relatively clean product, many liters can be filtered through a 47 or 50mm diameter, 0.45 micron RPD membrane filter such as is used for sterility testing. The disc filters are gridded with a nontoxic dye to facilitate colony counting, and most colony counting is done under a dissecting microscope, using epi-illumination. The number of colony-forming units per filter is controlled, not by sample dilution, but by the volume of liquid passed through the filter. One hundred milliliters might suffice, but a 300mL sample is preferable as 30 CFU, the allowable limit, can be counted readily, and some useful information may be obtained regarding lower levels of bioburden. However, if 300mL is to be sampled, then 100mL sample containers create problems.

Using a 6-place sterility test-type 47mm diameter disc filter holder, or something similar, which has been sterilized with the analytical membrane filter in place (the usual manner), then the sample(s) usually must be poured into the hydrosol-type filter holders. The sample(s) then are pulled through the membrane filter under negative pressure. The environment for this work need not necessarily be as scrupulously clean as that required for sterility testing. However, minimal precautions include sterile gloving and a HEPA hood (vertical or horizontal), the bench surface of which had been wiped down with antiseptic immediately prior to hood startup and the hood turned on 30 minutes prior to use.

Another method that provides more flexibility and fewer problems in the collection of the sample(s) involves coupling the sterile 47mm membrane filter directly to the outlet via a TC connection. Consider the case where a Valex sterile sampling valve is used, but the valve is different from the one shown in Figure 2. If the valve model has a 3.81cm (1.5 inch) TC outlet connection, one can flush the outlet in the usual way (2 to 3 minutes, full force), or even alcohol-flame (which is not much more effective). Separately, a 47mm holder and the enclosed analytical membrane filter are coupled to 3.81cm TC x 0.635cm (0.25 inch) national pipe thread (NPT) female and the assembly is wrapped in autoclave paper and sterilized, together with a TC gasket. The sterile filter assembly is attached, aseptically, to the TC outlet of the sampling valve. To the downstream side of the 47mm filter holder, nonsterile latex or Silastic™ (Dow-Corning) or other tubing is attached. The valve is opened and, through the downstream tubing, the desired sample volume (e.g., 300mL) is measured into a graduated cylinder. The valve is closed and the water in the graduated cylinder is discarded. The filter holder is brought to the HEPA hood and opened under laminar flow. Using sterile smooth forceps, the analyst removes the membrane filter and places the filter, upstream side facing upwards, on sterile plate count or soybean-casein digest agar in a 150mm petri dish. Several such discs can be placed on a single plate and labeled on the underside with a grease pencil. Incubation is as described above, as is the inspection and counting. Colonies of interest can be recovered with a flamed loop in the usual manner. Soybean casein digest agar, as with the other media, is detailed in the Difco Manual (Difco, 1984) and consists of

    Tryptone (pancreatic digest of casein . . . . 15 gram
    Soytone (papain digest of soybean meal) . . . . 5 gram
    NaCl . . . . 5 gram
    Agar . . . . 15 gram
    Distilled water to . . . . 1 Liter

Boil the preparation and sterilize by autoclaving for 15 minutes at 121°C. For blood agar, add sterile defibrinated bovine blood to the agar mixture at 45°C and mix well. Blood agar is well suited to the culturing of fastidious organisms, including human pathogens.

Another variation is applicable to the sterile sampling port. The 47mm disc filter is prepared as described above, but rather than 0.635 cm (0.25 inch) NPT to TC, the fitting is NPT to male Luer, on which a suitable needle is mounted (a needle is included with the sterile sampling port). On many of the 47mm filter holders, the upstream coupling is not only NPT but also female Luer, in which instance the parts sequence is filter holder, male Luer nipple, needle with female Luer (capped with a test tube so that the needle will not pierce the autoclave paper). Note: The sterile sampling port must be above the horizontal so that it drains completely and cannot harbor stagnant water.

Another variation on the theme is the 37mm microbial analysis monitor (Millipore; equivalent units now are available from Nuclepore, Sartorius and other vendors). These monitors are disposable polystyrene filter holders containing white gridded (or black gridded) 0.45 micron RPD membrane filter over fiberglass pads; filter holders and filters are sterile. The inlet and outlet ports are female Luer and are plugged with small plastic caps. Separately, one must prepare and sterilize short lengths of plastic tubing, each end of which is fitted with a male Luer. Stainless steel TC blanks are bored so as to be female Luers. These are autoclaved, with the male Luer tubing in place if the plastic tolerates stainless contact during autoclaving. After the customary 2 to 3 minute flush of the outlet, the apparatus (monitor, male-male Luer, female Luer x TC) is clamped in place and the valve is opened slowly (Luer fittings ideally will tolerate pressures greater than 7 bar, approximately 100 psig, but a pressure surge such as might occur when a valve is rapidly opened might cause problems). From the downstream side one recovers the desired volume into a graduated cylinder, shuts off the valve and discards the filtrate. The male-male Luer tubing is disconnected and the plastic plug is inserted into the upstream port of the monitor. Two milliliters of the appropriate sterile liquid medium ar added to the fiberglass pad from the downstream port and that port also is capped with a plastic plug. The medium wicks up into the membrane filter by capillarity, supplying the filter-trapped colonies with sufficient nutrient that they can grow to a discernible size. This is a mini-Petri dish ready for inverted incubation and inspection and counting at 24, 48 and 72 hours.

Many highly motile organisms are "spreaders" and are difficult to count. High counts pose a similar problem as the colonies tend to become confluent. Analytical membrane filters with hydrophobic grid markings solve these problems to a considerable degree (Sharpe, 1981; Sharpe and Michaud, 1975). Isogrid™ membrane filters are available from QA Laboratories, Toronto, Canada.

In summary, the advantages of the membrane method are:

i. The sensitivity of the method is dependent on the volume of liquid passed through the filter. One CFU per 10 liters is possible.

ii. Colonies can be recovered for subculture and identification. However, this also is possible using standard plate counts.

iii. Selective media can be used to aid in the detection and identification of particular organisms.

iv. Membrane methods are well described and accepted within the pharmaceutical and public health communities.

v. The membrane filter methods are rapid and less expensive than alternative methods such as most-probable number (MPN) due to reduced man-hour and medium requirements.

One additional membrane filter method cannot be grouped with the colony growth methods described above. The epifluorescence microscopy method entails collection of organisms onto the surface of a 25mm diameter, 0.2 or 0.4 micron RPD membrane filter (track-etch polycarbonate from Nuclepore Corp.); in-situ staining of the organisms with acridine orange; and examination and counting under oil immersion when the filter is illuminated with a UV source. The method was developed by Pettipher et al. (1980) for determining the microbial quality of milk, and has been adapted to intravenous solutions (Denyer and Ward, 1983; Denyer and Lynn (1987)) and to purified water (Mittelman et al., 1983; Mittelman et al., 1985). Filters are dipped in a 0.2% solution of irgalan black (Ciba-Geigy, Boston) in 2% (v/v) acetic acid that previously had been filtered through a 0.2 micron RPD membrane filter. The fluorescent dye is 20mg acridine orange per milliliter of a 0.1M phosphate buffer, pH 7.5, and contains a small amount of a wetting agent, e.g., 0.01% Triton X-100. The dye solution also must be filtered prior to use. There are claims that viable cells can be differentiated from nonviables on the basis of fluorescent color, but the more conservative approach is to count everything. This method can be rapid and results often can be made available within one or several hours after samples are taken. The major problems are fatigue of the microscopist(s) and nonuniform distribution of organisms on the filter surface, necessitating the counting of many fields. Epifluorescent antibody methods have been partially automated. Pettipher (1983) indicates that the direct epifluorescent technique can be automated by means of instruments reminiscent of those manufactured by American Optical and Cambridge Instruments. If this method can be automated for less than the cost of one or 1.5 technicians to do the microscopic counting, the equipment to automate the counting may be a worthwhile investment.

E. Luciferin-Luciferase (ATP)

Adenosine triphosphate (ATP) is the primary energy source found in all viable cells, whether eukaryote or prokaryote. The amounts of ATP vary according to cell type and phase, but are roughly approximate for most bacteria. Yeasts contain considerably more ATP per cell than do bacteria. When the enzyme luciferase, from fireflies, acts upon the substrate luciferin (from a variety of sources, each unique in composition), ATP is consumed and light is emitted. When luciferin and luciferase are present in excess, photon (light) emission is a function of the ATP concentration (Holm-Hansen, 1966). The system is capable of measuring the amount of ATP in 1,000 or more cells. Therefore, for measurement of microbes in WFI, some means of cell concentration is necessary. Centrifugation is possible in theory, but is impractical because of the difficulties in sterilizing a centrifuge, or handling aseptically the liquid from a large number of large containers in a bucket centrifuge. Filters are readily sterilized, and large volumes of WFI can be filtered through a 0.45 micron RPD membrane filter. For a conservative estimate of the sample volume required for WFI analysis using this method, we will assume that the minimal number of organisms for reliable quantitation is 2,000. Then one must filter about 20 liters through the membrane filter in order to estimate, with good accuracy, 10 organisms per 100mL. This can be done and is practical. Furthermore, the numbers are encouraging for another reason. If one couples a membrane filter via a TC connection to a valve and some organisms are on or in that valve, the adventitious contaminants are unlikely to be of the order of magnitude of the organisms in a quite large sample volume of water. Even an alcohol flaming of a valve does not necessarily make it sterile. For example, one may pass 20 liters of WFI through a 47mm diameter membrane filter. The water contains 5 CFU per 100mL. There would be, in theory, 1,000 organisms on the analytical filter from the sample containing 5 CFU per 100mL. If the valve contributed 300 CFU, then the estimated bioburden would be 1,300 CFU in 20 L, or 6.5 CFU per 100mL. That is to say, if the volume sampled is sufficiently large, low levels of contaminants from the valves can be tolerated.

Therefore, a 0.45 micron RPD membrane filter, is coupled to a WFI outlet and 20 liters of water are run through the filter. The filter is disconnected from the WFI loop and, in the lab, a $0.1N\ HNO_3$ rinse elutes the ATP into the reaction chamber where buffer, luciferin and luciferase are added. The light emission of the reaction is read as ATP (or organism) concentration. Some authors regard the initial burst of light as misleading, and advocate integration of the light-time continuum (Picciolo et al., 1978; Stevensen et al., 1979). Standardization can be with a variety of organisms, although *Bacillus subtilis, Pseudomonas cepacia,* and *Serratia marcescens* seem particularly appropriate as they are common contaminants in the manufacturing environment and in the water supply. Because yeasts have more ATP per cell than bacteria, any error in CFU on the basis of ATP concentration will be conservative in overestimating the bioburden. All things considered, set action limits at 8 CFU per 100mL.

Hyland experience has been with the 3M's Lumac system. Relative light units (RLU) are a function of the square root of bacterial counts trapped and replicating on a 0.45 micron RPD membrane filter (Webster and Lykke, 1985); r^2 is 0.965. Contrary to expectations, precision improves at lower counts, perhaps because (a) high counts are difficult to make, with accuracy, on a 47mm disc, in part due to the fusion of adjacent colonies; and (b) in large microbial populations, many organisms may be injured and unable to reproduce. Injured organisms might not form visible colonies on a conventional nutrient agar, yet could be a source of ATP for the luciferase test.

The track-etch polycarbonate membrane filter (Nuclepore), with pore size ratings of 0.2 or 0.4 micron can be used; they have very low extractables to interfere with the assay. However, filter extractables do not seem to be a major

Figure 4—**Schematic for estimation of bioburden in water.** *From Webster (1986), with permission.*

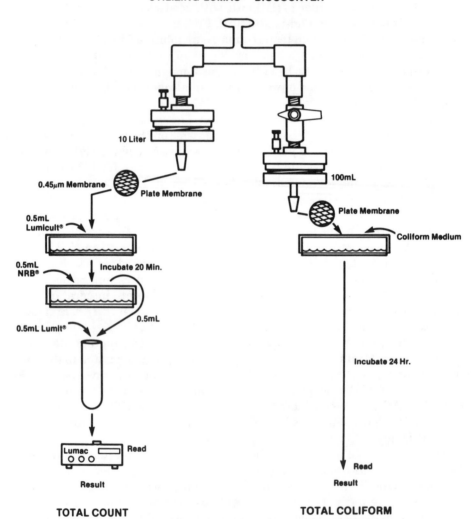

DUAL SWINNEX FILTER SYSTEM FOR DIRECT OUTLET SAMPLING
UTILIZING LUMAC® BIOCOUNTER

10 Liter

0.45μm Membrane   Plate Membrane   100mL

0.5mL Lumicult®   Plate Membrane   Coliform Medium

0.5mL NRB®   Incubate 20 Min.

0.5mL Lumit®   0.5mL

Lumac Read   Incubate 24 Hr.

Result   Read

TOTAL COUNT   Result

          TOTAL COLIFORM

Dual Swinnex Filter Allows Direct Sampling of 10L from Outlet. Sampling Time is
Approximately 3-5 Minutes Depending on Pressure of System.

Figure 5—Correlation of bioburden estimated by the luciferin-luciferase method with membrane filter counts of organisms. *From Webster (1986), with permission.*

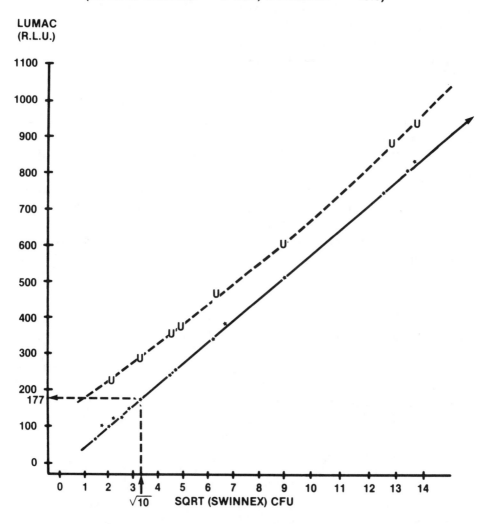

PLOT OF LINEARIZED LUMAC MODEL VS.
SQUARE ROOT OF SWINNEX
WITH UPPER 95% CONFIDENCE LIMIT ("U")
(LUMAC RANGE = 0-200, STD.DEV. = 48.5)

problem and many other types are also suitable. The luciferase is stabilized at a pH of 7.75 to 8.2 and dithiothreitol (Cleland's reagent) is added to stabilize sulfhydryl groups of the enzyme. Divalent Mg is added as a luciferase cofactor and 0.001% Triton X-100 acts as a wetting agent to ensure complete wetting and permeation of the filter. The sample is filtered through the membrane filter, 0.25mL of 0.1N HNO_3 run through the membrane filter to elute the ATP followed by 0.25mL of 85mM $NaSO_4$ (Chappelle et al., 1978).

The luciferin-luciferase assay also has been used to sharpen the endpoint of the sterility test, so as to eliminate bias in the readings (Bussey and Tsuji, 1986).

Non-luciferase luminescent methods may also merit attention. Oleniacz et al. (1968) added 37 mg% luminol (5-amino-2, 3-dihydro-1, 4-phthalazinedione) in 0.12N NaOH containing 2% pyrophosphate. The reaction likely is of iron porphyrins in bacteria with the luminol. Detection limits (sensitivity) are 3,000 to 5,000 cells. In this system, light is measured after the first 6 seconds, during which the free iron is consumed. The same method can be used when the bacteria are concentrated with membrane filter or with ultrafiltration hollow fibers. The organisms are backflushed from the hollow fibers (Chappelle, et al., 1978)

F. Impedance

If the resistance to current flow in a liquid containing viable microbes is measured as the cells respire and reproduce, the resistance will alter as the cells release organic acids. Therefore, if one passes several liters of WFI through a filter, then places the filter atop a suitable growth agar and two electrodes on the filter surface, the change in impedance with time can be observed. That impedance change would be plotted as a function of CFU during validation. The time required for a significant change in impedance is a function of the initial cell population (Wilkins et al., 1980).

This system has not been validated for pharmaceutical applications. The method resembles that of the commercial Bactomatic system in which liquid samples, e.g., apple juice, are put into small plastic cups containing electrode pairs (Cady et al., 1978). The use of membrane filter increases the sensitivity by several orders of magnitude and considerably reduces the time to a significant change in impedance. However, although data can be obtained in hours rather than 1 or 2 days required for normal culturing, measurements are not as rapid as the luciferin-luciferase technique.

G. Radiocarbon technique

The addition of ^{14}C-labeled glucose to growth medium results in the generation of $^{14}CO_2$ which can be counted in the gas phase or precipitated with $Ba(OH)_2$ and then counted. The generation of countable amounts of $^{14}CO_2$ requires and incubation time, and the amount of $^{14}CO_2$ formed at fixed time intervals is a function of the concentration of organisms. The technique is used in hospitals for the detection of organisms in blood samples (septicemia) (Bergen, 1982; Murray, 1982). The method can be applied to the detection and quantitation of organisms in water or product. It should be possible to concentrate organisms on a filter.

A particular advantage of this test is that the sensitivity can be increased by increasing the counting time. For example, if 1 minute counts are only 2× background, 10 minute counts can be done and such counts should be significant. The great drawback of the method is that even weak beta-emitters such as ^{14}C present a disposal nuisance of considerable proportion. For example, toluene-based cocktails cannot be poured down the sink and, even with disposable counting cocktails, only microCurie amounts can be disposed of in ordinary sewage. Furthermore, state licensing is required in the use of radioisotopes and the "hot" laboratory space usually must be dedicated, even if the area is used only once per week. For these reasons, the radiocarbon method is the least attractive.

8. Millipore samplers

Millipore produces the Sampler™ line, which imbibes 1mL of water through a dry gridded membrane filter into a dried medium beneath the filter. These units are suitable for order-of-magnitude microbial assay of grossly contaminated water or food (Richards, 1979), but are completely unsuitable for determining the microbial quality of WFI or liquid product. The Sampler does not imbibe sufficient water for accurate estimation of organisms below 30–50 per milliliter.

6. Microbiological Assessment of Air

A. Centrifugal sampling

The Reuter Centrifugal Sampler (RCS), distributed by BioTest, is a sterilizable, hand-held, battery-operated device (Figure 6) that pulls air at fixed rates through an orifice in such a way that particles in the air impact into a plastic strip on which sterile nutrient agar has been placed. The strip is incubated in its own container and the microscopic colonies that form within 24 hours can be counted under a dissecting microscope using epi-illumination. Because known volumes of air are sampled, the data are quantitatively meaningful. Because discreet colonies form on the nutrient agar, individual colonies can be selected for identification. The RCS is highly portable (hand-held), and can be used under the vertical laminar flow HEPA immediately above a filling line, or in the horizontal HEPA flow of a sterility test hood.

The RCS consistently gives higher recoveries than the slit-to-agar sampler (Placencia et al., 1982). The RCS is the most efficient system currently in use and is the present system of choice for monitoring the microbiological quality of air.

A slit-to-agar system is the model 200 of the Matson-Garvin Co., which samples air at 28.3 liters per minute. A similar unit is also manufactured by F.P. Thornton Associates of Newark, NJ.

Figure 6—The Reuter Centrifugal Sampler™. *Photo courtesy of BioTest.*

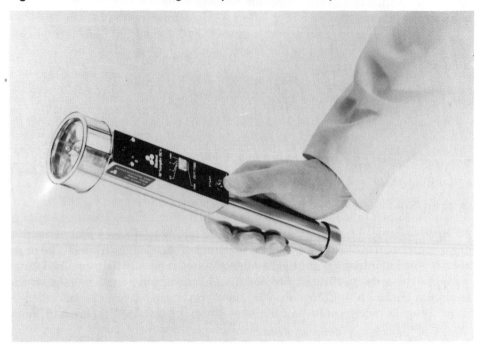

B. Cascade impaction

Traditionally, cascade impactors have been used for the separation and enumeration of airborne particles. Whether the system is driven under positive or negative pressure, the largest particles fall on the topmost plate. Particles able to follow the airstream pass to lower plates. The plates can be coated with nutrient or other suitable sterile agars so that organisms, impacting into the semi-solid medium, can be grown to a visible size, counted, and recovered for identification. This technique is used occasionally in pharmaceutical applications (Duberstein and Howard, 1978). As with the RCS, colonies can be sampled for identification, and sampling is volumetric. Unlike the RCS, the slit-to-agar machine (which uses any medium) is somewhat large and ungainly, hence difficult to maneuver. For example, it will not fit above the filling line. The advantage of the cascade impactor is that the system can be run slowly so that the effect of personnel, or equipment, entering the filling room can be shown. This is applicable especially to those few facilities that wheel a sterile bulk tank into the filling room.

The Anderson sampler, with the model 20-725 LPI Adaptor Kit, can sample to less than 0.23 micron particle diameter. The Anderson sampler allegedly gives higher bacterial counts than slit-to-agar or liquid impingers (Ludholm, 1982). However, because the Anderson unit (like the slit-to-agar system) is not highly maneuverable, it is not as effective a monitoring tool as the RCS.

C. Liquid Impingement

All of the foregoing methods utilize impinger technology, wherein particles, including bacteria, are driven, usually under negative pressure, into a nutrient agar surface. In the liquid impinger, bacteria are driven, under negative pressure, into a liquid, usually a nutrient broth containing a Dow antifoam. During sample collection, all organisms are mixed in the recovery liquid and some may increase in number while others reduce in numbers, if the sampling period is protracted. At the end of the sampling period, the liquid is run through a gridded 0.45 micron RPD membrane filter and placed on a suitable nutrient agar or a depth filter disc saturated in a suitable medium.

If the impinger medium is a nutrient broth solution, one of the Dow antifoams must be used to prevent a foam build-up that clogs the system. Phosphate-buffered saline (PBS) likely would prove to be more satisfactory than a peptide broth solution, as the problem of foam generation should be obviated. The most readily available impingers are the all-glass models from Millipore. The units would be far more popular if they were fabricated from polycarbonate, which is more difficult to break.

The liquid impinger system can be coupled to a filter system for a luciferin-luciferase assay. This system will be significantly faster for the generation of data than the RCS or slit-to-agar methods. However, a proper validation of the technique, coupled with the ATP assay, seems not to have been done.

D. Settling plates

The most common and cheapest method of monitoring clean room air is the settling plate method. The plates usually are 100×15mm petri dishes containing blood agar or nutrient agar, and the plates are exposed at various positions in a filling room during the filling process. Some plates are placed on or near the filling line. The presumption is that particles fall out of the air onto such plates.

For many years, there has been a widespread assumption that there is a correlation between airborne particles and bioburden. There is no correlation between total particle counts in a clean room and CFU on fall-out plates (Olson et al., 1983). There may be a correlation between airborne particles and bioburden, but it has not yet been shown. Further, one assumes a cumulative increase in counts with time, but that does not occur with settling plates (Lee et al., 1982). Rather, Lee's work indicates that microbial counts, on settling plates in clean rooms, follow the negative binomial regardless of the exposure time. The negative binomial formerly was called "contagious distribution," which essentially meant that because microbes are reproductive units, they are found infrequently but always in clusters. In a contagious distribution, most samples show a zero population. What Lee's statistical finding probably means is that if nonsterile equipment, or an improperly gowned operator, moves into the filling room near a settling plate, organisms may be found on the plate. Otherwise, the plate will remain sterile.

The settling plates do not act as suitable microbial monitors because there is no way of measuring the air volume that is sampled nor is the effect of airstream over the plates known. As discussed by Tsuji (1975) settling plates may be suitable for monitoring the air quality with vertical flow HEPA filtration units, but are unsuitable for monitoring air quality with horizontal HEPA filtration units; such as are typical for sterility test horizontal laminar work stations. The only reason that settling plates are still are in use is because a complete study, showing their inadequacies, has yet to be performed.

6. Microbiological Assessment of Surfaces

A. Contact plates
Contact plates (e.g. Rodac™) are small petri dishes containing a nutrient agar. The surface of the agar is convex and extends beyond the walls of the dish. The user removes the lid and presses the agar-containing surface against the surface to be analyzed. The lid then is replaced and the dish is incubated in the usual manner. This is the most widely accepted method for monitoring the microbiological quality of surfaces, However, more recent work at NASA and at the University of Utah suggest that better methods are available (see Sampler, and Synthetic Polymer Cloth Capture, below).

B Swab samplers
The Millipore Sampler™ that is inadequate for monitoring the microbiological quality of WFI has a counterpart that has been used fairly extensively in supermarkets to monitor the microbiological quality of meat-cutting instruments and surfaces before and after use (Bower, 1976). The sterile swab, attached to a small handle, is in sterile saline. Remove the swab by the handle and swab in parallel strokes a square 2.54 cm (one inch) on a side, first side-to-side, then top-to-bottom, and then, again, side-to-side. The swab is replaced into the sterile saline and the swab/saline is shaken vigorously to dislodge many, hopefully most, organisms from the swab. A sterile Millipore total count membrane filter paddle, which is dry and contains medium, then is inserted into the saline. The paddle imbibes 1mL of the saline. The paddle, in a separate container, is incubated and counted in the usual way under epi-illumination. Aside from Soucy et al. (1983), there appear to be no scientific evaluations in the literature, although the Sampler has been tested for the evaluation of dialysis fluid used in hemodialyzers (Favero and Petersen, 1977), an application that does not require high-purity water.

Craythorn et al. (1980) claim that Millipore Samplers, containing 3 to 5 micron RPD membrane filter, are more efficient in the recovery of microbes from surfaces than Rodac plates. The work was done only with moist surfaces, and the 3 to 5 micron RPD membrane filter paddles were prepared by Millipore as a special item. There is no mention of these in the current Millipore catalogue.

C. Synthetic polymer cloth capture

Sterile cloths, woven or nonwoven, of polyolefin or other synthetic materials, can be wiped across a surface and placed in sterile phosphate-buffered saline (PBS) or other suitable medium. The cloth and the medium are placed in an ultrasonic bath operating at 25 kHz for 2 minutes. The cloth is stirred briefly, then removed. Samples are plated as for standard plate counts. This method is claimed to be more efficient in the removal and recovery of microbes from surfaces than the use of swabs (Puleo and Krischner, 1981), although it would appear that the swabs were not ultrasonicated and the type of swabs, or swab systems, were not identified.

The PBS or broth medium in which the wiping cloth had been sonicated could be filtered through a 0.45 micron RPD membrane filter for subsequent plating on a suitable nutrient agar in a petri dish. This was not explored in the NASA article, Of the methods listed, this seems the most soundly based and rational.

The headcount in the filling room must be kept to a minimum in the interest of the cleanest possible environment (Shaughnessy, 1986). Therefore, whenever possible, filling room personnel should be trained in the monitoring methods so that QC people do not have to enter the filling room. Equipment like the RCS should enter and leave the filling room via a "pass-through."

7. Identification of Microorganisms

A. Introduction

The primary source of bacteria and fungi in aseptically-processed products is people. The organisms shed by humans are fairly predictable and include *Proteus* spp., *Staphylococcus aureus* and other *staphylococci*, *Streptococcus pyogenes* and other *streptococci*, *Escherichia coli* and other coliforms which are intolerable in WFI or autoclave cooling water and so forth. These organisms are shed on flakes of skin dandruff and hair; a veritable microbial cloud follows each worker (see data of Hooper et al., 1972, quoted in Beloian, 1983), and vigorous hand washing and capping, masking, gowning and gloving in sterile fabrics is essential to containment (Whyte et al., 1982; Whyte and Bailey, 1985).

The second significant source of microbial contaminants is the air in the manufacturing environment and the air in the filling room. Despite the pervasiveness of the HEPA air wash over the filling lines, the occasional organism is detected (see, for example, Lee et al., 1982). The airborne organisms not clearly associated with a human source include *Bacillus* spp., often *B. subtilis,* and the various pseudomonads such as *Pseudomonas cepacia. Ps. cepacia* is commonly observed in water systems, including distilled water lines, but almost certainly is acquired, in the pharmaceutical processing area from the air.

Raw materials seldom contribute significant microbial bioburden (Baggerman and Kannegieter, 1984) but biologicals should be monitored (Olson, 1985). However, cleaned equipment can present a problem if tanks, for example, contain standing water. *Pseudomonas cepacia* (Carson et al., 1973) and *Pseudomonas aeruginosa* (Favero et al., 1971) can grow to 10^5 to 10^6 per milliliter in distilled water, using trace organics in air as a carbon source.

When contaminants are found in the final product, e.g., during bulk testing or the sterility testing of the final container, it is appropriate to streak the microbe(s) on blood agar or a suitable nutrient agar to observe whether there is one contaminant or many, and to provide a source for colony isolation and identification. If there are many contaminants, a major incursion or break in sterility is likely, e.g., a faulty TC pipe connection or a holed hose. But if a pure culture of, for example, *Streptococcus pyogenes,* is observed, the likely source is the filling room or the sterility test room.

Furthermore, if media fills consistently show contamination levels of 0.1%, which is commonplace in a well-run facility, and *S. pyogenes* is found during the first sterility test of 20 final containers but a proteus is found when the second sterility test is done, the most likely conclusion is that the sterility test is not being done properly, and that these are false positives. The manufacturer still must withhold the product from the marketplace, but the identification of the contaminants provides the first clue in the location of the source of the contamination. However, identification of the source of contaminants is no substitute for good manufacturing practice that excludes microbes from the product during downstream manufacturing or testing.

There is no substitute for hands-on experience in practical microbiology. Anyone who has not practiced Gram stains with organisms of known reaction should not be performing such a test or attempting to identify organisms. The discussion is intended as a convenient source for some information on commercially available chemical and biochemical tests that can simplify and accelerate organism identification.

B. Biochemical tests

The conventional methods for identification of microbes include streaking on a nutrient agar, such as soybean-casein digest, so as to obtain a colony derived from a single organism, subculturing the organism on slants, and performing a Gram stain. For many organisms, the colonial morphology is known to the plant microbiologist. Then the colonial morphology, odor, Gram reaction, and shape, size and arrangement of the cells may provide sufficient information for probable identification.

Even for a commonplace pseudomonad such as *Ps. fluorescens,* a Gram-negative rod with a characteristic butyric odor and green color, the microbiologist may wish to confirm that the organism does not ferment glucose. Fairly extensive batteries of semisolid media, compartmented into sections that contain different sugars, are available as disposable trays to be inoculated with the unknown organism. These systems can be used alone, such as the various API systems (Analytab Products) (see Figure 7) or automated for the identification of particular genera and species within a given group, such as the *Enterobacteriaceae*. Several manufacturers supply reagents to this market, e.g., Becton Dickinson with the Minitek series; additional particulars can be found in Lenette et al. (1985).

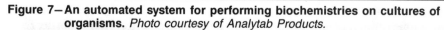

Figure 7—An automated system for performing biochemistries on cultures of organisms. *Photo courtesy of Analytab Products.*

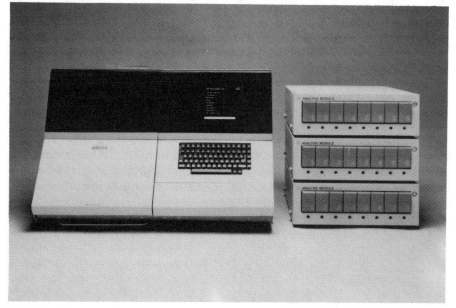

C. Gas chromatography and cellular lipids

Attempts to identify microorganisms from their pyrolysis products have had only limited success, and that effort, dating from the early 1960s, seems not to be in current use. However, Hewlett-Packard now markets an automated system for identification of microbes based on the composition of their cellular fatty acids. Cells from a streak colony are grown on soybean-casein agar, the fatty acids are extracted from the cells, saponified, methylated, and separated, identified and quantitated by gas chromatography. The automated system, designated HP 5898A Automated Microbial Identification System, is shown in Figure B-1 in Appendix B at the end of this book.

The concept is sound. Various organisms already are identified by the presence or absence of various enzymes or groups of enzymes, e.g., catalase positive or negative, glucose-fermenting, etc. Similarly, the generation of the various fatty acids in a given microbial species or strain is a reflection of the enzymes that construct those fatty acids. In turn, the synthesis of those enzymes is dictated by components of the genome. Therefore, identification of an organism from fatty acid composition should be as valid as any other technique. Sample chromatographic separations of the fatty acids (as the methyl esters) from two different *Bacillus* spp. are shown in Figure B-2. One sample printout is shown in Figure B-3. Identifications of bacteria are based on an extensive library, in the computer memory, of fatty acid compositions for many organisms. Identification is expressed as a percentage agreement with the fatty acid profile, from the computer memory, of the organism that most closely matches the unknown. Those familiar with the identification systems of Sneath (1962) will recognize the comparisons.

According to Hewlett-Packard personnel, enteric bacteria cannot be identified from their fatty acids. Apparently, the enterics share a common fatty acid profile, and must be further identified by conventional biochemistries.

D. Differential media

The inclusion of some compounds into a growth medium can inhibit the growth of groups of organisms, a desirable feature when total counts are not required. One of the critical instances in which the microbiologist in an industrial pharmaceutical setting may use differential media to advantage is in the detection and enumeration of coliforms in WFI or cooling water. Coliforms are taken to mean enteric organisms and include, for example, *Escherichia coli, Klebsiella pneumoniae, Enterobacter aerogenes, Citrobacter freundii,* etc.

LeChevallier et al. (1983) have indicated that a medium named m-T7 is more effective than m-Endo in the differential recovery of coliforms. The composition of m-T7 is:

Difco proteose peptone no. 3	5 gram
Lactose	20 gram
Yeast extract	3 gram
Polyoxyethylene ether W-1	5 mL
Bromthymol blue	0.1 mL
Bromcresol purple	0.1 mL
Agar	15 gram
Tergitol 7 (25%)	0.4 mL
Distilled water	1 Liter

Autoclave, and then aseptically, add

Penicillin G	199 micrograms

Some workers may prefer to collect organisms directly onto 47mm membrane filter, which filters then are cultured directly onto a selective medium such as m-T7 so as to provide information on coliforms as rapidly as possible. For coliforms, m-TEC gives the best combination of recovery and lowest false positives (Pagel et al., 1982). A good pseudomonas isolation agar, and other differential media, can be found in the Difco Manual (1984). A rapid method for confirming *P. Aerubinosa* on the basis of pigment production is given in Table III.

E. Rapid identification of Pseudomonas cepacia

Increasingly, *Pseudomonas cepacia* is identified as a contaminant of water supplies and bacteriostatic solutions (Gelbart et al., 1976; Mannielo et al., 1978; Richards and Richards, 1979). Unpublished comments from the pharmaceutical industry suggest that the organism is a source of concern to segments of the industry. A medium, selective for *P. cepacia* and *Serratia marcescens,* which are readily differentiated, was developed by Wu and Thompson (1984) and is the subject of this appendix. Ten *P. cepacia* strains have been examined by Wu and Thompson; they found recoveries on the selective medium of 67.8 to 94.1% of the colony-forming units on plate count agar. An *Alcaligenes* sp., *E. coli, K. pneumoniae, P. mirabilis,* eight other pseudomonads including 53 strains of *aeruginosa, S. aureus* and *S. faecalis* were inhibited and did not grow on the medium.

> Plate count agar . . . . 23.5 gram
> Distilled or DI water . . . . 1 Liter
>
> Boil to dissolve. Autoclave 15 minutes at 121°C;
> post-autoclave pH 7.0 ± 0.2 at 25°C.
>
> Per liter plate count agar add:
> C-390 . . . . 1 milligram
> Polymixin B sulfate . . . . 75 milligram

Mix and autoclave 15 minutes at 121°C. The final pH should be 6.95 ± 0.05. Polymixin B sulfate is available from Pfizer, Inc., Groton, Connecticut, USA. C-390 is the commercial name for 9-chloro-9-(4-diethylaminophenyl)-10-phenylacridan, available from Norwich Eaton Pharmaceuticals, Inc., Norwich, NY. The plate count agar is from Difco (Detroit, MI). The C-390 inhibits organisms other than *P. aeruginosa* and *P. cepacia*. Polymixin B sulfate inhibits the growth of *P. aeruginosa* but not *P. cepacia*.

On the Wu-Thompson agar, *P. cepacia* colonies are small, raised and cream colored, but the *S. marcescens* colonies were pink, large and convex. *P. cepacia* is oxidase-positive (as are all pseudomonads), whereas *S. marcescens* is oxidase-negative. The oxidase reagent is p-aminodimethyl-aniline oxalate (PADA). A 1% solution in DI or distilled water is heated gently and flooded onto plates containing isolated colonies. Alternatively, a filter paper may be wetted with the 1% PADA and a loopful of the colony of interest deposited onto the paper. Positive colonies turn pink, then maroon, and finally black.

All water sources exposed to environmental air contained some *P. cepacia* counts, including distilled water.

8. Robotics in Sterility Testing

Using robotic systems to perform sterility tests, Hoffmann-La Roche has reported no false-positive sterility tests in the last two years (Zlotnick, 1987). At Hyland, false-positive sterility test results have been reduced to a rate of about 0.02% by means of presterilized closed container filtration systems (Steritest and Sterisart).

Zlotnick and Franklin (1987) deployed a Puma 260 computer-controlled robot arm which, when adjusted by an operator, drove a Steritest needle (see Figures 1 and 2) into the final container under test, then into a bottle of the appropriate growth medium (soybean-casein digest or fluid thioglycollate). Accuracy of the robot arm movements (and needle placements) was to within 0.127mm. Fluid lines were opened and closed with computer-controlled pinchclamps.

The closed environmental cabinets housed adjacent sterility test units completely under laminar filtered (HEPA) air flow. Two adjacent cabinets each housed a Steritest system and shared a robot arm that moved on a rail between between chambers. The chambers were opened to place the sample vials and the vials containing growth medium, and to make minor adjustments to the robot prior to the onset of testing. During testing, the cabinets were closed; minimizing the potential for operator contamination of the samples or the test system.

References

Alegnani, W.C. (1979) Pharm. Technol. 3 (12), 44-49.

American Public Health Association (1981) "Standard Methods for the Examination of Water and Waste Water", 15th Ed., 789-793, American Public Health Association, Washington, D.C.

Anderson, R.L., Berkelman, R.J., Mackel, D.C., Davis, B.J., Holland, B.W. and Martone, W.J. (1984) Appl. Environ. Microbiol. 47, 757-762.

Baggerman, C. and Kannegeiter, L.M. (1984) Appl. Environ. Microbiol. 48, 662-664.

Beloian, A. (1983) In "Disinfection, Sterilization and Preservation, 3rd Ed.", (S.S. Block, ed.), pages 885-917, Lea and Febiger, Philadelphia, PA.

Berkelman, R.L., Anderson, R.L., Davis, B.J., Highsmith, A.K., Petersen, N.J., Bond, W.W., Cook, E.H., Mackel, D.C., Favero, M.S. and Martone, W.J. (1984) Appl. Environ. Microbiol. 47, 752-756.

Bergau, A. (1982) In "Rapid Methods and Automation in Microbiology", (R.C. Tinton, ed.), pages 36-40, Am. Soc. Microbiol., Washington, D.C.

Bitton, G. and Marshall, K.C. (1980) "Adsorption of Microorganisms to Surfaces", John Wiley and Sons, New York.

Blank, J. (1983) Appl. Environ. Microbiol. 45, 319-320.

Borick, P.M. and Borick, J.A. (1972) In "Quality Control in the Pharmaceutical Industry". (M.S. Cooper, ed.), pages 1-38, Academic Press, New York.

Bower, J. (1976) Personal communication with Mrs. Jacqueline Bower, presently at MicroFiltration Systems, Dublin, CA.

Bowman, F.W. (1966) J. Pharm. Sci. 55, 818-821.

Bowman, F.W. (1968) Bull. Parenteral Drug Assoc. 22, 57-63.

Bowman, F.W. (1969) Bull. Parenteral Drug Assoc. 22, 57

Bowman, F.W. (1969) J. Pharm. Sci. 58, 1301-1308.

Bowman, F.W., Knoll, E.W. and Calhoun, M.P. (1967) J. Pharm. Sci. 56, 1009-1010.

Bryce, D.M. (1956) J. Pharm. Pharmacol. 8, 561-572.

Bush, J.H. and Lomonier, J. (1977) U.S. Patent 4,036,698.

Bussey, D.M., Kane, M.P. and Tsuji, K. (1983) J. Parenteral Sci. Technol. 37, 51-54.

Bussey, D.M. and Tsuji, K. (1986) Appl. Environ. Microbiol. 51, 349-355.

Cady, P., Hardy, D., Martius, S., Dufour, S.W. and Kraeger, S.J. (1978) J. Food Protect. 41, 277-283.

Calhoun, M.P., White, M. and Bowman, F.W. (1970) J. Pharm. Sci. 59, 1022-1024.

Carson, L.A., Favero, M.S., Bond, W.W. and Petersen, N.J. (1973) Appl. Microbiol. 25, 476-483.

Carson, L.A., Petersen, N.J., Favero, M.S., Doto, I.L., Collins, D.E. and Levin, M.A. (1975) Appl. Microbiol. 3, 935-942.

Chappelle, E., Demine, J., Picciolo, G.L., Jeffers, E. and Thomas, R.R. (1978) NASA Tech Briefs Summer, 237-238.

Chappelle, E.W., Picciola, G.L. and Deming, J.W. (1978) Methods in Enzymol. LVII, 65-72.

Christiansen, G.G. and Koski, T.A. (1983) J. Biol. Stand. 11, 83-89.

Committee of Revision (1982) Pharm. Forum 8, 2239.

Cooper, M.S. (1982) J. Parenteral Sci. Technol. 36, 256-258.

Craythorn, J.M., Barbour, A.G., Mateen, J.M., Britt, M.R. and Garibaldi, R.A. (1980) J. Clin. Microbiol. 12, 250-255.

Denyer, S.P. and Ward, K.H. (1983) J. Parenteral Sci. Technol. 37, 156-158.

Difco (1984) "Difco Manual". 10th Ed., Difco Laboratories, Detroit, MI.

Duberstein, R. and Howard, G. (1978) J. Parenteral Drug Assoc. 32, 192-198.

Dupe, D. and Peters, K. (1984) In "Advances in Laboratory Automation Robotics 1984", (G.L. Hank and J.R. Strumaitis, eds.), 91-103, Zymark Corp., Hopkintown, MA.

Eskenazi, S., Bychkowski, O.E., Smith, M. and MacMillan, J.D. (1982) J. Assoc. Off. Anal. Chem. 65, 1155-1161.

Favero, M.S., Carson, L.A., Bond, W.W. and Petersen, N.J. (1971) Science 173, 836.

Felts, S.K., Schaffner, W., Melly, M.A. and Koenig, M.G. (1972) Ann. Int. Med. 77, 881-890.

Gee, L.W., Harvey, J.M.G.H., Olson, W.P. and Lee, M.L. (1985) J. Pharm. Sci. 74, 29-32.

Gee, L.W., Zeiner, R. and Olson, W.P. (1986) Pharm. Res. 3 (6) (in press).

Gelbart, S.M., Reinhardt, G.F. and Greenlee, H.B. (1976) J. Clin. Microbiol. 3, 62-66.

Gram, C. (1884) Fortschr. Med. 2, 185-189.

Hibbert, H.R. and Spencer, R. (1970) J. Hyg., Camb. 68, 131-135,

Holdowsky, S. (1957) Antibiot. Chemother. 7, 49-54.

Holm-Hansen, O. (1966) Limnol. Oceanogr. 11, 510-519.

LeChevallier, M.W., Cameron, S.C. and McPeters, G.A. (1983) Appl. Environ. Microbiol. 45, 484-492.

Lee, M.L., Kantrowitz, J.L. and Ellis, J.E. (1982) J. Parenteral Sci. Technol. 36, 237-241.

Lennette, E.H., Balows, A., Hausler, W.J. and Shadomy, H.J.(eds) (1985) "Manual of Clinical Microbiology". 4th Ed., Amer. Soc. Microbiol., Washington, D.C.

Ludholm, M. (1982) Appl. Environ. Microbiol. 44, 179-183.

Manniello, J.M., Heymann, H. and Adair, F.W. (1978) Antimicrob. Agents Chemother. 14, 500-503.

Marrie, T.J. and Costerton, J.W. (1981) Appl. Environ. Microbiol. 42, 1093-1102.

Mascoli, C.C. (1981) Med. Dev. Diag. Ind. 3 (4), 8-9.

Millipore Corp. (1971) "Sterility Testing with the Membrane Filter", AM201, Millipore Corp., Bedford, MA.

Mittelman, M.W., Geesey, G.G. and Hite, R. (1983) Microcontamination 1 (2), 32-37, 52.

Mittelman, M.W., Geesey, G.G. and Platt, R.M. (1985) Med. Dev. Diag. Ind. 7 (6), 144-148.

Mossel, D.A. and Beerens, H. (1968) J. Hyg., Camb. 66, 269-272.

Odlaug, T.E., Ocwieja, D.A., Purohit, K.S., Riley, R.M. and Young, W.E. (1984) J. Parenteral Sci. Technol. 38, 141-147.

Oleniacz, W.S., Pisano, M.A., Rosenfeld, M.H. and Elgart, R.L. (1968) Environ. Sci. Technol. 2, 1030-1033.

Olson, W.P. (1979) Pharm. Technol. 3 (11), 85-92, 120.

Olson, W.P. (1983) Process Biochem. 18 (5), 29-33.

Pagel, J.E., Qureshi, A.A., Young, D.M. and Vlassoff, L.T. (1982) Appl. Environ. Microbiol. 43, 787-793.

Pettipher, G.L., Fulford, R.J. and Mabbitt, L.A. (1983) J. Appl. Bacteriol. 54, 177-182.

Pettipher, G.L., Mansell, R., McKinnon, C.H. and Cousins, C.M. (1980) Appl. Environ. Microbiol. 39, 423-429.

Picciolo, G.L., Deming, J.W., Nibley, D.A. and Chappelle, E.W. (1978) Methods in Enzymol. LVII, 550-559.

Pickett, M. and Litsky, W. (1981) Pharm. Technol. 5 (5), 63-68.

Placencia, A.M., Oxborrow, G.S. and Danielson, J.W. (1982) J. Pharm. Sci. 71, 704-705.

Placencia, A.M., Peeler, J.T., Oxborrow, G.S. and Danielson, J.W. (1982) Appl. Environ. Microbiol. 44, 512-513.

Puleo, J.R. and Krischner, L.E. (1981) NASA Tech Briefs 6 (2), Item 47, Jet Propulsion Lab., Pasadena, CA.

Richards, G.P. (1979) Appl. Environ. Microbiol. 38, 341-342.

Richards, R.M.E. and Richards, J.M. (1979) J. Pharm. Sci. 68, 1436-1437.

Riggs, T.H. (1979) Med. Dev. Diag. Ind. 1 (6), 18-19.

Rycroft, J.A. and Moon, D. (1975) J. Hyg., Camb. 74, 17-22.

Sautter, R.L., Mattman, L.H. and Legaspi, R.C. (1984) Inf. Control 5 (5), 223-225.

Sharpe, A.N. (1981) In "Membrane Filtration Applications, Techniques, and Problems", (B.J. Dutka, ed.), pages 513-535, Marcel Dekker, New York.

Sharpe, A.N. and Michaud, G.L. (1975) Appl. Microbiol. 30, 519-524.

Soucy, K., Randal, C.J. and Holley, R.A. (1983) Poultry Sci. 62, 298-309.

Standard Methods (1980) "Standard Methods for the Evaluation of Water and Wastewater, 15th Edn.", Am. Publ. Hlth Assoc., Washington, D.C.

Stevenson, L.H., Chrzanowski, T.H. and Erkenbrecher, C.W. (1979) In "Native Aquatic Bacteria: Enumeration, Activity, and Ecology, ASTM STP 695", (J.W. Costerton and R.R. Colwell, eds.), pages 99-116, Amer. Soc. Testing and Materials, Philadelphia, PA.

Tsuji, K. (1975) In "Automation in Microbiology and Immunology", (C.G. Heden and T. Illeni, eds.), pages 157-167, John Wiley and Sons, New York.

Tsuji, K., Stapert, E.M., Robertson, J.H. and Waiyaki, P.M. (1970) Appl. Microbiol. 20, 798-801.

Webster, W.A. (1986) "Application of ATP: Process Water", Amer. Soc. Microbiol. Workshop, Industrial Applic. Rapid Microb. Detect. Methods, May 30, Philadelphia, PA.

Whyte, W. and Bailey, P.V. (1985) J. Parenteral Sci. Technol. 39, 51-60.

Whyte, W., Bailey, P.V., Tinkler, J., McCubbin, I., Young, L. and Jess, J. (1982) J. Parenteral Sci. Technol. 36, 102-107.

Wilkins, J.R., Grana, D.C. and Fox, S.S. (1980) Appl. Environ. Microbiol. 40, 852-853.

Winstead, M. (1967) "Reagent Grade Water: How, When and Why?", Amer. Soc. Med. Technologists, Houston, TX, 42, pages 57-58.

Zlotnick, B.J. (1987) Personal communication with Dr. Barbara Zlotnick at Hoffmann-La Roche, Nutley, NJ.

Zlotnick, B.J. and Franklin, M.J. (1987) Pharm. Technol. 11 (5), 58-64.

13

Viruses in Therapeutics from Human Plasma: Upstream and Downstream Process Strategies

Wayne P. Olson
Hyland Therapeutics, Los Angeles, CA, USA

1. Introduction

The human immunodeficiency virus (HIV), also termed HTLV-III or AIDS virus, is a retrovirus (RNA-containing virus) surrounded by a cell membrane-like envelope. The virus largely proliferates in T-cells, a critical portion of the immune system. Without a functional immune system, the host eventually succumbs to one or more of myriad diseases that the immune system routinely controls, such as newly arising cancers and pneumonias caused by rarely encountered organisms.

At this writing, the greatest concern of the American medical community is the spread of HIV, primarily by sexual contact among homosexuals but also by the sharing of needles among IV drug users. About 50,000 cases have been diagnosed of which about 20,000 have died to date. Some cases have been attributed to AIDS via whole blood transfusion, and a relatively small number of cases to hemophiliacs receiving concentrates of clotting factor VIII (F-VIII). This chapter cannot address the issues of sexual contact and drug use, nor HIV in whole blood. However, that virus and others in plasma fractions of human source is addressed. The viruses of greatest concern are HIV, hepatitis B, non-A non-B hepatitis and a parvovirus. Polio virus, hepatitis A, HTLV-I, and other viruses mentioned in this chapter are not transmitted in human plasma and are studied largely as markers and models.

2. Sources

A. Raw materials

The ultimate source of any viruses in human source material is the donor. Where single-donor F-VIII is prepared, e.g., Dutch Red Cross, the probability of AIDS or other viral infection relates to the infection level of the donor population. Where donations (400–500 mL each) are pooled, the probability can be much higher unless viral elimination or inactivation strategies, or both, are invoked.

B. Process

Viruses, like bacteria, can be adsorbed to a wide variety of surfaces (see Olson and Greenwood, 1986 for a discussion). These include stainless steel tanks and components (pipes, valves, etc.). Ion-exchange matrices, e.g., DEAE-substituted materials, also are used in the purification of clotting factor IX (F-IX) (Brummelhuis, 1980) and IgG (Suomela, 1980). Viruses might be concentrated on the matrices leading to the contamination of subsequent lots. A minor consideration, unlikely to be of consequence, is that manufacturing personnel might contribute virions to the process stream. There is no record of such contamination.

3. Strategies that Work

A. Screening donors and plasma

The proportion of virus-infected donors contributing to the plasma pool can be reduced by questioning and physically screening donors, and by testing the individual plasma donations by state-of-the-art techniques. The maintenance of records on all donors also is essential, especially because a donor without a history of, for example, hepatitis may develop the disease and later seek again to donate plasma or whole blood. Any donor who has had hepatitis is rejected permanently from the Hyland network of donor centers, as is any prospective donor who has AIDS or AIDS-related complex (as defined by the U.S. Centers for Disease Control) which includes unexplained weight loss, fever, persistent cough and shortness of breath, persistent diarrhea, drenching night sweats, lesions typical of Kaposi's sarcoma, etc. Plasma may not be donated by a person who is or ever has been a drug addict involving the injection of drugs. These judgments are made by physicians at the donor centers. Plasma may not be donated within six months of receiving whole blood or one of the clotting factors. (Recipients of normal serum albumin, or plasma protein fraction, or the various immune serum globulins are excepted, as these products have a history of viral safety.) There are many additional causes for donor rejection. For example, persons currently taking adrenergic blocking agents (alpha or beta) or antibiotics (other than small doses of tetracycline or erythromycin for acne vulgaris) also are excluded, whereas donors currently receiving vitamins or mild analgesics are not. The screenings represent medical histories and physical inspection by physicians. There are two levels of safeguards within the screening system, as used at Hyland, and safeguards during the preparation of the plasma fractions.

The first safeguard or backup to the screening procedure at the donor center is the testing of every individual plasma donation. Among the tests in use by the Hyland Plasma Screening Laboratory in Illinois are:

> HIV antibody (test for antibody to the AIDS virus; the test is obtained from Electronucleonics, Inc.)

> Hepatitis-B surface antigen (an immuno-assay for hepatitis virus, supplied by Connaught and distributed by Travenol Laboratories)

> Alanine amino transferase (ALT); this enzyme often is found in the plasma of people with non-A non-B hepatitis)

> Syphilis testing (the rapid plasma reagent screen (RPR), is used; a positive test is followed with a more specific test, e.g., FTA, MHA-TP or TPI).

If the results of the preliminary screening at the donor center allow for a donation, but are contradicted by results from the plasma screening lab, the means must exist to exclude the donated plasma from the pooling system. The lifestyle or state of health of any donor, paid or volunteer, can change. A donor may attempt to continue donation of plasma after becoming unsuitable as a donor. Some method is required for ensuring that the plasma of unacceptable donors, who might previously have been acceptable, does not enter the plasma pool. The Hyland system codes each donation into a central memory (computer) that also keys each donation to the medical history and to the results of the laboratory testing. This computerized network also makes possible the immediate rejection of any donor noted to be unacceptable at any other Hyland donor center. This is the second safeguard or backup system.

B. Cohn fractionation

The cold ethanol plasma fractionation method of Cohn et al. (1946) is used throughout the world as the primary method for the preparation of normal serum albumin, immune serum globulins and related products, all of which are viral safe and have been known for many years to be safe and effective. Ethanol inactivates HIV as a function of time and of concentration, and human immunoglobulins prepared by the Cohn process are free of HIV as can be shown by existing analytical methods (Piszkiewicz et al., 1985; Wells et al., 1986; Zuck et al., 1986). Forty percent ethanol rapidly inactivates HIV (Wells et al., 1986), thus albumin prepared by the Cohn process likely would be AIDS-free even in the absence of the pasteurization step (see below). Plasma products under scrutiny with regard to the potential for contamination with viruses are the clotting factors intended for intravenous use by hemophiliacs. Human clotting factor IX, prepared with an ethanol step but not heated, is also said not to cause a positive seroconversion in patients administered this product only (Gazengel and Larrieu, 1985).

C. Pasteurization

Human serum albumin is 100% virus safe because it is pasteurized at 60°C for 10 hours (Shikata et al., 1978). This occurs in the final container and the albumin is stabilized by 4mM caprylate (Edsall, 1984). Pasteurization of F-VIII in the absence of stabilizers is successful but results in 75 to 80% loss of activity. The D-value for HIV (time for 1 log of kill at the indicated temperature) is 32 minutes for freeze-dried preparations at 60°C, but 24 seconds in the liquid state (McDougal et al., 1985). Consequently, protracted heating of dried F-VIII also can be successful in the destruction of HIV (a heat-labile virus) where the F-VIII preparation is quite stable. However, non-A non-B hepatitis virus is not readily destroyed by heat.

Bovine leukemia virus (BLV), like the HTL viruses, proliferates in lymphocytes; infected cells can be found in raw milk. Pasteurization at 63°C for 30 minutes inactivates BLV-infected lymphocytes as well as free BLV (Rubino and Donham, 1984). The agent of adult T-cell leukemia (HTLV-1), in T-cells, is inactivated by 56°C for 30 minutes but not by 10 kRad X-rays (Yamato et al., 1986). Over 7 logs of mouse xenotropic type C retrovirus, added to human F-VIII, were inactivated in 1 hour at 56°C (Levy et al., 1984). At least 5 logs of Sindbis, Mahoney strain of polio, and Pseudorabies viruses were inactivated in hemoglobin solution (1 g/dL) held at 60°C for 30 min, without significant denaturation of the hemoglobin (Estep et al., 1987). Heating may prove to be a highly satisfactory method for virus inactivation in solutions of hemoglobin; additional data are needed for evaluation.

D. Solvents and detergents

A successful and widely-proven method for virus kill is the disruption of the virus envelope by means of detergents. Tri(n-butyl)phosphate and Tween 80 or sodium cholate kill Sendai, Sindbis, and vesicular stomatitis viruses within 18 hours at 4°C and very rapidly at 20°C (Horowitz et al., 1985). This work has since been verified with nonoxynol-9, a nonionic detergent (over 5 logs of HIV inactivated at concentrations greater than 0.05%–Hicks et al., 1985). Mitra and Wong (1986) also verified the solvent/detergent work using 20% amyl acetate with 0.1% deoxycholate. This general approach inactivates non-A and non-B hepatitis (Feinstone et al., 1983; Prince et al., 1984) as well as simian AIDS (Marx et al., 1984). Influenza and mumps viruses, for example, are destroyed by fluorocarbons (Hamparian et al., 1958), and will be destroyed by solvents and detergents of the types mentioned above. Aside from the viruses of primary interest (HIV, hepatitis B, non-A non-B hepatitis), the solvent/detergent strategy also will inactivate herpesviruses, measles and mumps viruses, influenza and rabies viruses, none of which have been known to be transmitted via plasma fractions. The Picornavirus group probably is not affected by these reagents.

E. Alkylation

Alkylation with beta-propiolactone also seems successful in the killing of viruses when applied to plasma (Stephan, 1982; Prince et al., 1985). However, plasma proteins also must be alkylated (Brusick, 1977), and the prospect emerges of the creation of unique antigens to which the recipient might become hypersensitive. Some of the more powerful alkylating agents, such as beta-propiolactone, are carcinogens and all such agents represent some hazard to the workers handling them routinely.

F. Virus and bacterial kill in ion-exchange and other chromatographic processes

Where one uses an ion-exchange matrix repeatedly for isolation of a plasma protein, e.g., F-IX, or transferrin, or IgG, presumably the best method for ensuring the kill of any virus sorbed onto the matrix would be steam autoclaving or steam-in-place sterilization (discussed in detail in another chapter of this book). There is no question of virus survival on a matrix that has been autoclaved or steamed-in-place (SIP). The gel media (agarose, cellulose, controlled-pore glass, Sephadex™, silica, etc.) are not well-suited to steam autoclaving or SIP, but a highly efficient new medium based on cellulose is suitable for SIP or steam autoclaving: Zeta-Prep (Cuno, Inc.). A Zeta-Prep system is shown in Figure 1 and a schematic of the cartridge assembly is shown in Figure 2. Unlike the gel-type systems, the Zeta-Prep cartridge behaves in cleaning and autoclaving like a depth filter which (devoid of the ion-exchange groups) it is. Because ion-exchange chromatography is the most efficient non-affinity purification step for a protein or peptide of interest, it is important that the matrix can be made virus clean with a very high level of assurance.

The Sephadex™ and Sepharose™ beaded gel supports, proposed for chromatographic purification of plasma proteins (Curling, 1980; Suomela, 1980), cannot be autoclaved or steamed-in-place in the columns in which they are packed. However, some chemical strategies have been developed for cleanup of such columns. 0.5M NaOH has been shown to kill *Pseudomonas aeruginosa* at 20°C in 5 hours and 1.0M NaOH kills the organism in 4 hours (Pharmacia, 1986). The same time-temperature relation is required to eliminate 65ng *Escherichia coli* endotoxin/mL of gel bed taken to 1.0M NaOH. Sodium hydroxide (1 M) for 2 hours at 20°C kills 2 logs of *Bacillus subtilis* spores (Whitehouse and Clegg, 1963). However, 0.1M NaOH for 10 minutes at about 20°C inactivates HIV (Martin et al., 1985). Presumably, other viruses also would be destroyed by the alkali.

Ultrafilters (UF) with polysulfone matrices (the most popular in current use) most often are cleaned with 0.5 or 1.0M NaOH, with or without a nonionic detergent, or with 50 to 200 ppm NaOCl, or both in series (with distilled water rinses between), and are stored in 0.1M NaOH. Provided the ultrafiltration systems are properly validated, such cleaning ensures viral and bacterial kill.

Because most of the equipment that is used with human-source material

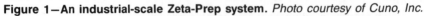

Figure 1—**An industrial-scale Zeta-Prep system.** *Photo courtesy of Cuno, Inc.*

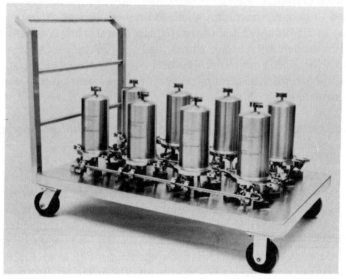

Figure 2—**Assembly of the Zeta-Prep cartridge. The substituted cellulose strip is fixed at one end to a long porous core, then is wrapped around the core; a plastic cage and endcaps are attached.** *Photo courtesy of Cuno, Inc.*

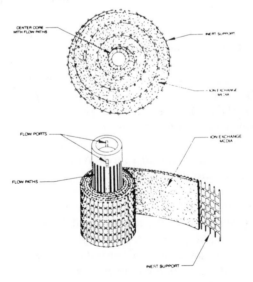

can be autoclaved, carry-over of putatively infectious material generally is not a consideration. However, because spills sometimes are a concern, the effectiveness of disinfectants against HIV is of particular interest. Spire et al. (1984) indicate that 25% ethanol, 1% glutaraldehyde, and 0.2% NaOCl are adequate. Wallbank (1985) recommends 2% glutaraldehyde. These recommendations ignore the powerful ability of detergents and solvents to destroy herpesviruses, arboviruses, myxoviruses, paramyxoviruses, and rhabdoviruses, in addition to the leukemia viruses.

4. Strategies that are Partially Successful

A. Heating of stabilized liquids

Fernandez and Lundblad (1982) patented a method that seemed to be the answer to viral contamination. For example, F-VIII was reconstituted with water for injection saturated with sucrose, then pasteurized (heating to 60°C for 10 hours); over 60% of the initial F-VIII activity was recovered. Regrettably, these steps in the heat-stabilization of human plasma proteins also protected viral contaminants (Ng and Dobdin, 1985). In cryoprecipitate or F-VIII solutions stabilized with sucrose and glycine, the following viruses are inactivated to nondetectable levels at 60°C for the indicated times: Rous sarcoma (1 hour), feline sarcoma (0.5 hours), simian sarcoma (0.5 hours) (Hilfenhaus et al., 1985), polio (10 hours), Epstein-Barr (1 hour), herpes simplex (4 hours) and cytomegalovirus (8 hours) (Hilfenhaus et al., 1986). What is not clear from the work of Hilfenhaus and coworkers is the apparent inconsistencies between their work and the work of Ng and Dobdin.

B. Heating of dried proteins

It would appear that the heating of dried proteins destroys HIV (see above). However, rigorous studies indicate that such strategies are effective to 4 or 5 logs for hardy viruses such as hepatitis B (Heldebrant et al., 1985). For example, about 5 logs of mouse xenotropic type C retrovirus, added to human F-VIII prior to freeze-drying, is inactivated after 96 hours at 68°C (Levy et al., 1984). The theory is that, in a dried preparation, there is more residual water in a virion than with a protein, and that heating will selectively destroy the water-binding structure (Holst, 1982).

 The concept was excellent and there is a good prospect that the AIDS virus is killed by this procedure.

C. Conventional ultrafiltration

Conventional ultrafilters have been used to depyrogenate human chorionic gonadotropin (Johnson et al., 1980). Presumably, UF could remove viruses from proteins small enough to pass readily through the UF pores. In point of fact, ultrafilters (independent of pore size rating) remove about 2.5 to 4 logs of endotoxin and show about the same performance with viruses (Bechtel et al., 1987).

This level of performance almost certainly relates to the presence of gaps ("holidays") in the thin (0.2 to 2mm-deep) skin of dense membrane matrix that accounts for the rejection behavior of ultrafilters. The holidays also account for the passage of bacteria through ultrafilters, which occur more slowly than do the endotoxin and virus passages.

D. Sorption
A technique that showed early promise was sorption to alkyl ligands with or without distal ω-NH$_2$ groups (Einarsson et al., 1981; Andersson et al., 1979; Neurath et al., 1975; and discussion in Olson and Greenwood, 1986). The theory was that a positively charged ligand would attract virions and that the alkyl ligand would bind to hydrophobic entities in the viral envelope.

E. Precipitants
Usually, this means polyethylene glycol 3500 molecular weight or higher (see Cole et al., 1983; Chandra and Wickerhauser, 1978; Wickerhauser et al., 1979; Hao et al., 1980), but also can refer to dextrans (Polson et al., 1964), ammonium sulfate (Dixon and Webb, 1964) and to various solvents (Scopes, 1982). Precipitation methods are never quite clean and leave behind a proportion of the material precipitated out. This includes viruses. Therefore, such methods are suitable for reducing viral burden but are not suitable for fail-safe elimination of any given virion.

   One system may prove to be the exception. Human leukocyte interferon now is produced, large-scale, in the following manner: The crude lysate is taken to 0.5M in KSCN and a pH of 3.5. The precipitate that forms is sedimented by centrifugation. The paste is redissolved in 94% ethanol and cooled to -20°C with intensive mixing; the precipitate is discarded. The interferon precipitates when the pH is raised to 7.4 (Cantell and Hirvonen, 1979). The KSCN step may disrupt the viral envelope in much the manner of the solvents and detergents that disrupt the envelopes (see above). However, the effectiveness of the KSCN remains to be established.

F. Serum inactivation
Human F-VIII concentrates slowly kill off many types of bacteria (Gee et al., 1986). Human serum inactivates murine, feline, and some primate retroviruses (Welsh et al., 1975; Cooper, 1979), but does not inactivate HTLV-1 (Hoshino et al., 1984) or HIV (Banapour et al., 1986).

5. Are We Safe?

Whole blood is as safe as the donor is free from infection. At this writing, massive loss of circulating red cells must be corrected either with packed red cells and saline or albumin, or with whole blood. Either the packed red cells or the whole blood may be contaminated; the risk exists to the extent and sensitivity of the screening process and the tests made on donor blood. At this writing, virus-safe or virus-free hemoglobin, either as a solution or encapsulated, is not readily available and the literature does not indicate clearly that intravenous-grade hemoglobin can be prepared that does not shut down the kidneys. Consequently, where hematocrit is lost by trauma, a risk of infection from whole blood or packed red cells must be taken.

Plasma fractions, pasteurized at 60°C for 10 hours with as little as 4mM caprylate as a protectant (albumin, HPPF), have been and continue to be free of any functional virus. Plasma fractions that are treated with organic solvents or detergents or both, by a validated method, will be free of any functional virus that contains significantly more than 10% lipid. Therefore, new reports of AIDS and other viral infections in hemophiliacs should commence a sharp decline in 1988 (or, most pessimistically, 1989) as a result of the heat treatment of dried clotting factors initiated by Hyland in 1983 and soon after by other plasma processors. The incidence of new reports of AIDS attributable to clotting factors should become nil before 1992 (the lag time is attributable to the incubation period of the disease, here taken as about five years).

The incidence of AIDS and other viral disease transmission attributable to whole blood or packed red cells from blood banks should commence a sharp decline due to screening methods now in place, and should not exist when a stable and effective intravenous hemoglobin solution is available in the marketplace.

ACKNOWLEDGMENTS: I would acknowledge the helpful comments provided by John Bacich, Keith Dillon, Emily Giustino, Dr. Henry Kingdon, and Johan van der Sande of Hyland Therapeutics. They provided the climate to respond to well-intended but poorly-informed critics of the plasma fractionation industry.

6. References

Andersson, L.O., Borg, H.G. and Einarsson, G.M. (1979) U.S. Patent 4,168,300, September.

Banapour, B., Sernatinger, J. and Levy, J.A. (1986) Virology 152, 268-271.

Bechtel, M., Bagdasarian, A., Olson, W.P. and Estep, T. (1987) Virus inactivation in hemoglobin solutions by ultrafiltration or detergent/solvent treatment. Paper to be presented at the 3rd Intl Symp. on Blood Substitutes, held May 26-28, Montreal, Canada.

Brummelhuis, H.G.J. (1980) In "Methods of Plasma Protein Fractionation", (J.M. Curling, ed.), pages 117-128, Academic Press, London.

Brusick, D.J. (1977) Mutation Res. 39, 241-256.

Cantell, K. and Hirvonen, S. (1979) Texas Rpt Biol. Med. 35, 138-141.

Chandra, S. and Wickerhauser, M. (1978) Thromb. Res. 12, 571-582.

Cole, S.C., Christensen, G.A. and Olson, W.P. (1983) Anal. Biochem. 134, 368-373.

Cohn, E.J., Strong, L.E., Hughes Jr., W.L., Mulford, D.J., Ashworth, J.N., Melin, M. and Taylor, H.L. (1946) J. Am. Chem. Soc. 68, pages 459-475.

Cooper, N.R. (1979) Comp. Virol. 15, 123-170.

Curling, J.M. (1980) In "Methods of Plasma Protein Fractionation" (J.M. Curling, Ed.), pages 77-91, Academic Press, London.

Dixon, M. and Webb, E.C. (1964) "Enzymes", pages 39-41, Longmans, London.

Edsall, J.T. (1984) Vox Sang. 46, 338-340.

Einarsson, M., Kaplan, L., Nordenfelt, E. and Miller, E. (1981) J. Virol. Methods 3, 213-228.

Estep, T.N., Bechtel, M., Miller, T.J. and Bagdasarian, A. (1987) Virus inactivation in hemoglobin solutions by heat. Paper presented at the 3rd Intl Symp. on Blood Substitutes, held May 26-28, Montreal, Canada.

Feinstone, S.M., Mihalik, K.B., Kamimura, T., Alter, H.J., London, W.T. and Purcell, R.H. (1983) Infec. Immun. 41, 816-821.

Gazengel, C. and Larrieu, M.J. (1985) Lancet ii, 1189.

Gee, L.W., Zeiner, R. and Olson, W.P. (1986) Pharm. Res. 3, 364-365.

Hamparian, V.V., Muller, F. and Hummeler, K. (1958) J. Immunol. 80, 468-475.

Heldebrant, C.M., Gomperts, E.D., Kasper, C.K., McDougal, J.S., Friedman, A.E., Hwang, D.S., Muchmore, E., Jordan, S., Miller, R., Sergis-Davenoport, E. and Lam, W. (1985) Transfusion 25, 510-515.

Hicks, D.R., Martin, L.S., Getchell, J.P., Heath, J.L., Francis, D.P., McDougal, J.S., Curran, J.W. and Voeller, B. (1985) Lancet ii, 1422-1423.

Hilfenhaus, J., Herrmann, A., Mauler, R. and Prince, A.M. (1986) Vox Sang. 50, 208-211.

Hilfenhaus, J., Mauler, R., Fiis, R. and Bauer, H. 1985) Proc. Soc. Exp. Biol. Med. 178, 584.

Holst, S. (1983) Personal communication.

Horowitz, B., Wiebe, M.E., Lippin, A. and Stryker, M.H. (1985) Transfusion 25, 550-522.

Hoshino, H., Tanaka, H., Mina, M. and Okada, H. (1984) Nature 310, 324-325.

Johnson, D.S., Lin, K., Fitzgerald, E. and LePage, B. (1980) In "Ultrafiltration Membranes and Applications", (A.R. Cooper, ed.), p. 475, Plenum Press, New York.

Levy, J.A., Mitra, G. and Mozen, M.M. (1984) Lancet ii, 722-723.

Martin, L.S., McDougal, J.S. and Loskowski, S.L. (1985) J. Inf. Dis. 152, 400-403.

Marx, P.A., Maul, D.H., Osborn, K.G., Lerche, N.W., Moody, P., Lowenstine, L.J., Henrickson, R.V., Arthur, L.O., Gilden, R.V., Gravell, M., London, W.T., Sever, J.L., Levy, J.A., Munn, R.J. and Gardner, M.B. (1984) Science 223, 1083-1086.

McDougal, J.S., Martin, L.S., Cort, S.P., Mozen, M., Heldebrant, C.M. and Evatt, B.L. (1985) J. Clin. Invest. 76, 875-877.

Mitra, G. and Ng, P.K. (1986) Thromb. Res. 37, 291-300.

Mitra, G. and Wong, M. (1986) Biotechnol. Bioeng. 28, 297-300.

Neurath, A.R., Lerman, S., Chen, M. and Prince, A.M. (1975) J. Gen. Virol. 28, 251-254.

Olson, W.P. and Greenwood, J.R. (1986) In "Fluid Filtration: Liquid, Vol. II, ASTM STP 975", (P.R. Johnston and H.G. Schroeder, eds.), 90-99, Am. Soc. Testing Materials, Philadelphia, PA.

Pharmacia (1986) Downstream/Upstream No. 2, Pharmacia Process Separation Div., Uppsala, Sweden.

Piszkiewicz, D., Kingdon, H., Apfelzweig, R., McDougal, J.S., Cort, S.P., Andrews, J., Hope, J. and Cabridilla, C.D. (1985) Lancet ii, 1188-1189.

Polson, A., Potgieter, G.M., Largier, J.F., Mears, G.E.F. and Jourbet, F.J. (1964) Biochim. Biophys. Acta 82, 463-475.

Prince, A.M., Horowitz, B., Brotman, B., Huima, T., Richardson, L. and van den Ende, M.C. (1984) Vox Sang. 46, 36-43.

Prince, A.M., Stephan, W., Dichtelmuller, H., Brotman, B. and Huima, T. (1985) J. Med. Virol. 16, 119-125.

Rubino, M.J. and Donham, K.J. (1984) Am. J. Vet. Res. 45, pages 1553-1556.

Scopes, R.K. (1982) "Protein Purification, Principles and Practice", 52-59, Springer-Verlag, New York.

Shikata, T., Karawawa, T., Abe, K., Takahashi, T., Mayumi, M. and Oda, T. (1978) J. Infect. Dis. 138, 242-244.

Spire, B., Barre-Sinoussi, F., Montagnier, L. and Chermann, J.C. (1984) Lancet ii, 899-901.

Stephan, W. (1982) Arzneim.-Forsch./Drug Res. 32 (11), Nr. 8, 799-801.

Suomela, H. (1980) In "Methods of Plasma Protein Fractionation", (J.M. Curling, ed.), pages 107-116, Academic Press, London.

Wallbank, A.M. (1985) Lancet i, 642.

Wells, M.A., Wittek, A.E., Epstein, J.S., Marcus-Sekura, C., Daniel, S., Tankersley, D.L., Preston, M.S. and Quinnan, G.V., Jr. (1986) Transfusion 26, 210-213.

Welsh, R.M., Jr., Cooper, N.R., Jensen, F.C. and Oldstone, M.B.A. (1975) Nature 257, 612-614.

Whitehouse, R.L. and Clegg, L.F.L. (1963) J. Dairly Res. 30, 415-322.

Wickerhauser, M., Williams, C. and Mercer, J.E. (1979) Vox Sang. 36, 281-292.

Yamato, K., Taguchi, H., Yoshimoto, S., Fujishita, M., Yamashita, M., Ohtsuki, Y., Hoshino, H. and Miyoshi, I. (1986) Jpn. J. Cancer Res. 77, 13-15.

Zuck, T.F., Preston, M.S., Tankersley, D.L., Wells, M.A., Wittek, A.E., Epstein, J.E., Daniel, S., Phelan, M. and Quinnan, G.V. (1986) N. Eng. J. Med. 314, 1454-1455.

14

FDA Regulatory Inspections of Aseptic Processing Facilities

Ronald F. Tetzlaff
U.S. Food and Drug Administration, Atlanta, GA, USA

1. Introduction

Aseptic processing is used for manufacturing a wide array of sterile pharmaceuticals and medical devices. There have been tremendous advances in aseptic processing technology, especially in the methods used to demonstrate that products have adequate assurances of sterility.

The firms that employ aseptic processing methods to produce sterile drugs or medical devices are subject to the regulatory authority of the US Food and Drug Administration (FDA). In regulating the industries utilizing aseptic processes, the FDA is responsible for making certain that such products are safe for the user and have been manufactured using good manufacturing practices in conformance with the appropriate laws and regulations. The FDA is responsible for enforcement of the Food, Drug and Cosmetic Act (FD&C Act) and the Current Good Manufacturing Practices Regulations for Finished Pharmaceuticals and the Good Manufacturing Practice for Medical Devices (21 CFR, Parts 211 and 820, respectively). The FDA conducts routine inspections of the aseptic production facilities where sterile drugs and devices are made to insure appropriate controls are in place to assure that the products distributed to the public are safe, effective, and of suitable quality. Noncompliance with the FDA laws or regulations can result in administrative sanctions such as product recalls or nonapproval of New Drug Applications (NDA's), or regulatory actions (such as regulatory letters, seizures, injunctions or prosecutions).

The aseptic processing method is used for manufacturing the diverse sterile pharmaceuticals and devices that are adversely affected by the severe stresses of thermal sterilization. This method usually involves filtration sterilization of a bulk solution, aseptic transfer into sterile containers that have been previously sterilized by conventional methods (such as steam, dry heat, ethylene oxide, or radiation), and subsequent container sealing with previously sterilized closures. Once sterilized, the containers, closures, bulk products, and all product contact surfaces must be maintained under aseptic conditions to prevent microbiological contamination. Aseptic processing involves all of these steps, procedures, and controls, which must be employed to effectively sterilize the product and components, as well as those steps necessary to prevent microbiological contamination during the various manufacturing and packaging operations.

Aseptic processing differs from terminal sterilization methods in the relative lack of standardized manufacturing and validation techniques. Aseptic processes are extremely complex, and are almost as varied as the number of firms employing this method. Standardized manufacturing methods, official guidelines, and widely recognized validation methods are largely undeveloped or are limited in scope. Probably the most significant difference from terminal sterilization methods is the frequency and extent to which the conditions may change in an aseptic environment. Demonstrating that adequate aseptic conditions are maintained while numerous interrelated variables may be changing under dynamic conditions is difficult at best. The potential presence of viable organisms in the manufacturing environment, and the prevalence of such organisms associated with personnel produce avenues of product contamination during virtually all stages of processing where sterile products and components are exposed. The possibility of adventitious microbiological contamination during any phase of aseptic transfer poses potentially serious health hazard consequences.

FDA regulatory inspections of aseptic processes involve special considerations that differ from the processes which include terminal sterilization. For terminal sterilization methods (eg. steam, dry heat, radiation, and chemicals), it is possible to quantify microbial death rate kinetics, allowing probabilities of microbial survival to be determined for a given sterilization process. Furthermore, it has become current good manufacturing practice for terminally sterilized products to have sterility assurance levels (SAL's) of 10^6 or better. Such SAL's are not realistically obtainable for aseptically produced products.

There are severe limitations with the validation methods used to predict the probability of products becoming contaminated during the aseptic manufacturing and packaging process. The probability that the product may become contaminated during the assembly process, must be maintained at a sufficiently low level to assure the safety for the users. These assurances can be achieved with available technology if the facilities, equipment, and processes have been properly designed and maintained and personnel properly trained, but only if sufficient validation testing and environmental monitoring confirm that the probability of microbiological contamination is held at acceptably low levels.

These inherent limitations have contributed to a number of controversies that remain unresolved or subject to debate within the industry, the scientific community, and the FDA. Experience has shown that some firms continue to have difficulty in satisfying FDA regulatory requirements as evidenced by recalls, nonapproval of NDA's, injunctions, regulatory letters, and product seizures. It is the objective of this chapter to discuss some of the objectionable conditions and practices that are commonly observed during FDA inspections of aseptic processes from the perspective of an FDA investigator. It should be noted that there are far more technical areas of regulatory significance than can be discussed in this limited presentation.

2. Scope and Definitions

A. Scope

The validation program for an aseptic process must consider all of the production and control systems that affect a manufacturer's ability to assure that aseptic conditions are maintained during the assembly/filling operations. The large number of variables that influence sterility assurances are found in virtually every manufacturing system involved with aseptic processing. Many of the sterilization validation systems for equipment, materials, components, and product have received considerable attention by the Food and Drug Administration (FDA, 1983 and 1985), industry and academia, and the various trade associations, such as the Parenteral Drug Association (PDA, 1978, 1980a,b, 1981, and 1984), the Health Industries Medical Association (HIMA, 1978), and the Association for the Advancement of Medical Instrumentation (AAMI, 1981 and 1984). These efforts have led to an improvement in industry conditions and practices, and have resulted in the standardization of many sterilization practices. This standardization and the recognization of the potential problems associated with aseptic processing has reduced but not eliminated the incidence of major problems during FDA inspections.

While this chapter does not emphasize sterilizer validation or the phases of production before or after the aseptic assembly process, their importance cannot be over emphasized. It is essential that these systems be properly designed, maintained, controlled, and validated if suitable assurances of sterility are to be provided.

The literature is replete with descriptions of the numerous problems associated with maintaining aseptic conditions and the potential origins of product contamination; however, there is a relative paucity of information about the specific quality control elements for aseptic processing. There are even fewer publications describing the FDA regulatory requirements of the current Good Manufacturing Practices (GMPs) for aseptic processes (FDA, 1985; Fry, 1985; Tetzlaff, 1983 and 1984; Avallone, 1984). This is especially true in the area of aseptic process validation for pharmaceuticals and medical devices where alternative approaches are frequently employed. Controversies continue to exist, and FDA inspections continue to reveal significant problems (Avallone, 1983, 1984, 1985; Tetzlaff, 1983 and 1984). Some of these problems are serious enough to compromise sterility assurances and result in FDA regulatory actions or administrative sanctions. This presentation is devoted almost exclusively to the actual aseptic assembly or transfer process itself. Particular emphasis is given to those areas where industry standards or guidelines may be lacking or are being established, and firms continue to have difficulty in satisfying the aseptic process validation and environmental control requirements of the FDA.

B. Definitions

Some of the commonly used aseptic processing terms have different meanings when used in the widely diverse industries ranging from aerospace and electronics to pharmaceuticals and medical devices. The following terms used in this chapter are defined in context of applications in the pharmaceutical or medical device industries where the primary objective of aseptic processing is to prevent microbiological contamination during assembly of the previously sterilized product, containers, and closures.

Aseptic: The absence of microorganisms capable of causing infection or contamination.

Aseptic processing: Manufacturing methods for sterile products that are not subjected to terminal sterilization. The objective of aseptic processing methods is to assemble previously sterilized product, containers, and closures within specially designed and controlled environments intended to minimize the potential of microbiological or particulate contamination. While aseptic techniques may also be employed during the manufacture of terminally sterilized products to control product bioburden or particulate levels, the term aseptic processing will herein be reserved for the manufacturing of products or components which are not terminally sterilized.

Related terms: Aseptic Filling, Sterile Filling, Aseptic Transfer, Aseptic Assembly.

Cleanrooms: Specially designed areas equipped with high efficiency particulate air (HEPA) filters which are intended to deliver air that is essentially free of particles and viable microorganisms. In the pharmaceutical related industries there are currently no official or recognized standards or regulations which specifically define the particulate and microbiological quality criteria for cleanrooms used for aseptic processing. The absence of such standards has contributed to misunderstandings and controversies which led in part to the FDA Guideline on Sterile Drug Products Produced by Aseptic Processing (1987) which is discussed below. Commonly the term cleanroom is restricted to those areas which meet the class 100 requirements of Federal Standard 209b, but individual firms have used the term with differing quality standards.

Controlled environments: Specially constructed/controlled processing areas designed to minimized particulate and microbiological contamination, but are not intended to provide aseptic conditions; such areas do not include those where sterile products or components are exposed to the environment. Controlled environments used in aseptic processing of pharmaceuticals and medical devices include the non-sterile manufacturing areas such as those used for weighing, mixing, formulation, container/closure washing, parts and equipment washing, etc.

Process validation: A documented program which provides a high degree of assurance that a specific process will consistently produce a product meeting its predetermined specifications and quality attributes (FDA definition in Guideline on General Principles of Process Validation, 1987).

Sterile: The absence of living organisms. In the field of aseptic processing, this term commonly creates misunderstandings because of differing definitions and statistical limitations. However, for this discussion, the term sterile describes the condition of equipment, materials, and products that are intended to be free of viable microorganisms.

Sterility Assurance Level (SAL): The probability that a product following sterilization may contain viable microorganisms that survived the sterilization process. For terminally sterilized pharmaceuticals or invasive medical devices, the FDA expects SAL's of 10^{-6} or better. The FDA recognizes the limitations of the currently available aseptic validation methods, and considers SAL's of 10^{-3} to be releastic and acheivable (Tetzlaff, 1984 and Fry, 1985).

3. FDA Historical Perspectives on Aseptic Processing

A. Early technological developments

The aseptic processing method, probably as old as the parenteral route of administration, was employed even before the principles of sterilization had become fully developed. Aseptic processing technology had its beginings in the 1860's with Louis Pasteur's discovery that viable microbes were carried in the air on dust particles. His early experiments revealed that heat treated liquids in U-neck flasks with cotton plugs (to prevent dust particles from entering the liquid) remained free of microorganisms as long as dust was not permitted to enter. His findings disproved the spontaneous generation theories that had persisted for nearly 200 years following the microscopic discovery of bacteria in 1674 by Leeuwenhoek (Pelczar, 1977).

While the work of Pastuer represented the beginnings of modern microbiology, it was John Tyndall who performed some of the earliest systematic experiments to determine the relationship between airborne particulate levels and microbiological contamination rates. In 1882, following a decade of investigations into airborne particulates and related microbiological contamination, Tyndall published his "Essays On The Floating Matter Of The Air." He devised an instrument to detect subvisible particles, and was able to demonstrate convincingly that microbiological contamination was a result of viable microbes being carried on dust particles in the air. For these early experiments, he utilized a rudimentary "aseptic" chamber to control the dust particles (Tyndall, 1882).

During the 1930s and 1940s, the aseptic processing methods became more prevalent in the pharmaceutical industry, largely due to the discovery of penicillin and other antibiotics which were sensitive to the heat of autoclaving. This coincided with the development of the commercial freeze drying processes used for making dried plasma during World War II (Flosdorf et al, 1940, Flosdorf, 1949, and Strumia, 1954). During the past two decades, there have been dramatic improvements in aseptic processing technology and increases in the knowledge about routes of airborne contamination. This can be attributed largely to the efforts of the U.S. Air Force and the National Aeronautics and Space Administration (NASA). HEPA filters were first introduced in the 1950's, and much of the impetus for the improvements in clean rooms and aseptic processing techniques was the result of the U.S. military in developing clean rooms for manufacturing aircraft instruments. By 1963, the Air Force Technical Order 00-25-203 (US Air Force, 1963) had received acceptance and laminar air flow principles were becoming recognized as an effective way to improve air cleanliness levels in clean rooms (Austin, 1970). Much of the current knowledge about clean room technology, microbial sampling methods, and mechanisms of microbial death was the result of the efforts of NASA in the spacecraft development program.

B. Recognition of aseptic processes in compendial standards

One of the earliest injectable drugs to receive official recognition was the hypodermic morphine solution which appeared in the 1874 addendum to the 1867 British Pharmocopeia (Groves, 1973). The 15th edition of the U.S. Dispensatory in 1833 described hypodermic morphine solution as being processed by a rather primative aseptic method; "filter and preserve the product in a stoppered bottle, excluded from light." By 1888, the first edition of the U.S. National Formulary (NF) included a monograph for hypodermic morphine solution. This early monograph recognized the potential for microbial contamination and offered one of the earlier recorded preservative systems for injectable drugs produced by aseptic processing. The monograph included the following instructions: "The development of fungoid growths or micro-organisms in this and similar solutions used hypodermically may be prevented, or at least greatly retarded, by using Chloroform Water instead of plain Distilled Water as a solvent . . . Another efficient method to preserve such solutions is to sprinkle a little Benzoic Acid on the surface of absorbent cotton through which the solutions are filtered" (NF I, 1888).

According to Groves (1973), some of the earlier fundamental studies into the applications of sterilization processes for pharmaceuticals by heat and filtration were done by Lesure in 1909 to 1911. By 1911, Lesure concluded that most parenteral solutions could be sterilized by autoclaving. In the same year, the British Pharmaceutical Codex described aseptically produced hermetically sealed ampules which were not termially sterilized. During this period, the aseptic processing method was begining to receive common official recognition in the various compendia such as the United States Pharmacopia (USP), National Formulary (NF), and British Pharmacopoeia (BP). For example, USP, 9th revision (1916) included a section devoted to solution sterilization (filtration) with aseptic transfer to sterilized containers which were to be sealed with sterilized stoppers. The compendium included a requirement that the "filtration must be conducted in such a manner that no contamination will result."

The 1926 National Formulary described in detail the Tyndallization Method for "sterilizing" ampules by alternate heating at 60–100°C for 20 minutes on three consecutive days to kill vegetative cells, while permitting germination of spores (NF V, 1926). Heat sensitive products could be processed by such aseptic methods using a "germ proof filter" if the filter had been tested and found to be free from leakage or defects and to be actually germ proof and if operations were conducted under aseptic conditions. However, there was no description in the compendium for methods used to prove filter integrity or methods/equipment used to assure aseptic conditions.

Similarily, the 1932 British Pharmacopoeia (appendix XVI) described another early official method for preparing injectable solutions by aseptic techniques which included solution sterilization by filtering the product through a sterile "bacteria-proof filter" and aseptic distribution of sterile solution into previously sterilized containers. This method remains largely unchanged in subsequent editions of the BP until as recently as 1980 (BP, 1980). The 1960 edition of USP XVI includes a section devoted to aseptic filling areas and specifies some of the methods employed to prevent product contamination as well as control checks for the aseptic filling environment such as environmental agar plates and the use of simulated filling with media (media fills). More recent USP editions (IXX, 1975; XX, 1980; and XXI, 1985) contain sections with detailed procedures for assuring aseptic conditions.

4. Perspectives on FDA Laws and Regulations

A. Establishment of applicable FDA laws and regulations

Virtually all laws and regulations governing the pharmaceutical industry were enacted in reaction to hazardous, defective, or substandard products found in the market place. A brief review of some of the significant incidents that resulted in major legislation or regulations is helpful in understanding the development by the FDA of regulatory controls for aseptic processing (Krzyzyk, 1977). The first federal drug law, the Import Act of 1848, was enacted because the antimalarial drug, quinine, used by the U.S. Military in the Mexican War was found to be found sub-potent and grossly contaminated (Janssen, 1975). The impetus for Congress passing the orginal Food and Drug Act (1906) was the disclosure of insanitary conditions in food plants and the cure-all claims of worthless and dangerous patent medicines. In 1937 the drug, Elixir of Sulfanilimide, killed

107 persons (US Government Printing Office, 1937) which prompted Congress to pass the Federal Food Drug and Cosmetic Act (FD&C Act) of 1938. This law enacted important new provisions such as pre-clearance of the safety of new drugs prior to distribution, authorization of factory inspections, and authorization of Federal courts to restrain violations by injunctions (US Government Printing Office, 1974).

Since the passage of the FD&C Act, there have been various drug related amendments, but none has had the impact of the 1962 Kefauver-Harris Amendments. These were passed in reaction to the births in Europe of thousands of malformed babies from mothers that had used Thalidomide (FDA Consumer Memo, March 1984). These sweeping legislative changes included new provisions for drug manufacturers to prove their products were both safe and effective before marketing them. Of particular relevance to drug manufacturers (including aseptic processes) was the new provision, section 501, that deemed a drug to be adulterated if the facilities, methods, and controls used for making drugs were not in conformance with the current good manufacturing practices.

The following year, the FDA promulgated the first drug GMP regulations (Federal Register, June 20, 1963). These have been updated during the intervening years in light of changes in technology and to better reflect the upgrading of drug quality assurance programs used by most manufacturers. Between 1963 and 1976, these drug GMP regulations were applicable to aseptic processes, but they failed to define specific elements of equipment and facility construction or methods to control aseptic processes. In 1976, a revision was proposed under part 211.42 (Federal Register, February 13, 1976) which added specific design and construction requirements for buildings and facilities used for aseptic processing. These new provisions included requirements for separate aseptic processing areas designed to prevent contamination including:

Smooth, hard, cleanable surfaces
Temperature and humidity control
HEPA filtered air supply
Systems for environmental monitoring
Systems for cleaning and disinfection to produce aseptic conditions
Systems to maintain equipment used to control aseptic conditions.

This 1976 proposed revision included the first use of the term validation in the Regulations by the FDA under Part 211.113 (b) for sterilization processes. These proposed changes, adopted in the 1978 revision (Federal Register, September 29, 1978), became effective on March 1, 1979, and have not been substantially changed for any aseptic related requirements. While these regulations contain some of the minimum acceptable aseptic practices, they fail to identify the specific physical or microbiological validation and monitoring requirements for aseptic equipment and processes.

B. FDA enforcement of current laws and regulations

During the past decade, the pharmaceutical and medical device manufacturers that are regulated by the FDA have had ample opportunity to become familar with FDA policies, procedures, and expectations through various public forums, scientific meetings, and publications. Despite the Agency's attempts to articulate its positions on aseptic process validation, some firms continue to have problems satisfying the FDA requirements. It has been necessary for the FDA to issue a number of regulatory letters, initiate seizure actions, or to bring injunctions against firms for the failure to adhere to reasonable current good manufacturing practices for aseptic processes for both drugs and medical devices. It seems unlikely that such occurences would happen if responsible management were aware of the FDA legal authority, regulatory policies, and guidelines and fully appreciated the consequences of non-conformance.

The principle law enforced by the FDA is the FD&C Act (U.S. Code, Title 21). This law gives the FDA authority to conduct factory inspections, defines the prohibited acts, and provides for FDA regulatory and administrative sanctions to enable the FDA to bring noncomplying firms or individuals into compliance with the law. The following is a brief review of a few important legal issues of concern to aseptic processing that may be helpful in dispelling misunderstandings about the FDA regulatory jurisdiction.

The FDA authority to conduct inspections of drug and medical device manufacturers is found in Section 704(a) of the FD&C Act. The law authorizes officers of the FDA to enter drug or device manufacturing plants at reasonable times, within reasonable limits, and to inspect in a reasonable manner all pertinent equipment, finished and unfinished materials, containers, and labeling. Particular statutory authority is provided for inspections of prescription (Rx) drug and restricted medical device manufacturing plants. In the case of Rx drug or restricted device inspections, the law specifically authorizes the inspection to extend to all things therein (including records, files, papers, processes, controls, and facilities) that would indicate whether the drugs or devices are adulterated or misbranded. This authority permits FDA investigators access to virtually all production and laboratory facilities including inspection of all manufacturing and control records that are maintained by firms in accordance with the Current Good Manufacturing Practices Regulations (CGMP's). The law does not extend to financial data, sales data other than shipment data, pricing data, personnel data (other than personnel qualification data), and research data (other than new drug or device data pursuant to sections cited in the law).

The primary objective of FDA inspections of aseptic processing facilities is to observe conditions and practices that may have a bearing on whether the drugs or devices may be adulterated or misbranded within the meaning of the FD&C Act. Sections 301(a), 301(k), and others, prohibit the introduction into interstate commerce (or receipt) of any adulterated or misbranded drug or device. Of particular relevance to aseptic processing is the statuatory definition of adulteration under Section 501. This law deems a drug or device to be adulterated if the facilities used for its manufacture do not conform to or are not operated in conformance with current good manufacturing practice to assure purity, quality, and safety. If the manufacturing or control procedures do not conform to the GMP's the FDA may deem the products made under these conditions to be adulterated and these may become subject to regulatory sanctions. It is important to recognize that for aseptic processes, any condition or practice which jeopardizes SAL's may result in the FDA deeming as adulterated any products made under such conditions, and the FDA has the authority to initiate regulatory sanctions as provided by the FD&C Act.

Some manufacturers have failed to fully appreciate the fact that it is not necessary for the FDA to find products actually contaminated before initiating legal procedings. The FDA has in recent years utilized this powerful statuatory authority, through seizures (Section 301), injunctions (Section 302) and prosecutions (Section 303), to bring noncomplying firms or individuals into compliance with the law and GMP Regulations. While the law enables the FDA to enforce strict adherence to the GMP's, the FDA does not have the power to actually impose these penalties. It is necessary for the FDA to initiate such procedings through the federal judicial system, and only the federal courts may actually invoke these penalties. However, the FDA has the mechanisms at hand to insure that drugs or devices made by aseptic processing methods have been manufactured under suitable assurances of safety, quality, and purity.

C. FDA expectations for aseptic process validation

i. Regulatory policies

During FDA inspections of aseptic processes where firms are found to be in noncompliance with the GMP regulations, it is not uncommon for management to profess unfamiliarity with FDA expectations or to claim that the GMP regulations fail to include specific or detailed aseptic processing requirements or are vague. Responsible management must appreciate that the GMP regulations are not intended to be specific or detailed in nature. Instead, while they are considered to be binding requirements, the courts have upheld they have the effect of law, and have recognized the need for flexible language.

It is not the objective of this limited presentation to support or defend the legal precedents that have reaffirmed the FDA authority to promulgate and enforce regulations; a detailed treatment of this subject can be found in the preamble to the current GMP regulations (Federal Register, Volume 43, 1978, Pages 45020-45026). Instead, the following is meant to emphasize the importance of knowing the FDA expectations and recognizing the consequences of nonconformance. The FDA authority to promulgate regulations for the enforcement of the FD&C Act is found under Section 701(a). The FDA considers the current GMP regulations to be binding (Michels, 1985), and the failure to comply will render a drug product to be adulterated under Section 501(a)(2)(B) of the FD&C Act. The FDA legal authority to promulgate binding regulations has been repeatedly upheld in federal courts, but one case deserves special mention because it involved aseptic processing. In "U.S.A. v Morton Norwich Products, Inc., et. al.," the U.S. District Court for the Northern District of New York (opinion 75-CR-114, decided 5/11/76) upheld the constitutionality of the GMP statute and regulations (Food, Drug, Cosmetic Law Reporter, 38,068, 1976). In this decision, the court ruled on the challenge that the term "current good manufacturing practice" (CGMP) was unconstitutionally vague. The court noted that this term must be flexible in its application and pointed out that drug manufacturers had participated in the legislative hearings from which this term eminated. The court further ruled that the drug industry had ample opportunity to become familiar with the current GMP's through various government and trade association seminars, college courses, and other printed publications, and that it was not necessary for the FDA to provide specific detailed regulations. In effect, the court considered the term, good manufacturing practice, to be generally recognized.

ii. FDA Guidelines

The FDA has considered the GMP Regulations to be binding and has expected the aseptic processing industries to utilize sound scientific principles and practices (Byers, 1978; Loftus, 1977; Avallone, 1980, 1982, 1983, 1984, and 1985; Tetzlaff, 1983 and 1984; Fry, 1982 and 1985; and Michels, 1985). However, in recent years there have been dramatic changes in the technologies utilized in aseptic processing and legitimate areas of controversy have developed especially relating to the methods used to validate and monitor aseptic processes. Recognizing the benefit in communicating its expectations to the regulated industry, the FDA has recently published two guidelines of particular relevance to aseptic processing. Both were published under the procedural provisions of 21 CFR Part 10.90 to permit comments from interested individuals or companies. This Regulation provides for the establishment of guidelines that are of general applicability, but are not legal requirements. A person who follows a guideline is assured that this conduct will be acceptable to the FDA, but alternate procedures may also be followed. These two guidelines were finalized and published in 1987, based upon the comments received. The following is a brief review of these two guidelines to illustrate areas of current concern to the FDA.

A. General guidelines on principles of process validation

This guideline was published by the FDA in recognition that the GMP regulations specified only broad objectives and included terms such as "adequate" and "appropriate" (Federal Register, March 29, 1983). Since good manufacturing practices must evolve with changes in technology, there is a need to communicate FDA expectations in a manner that will not freeze technology (Michels, 1985). This final guideline discusses the broad concepts and elements of process validation as currently viewed by the FDA. The FDA recognizes that the widely diverse drug and device industries employ such a variety of different manufac turing and control processes that it is not practical to include in a single document all elements of validation. However, this guideline document does provide some important insight into FDA philosophies about validation and offers useful background, definitions and concepts.

B. Guideline on sterile drug products produced by aseptic processing

The FDA has observed a wide variation in the degree of GMP compliance within the aseptic processing industry. These variations have been apparent for years: in 1981 the FDA convened a task force to draft a guideline on aseptic processing addressing issues that were subject of current controversy and had not been specifically covered in the regulations or other FDA publications. The objective of this guideline was not to provide the only acceptable way(s) of complying with the FDA expectations, since the FDA acknowledges alternative methods may be acceptable or may become preferable as technologies improve.

This proposed guideline was published (notice of availability), on February 1, 1985 (Federal Register, 1985) and provided for a 90 day comment period. The final guideline incorporated changes based on comments received and was published in 1987. It is beyond the scope of this chapter to discuss this guideline in detail: recent reviews provide further insight into the background and development (Fry, 1985), content (Gold Sheet, 1985), and the regulatory status (Michels, 1985). However, emphasis is given to the fact that this guideline was developed to provide guidance in areas where pertinent questions have been raised and GMP problems have been found during FDA inspections. Examples of such problems have been discussed in detail by Avallone (1980/1985) and Tetzlaff (1983/1984). The Gold Sheet (1985) cites at least 17 instances during 1984/1985 of FDA issuing regulatory letters to firms having problems with sterile product manufacturing processes.

5. Examples of GMP Problems Found During FDA Inspections

A. Validation of related systems

Aseptic process validation involves many disciplines and impacts upon virtually every major department including engineering, production, and quality control/quality assurance (QC/QA). Besides the actual aseptic assembly process itself, numerous other potential avenues of product contamination need to be subjected to sufficient validation testing to establish adequacy of performance. This includes component sterilization, personnel training and performance, and the various related manufacturing and utility systems. A comprehensive treatment of systems validation is beyond the scope of this presentation: these systems have all recently received considerable attention in the literature. The following is a brief review of some of the typical problems during FDA inspections to stress the importance that FDA places on these elements of validation.

i. Component and Equipment Sterilization

All of the various materials which come into direct contact with a parenteral drug product or medical device such as containers, closures, filling equipment, bulk holding vessels, pipes, pumps and other equipment used to produce sterile products should be sterilized. The equipment used to sterilize the components and equipment shall have been shown by validation testing to provide uniform and reproducible sterilizing environments using cycles and loading patterns/configurations of proven effectiveness. The well established validation principles for the various component and equipment sterilization methods such as steam (PDA, 1978), dry heat (PDA, 1981), ethylene oxide (AAMI, 1984), radiation (AAMI, 1981), and chemicals (Block, 1984) would seem to need no further elaboration. However, FDA inspections frequently find that component and equipment sterilization systems have not been adequately validated, including, but not limited to the following examples;

a. Validation protocols
- absence of written protocols
- absence of formal written review/approval
- lack of written acceptance criteria such as:
    number of runs necessary to demonstrate reproducibility
    uniformity of process parameters, (e.g. times, temperatures, pressures, etc.)
- inappropriate acceptance criteria
- too few runs to demonstrate reproducibility
- parameter limits too wide, (i.e. excessive variation)

b. Validation test data collection
- original data unavailable (lost or missing)
- original data not maintained at site where testing performed
- failure to record important data
- insufficient testing to establish reproducibility (i.e. too few tests)
- data failed to demonstrate uniformity (i.e. excessive variations)
- inadequate/inappropriate instrument calibration (e.g. lack of reference standard traceability)
- inadequate sensitivity of test instrumentation
- erroneous data obtained/recorded in validation reports
- insufficient microbiological data

c. Validation data review
- absence of formal review of data accuracy
- failure to detect errors or discrepancies
- lack of written investigation/justification for validation failures
- lack of documented corrective action following validation failures

- failure of validation reports to show written approval
- validation reports fail to show specific acceptance criteria

ii. Personnel

Employees working in aseptic processing areas are a major source of microbiological contamination. The need for thorough ongoing training of personnel may seem obvious, but FDA experience has shown this is not always the case. The FDA, recognizing the importance of personnel training, has included specific training provisions in the drug and device GMP Regulations, Parts 211.25 and 820.25, respectively. These regulations require not only that personnel have suitable education, experience, and training in the duties they perform, but also that training be on a continuing basis to assure employees are familiar with applicable GMP's and appropriate company procedures. The FDA expectations relating to the specific topic of employee GMP training was addressed by Tetzlaff (1982). The value of performing training in a formal systematic fashion with appropriate documentation and certification of proficiency cannot be overstated. A large body of literature is available on the specific topic of GMP's and employee training for aseptic processes such as, DeLuca, 1983; DeVecchi, 1978; Schmitt, 1983; Kitt, 1979; Luna, 1984; Loughhead, 1969; Hall, 1982; and Betts, 1981.

iii. Product filtration sterilization

Most drugs produced by aseptic processes utilize filtration sterilization of solutions followed by aseptic transfer to previously sterilized containers. The sterilization of these solutions is one of the most critical of all sterilization processes, but is often not afforded a suitable degree of control by some manufacturers, especially in determining the adequacy of the sterilization process or suitability of filters being used. The drug GMP's, Part 211.72, Filters, require that filters used for making injectable drugs for human use shall not be fiber releasing (unless there exist no alternatives). If the use of fiber releasing filters is unavoidable, then the drug products must receive additional filtration with 0.22 micron nonfiber releasing filters. The use of asbestos filters is contraindicated, and is permitted only after submission of proof to the FDA that the use of a non-fiber releasing filter will compromise the safety or effectiveness of the drug product.

The GMP's, Part 211.113, Control of Microbiological Contamination, require that all sterilization processes be validated. This requirement applies to membrane filtration sterilization, but the GMP regulations do not specify methods. There continue to be controversies about filtration sterilization validation; in particular, questions persist about whether the filter manufacturer or the user is responsible for validation. It is the FDA position that the manufacturer of drugs and devices is responsible for assuring the quality and safety of the products they produce. The filter user is ultimately responsible for assuring that whatever filtration system is utilized will be capable of reproducibily sterilizing the product including the demonstration of adequate SAL's.

The FDA is aware that some firms do not have the in-house capabilities to perform microbiological challenge testing (FDA Guideline on Sterile Drugs Produced by Aseptic Processing, 1985). In such cases it may be appropriate to rely upon the filter manufacturer or outside testing laboratories to perform the actual validation testing (Leahy et al, 1978; Pall et al., 1980; Reti, 1977). However, if the testing is performed by outside facilities, it is still the responsibility of the filter user to have the validation test data available at the location of use. FDA inspections have revealed instances of firms utilizing commercially produced filters without having filter validation data, usually under the erroneous assumption that the filter manufacturer was responsible for validation testing. The FDA considers it appropriate that filtration validation be specific to each product, process, and filter. This is particularily significant to firms with many products having different chemical/physical properties that may influence filtration performance (including filtration effectiveness, compatibility, and integrity). If the filter manufacturer used water or other common solvents (eg. alcohol) to wet the filters for microbial challenge or integrity validation testing, this data may not apply to different solvent/solute systems actually used in pharmaceutical production applications. FDA inspections would include a careful evaluation of correlations between filter effectiveness data (microbial challenge) and filter integrity test data(minimum bubble point values).

It is not uncommon for this testing to be performed by the filter manufacturer. However, if this testing is done with filters that have been wetted with water or alcohol, then this data is specific to the system tested. In practice, many firms perform integrity testing during production using the drug product solution as the wetting agent. In such cases, the filter integrity test may not be considered as being validated, particularily if the surface tension of the drug solution differs appreciably from the solution used by the filter manufacturer to establish integrity test values. In addition, physical/chemical incompatibilities may exist between the filter and drug solution. It is incumbent upon the user to demonstrate that there are no incompatibilities. Since membrane filters themselves may be a source of particulate matter or extractables when placed into service, it is customary to pre-flush the filters with a solvent or drug solution prior to actual use. It is the user's responsibility to determine by validation testing that the flushing process is proven to be effective in reducing such contaminants.

The FDA considers it appropriate for filter validation to simulate to the extent practical worst case production conditions. For example, this would include microbial challenge with microorganisms small enough to represent a challange of the filter pore size being tested. *Pseudomonas dimuta* is commonly used since its nominal diameter is approximately 0.3 micron size range, but it has been reported that under certain conditions this organism may pass through a 0.22 rated membrane filter (Leahy and Sullivan, 1978). The microbial challenge levels as well as other factors that may be involved in the conditions of actual use (such as surface tension, pH, viscosity, pressure, flow rates, etc.) should be demonstrated to represent those conditions that may be encountered during use.

iv. Manufacturing equipment

There are a large number of related manufacturing systems which, if not properly installed and suitably maintained to assure proper performance, may adversely affect aseptic conditions. These systems need to be validated separately at the time of installation and revalidated following any major changes or modifications that may impact upon the aseptic environmental conditions. Such systems include, but are not limited to, the following important examples:

The High Efficiency Particulate Air (HEPA) filters should be integrity tested using a suitable challenge test method, e.g. dioctyl-phthalate (DOP) to demonstrate absence from leaks (Federal Standard 209b, 1973). This integrity testing should be performed following installation of new HEPA filters, and afterwards at regular intervals to insure continued performance. The frequency of integrity retesting will depend upon the data obtained during the regular periodic environmental monitoring, and if data shows suitable microbiological and physical conditions this retesting is commonly performed at biennial or annual intervals. Also to be tested initially and periodically thereafter are the other related air quality conditions such as particle counts, air flow patterns to establish lack of turbulence, pressure differentials, temperature, and relative humidity (Rh). This testing should be performed at representitive sites and at a frequency that will be sufficient to insure that suitable environmental control is being maintained.

Any other systems that are in direct contact or in close proximity to the aseptic environment must be validated when the system is initially installed and monitored frequently enough to assure adequate conditions are being maintained. This would include utility systems such as Purified Water, Water for Injection (WFI), compressed gasses (air, nitrogen, carbon dioxide, argon, etc.), filter systems (e.g. compressed gas and vacuum breaker filters on lyophilizers and sterilizers), and cleaning, sanitization, and disinfection systems. Of course, all major equipment systems such as filling machines, container capping/sealing equipment and lyophilizers need to be subjected to validation testing to insure proper performance (FDA, 1986 and Gold Sheet, 1986). While these systems are not being emphasized in this presentation, experience during FDA inspections has revealed that problems continue to exist in these areas, and it is unrealistic to consider an aseptic process to be validated unless and until these related manufacturing systems have been documented as operating under a state of control.

B. Validation of aseptic assembly processes

Unlike terminally sterilized products that can provide SAL's on the order of 10^{-6} or better, it is not possible to provide such SAL's for aseptically produced products. In fact, with current technology and validation methods, it is possible only to provide sterility assurance levels on the order of 10^{-3}. It is not the objective of this presentation to provide a rigorous treatment of the limitations of aseptic process validation. Instead, these limitations are being acknowledged with special emphasis being given to those areas where FDA inspections continue to find firms that do not meet FDA requirements. FDA is well aware of the limitations with aseptic process validation, and permits firms to take these factors into account when validating these systems. However, too commonly FDA investigators find that firms have not adequately validated their processes based upon the erroneous arguments that recognized validation methods do not exist, methods are impractical, costly, or otherwise unattractive. The FDA does expect that each aseptic process be validated in a manner that provides adequate assurances of sterility to the ultimate user of such products. Media fills, or process simulation tests, are used extensively by the pharmaceutical industry for validating aseptic processes (PDA, 1980). Media fills are simulated tests conditions in which open containers with sterile media capable of supporting microbiological growth are exposed to the aseptic environment and manufacturing manipulation processes. Following exposure to the aseptic environment, the containers are sealed and then incubated to detect microbiological growth. Following incubation, the number of containers exhibiting growth is determined, and the observed contamination rate can be calculated by the following equation (PDA, 1980):

% Contamination level =

$$\frac{\text{No. of undamaged containers with microbial growth}}{\substack{\text{(Total no. containers filled} - \\ \text{no. contaminated damaged containers)}}} \times 100$$

The principal objective of these simulations is to quantitatively demonstrate the contamination rates resulting from the aseptic assembly operations. The use of media fills has become accepted industry practice, but not without controversies (some of which remain unresolved). This is especially true with respect to interpretation of results and methods used to statistically treat media fill test data. The FDA does not consider media fills to be an absolute GMP requirement per se. The FDA is aware that even better methods may eventually be developed and would not likely restrict the use of preferable methods. However, at the current time media fills are realistically the only practical validation approach that allows contamination rates to be determined quantitatively. While such tests can provide valuable quantitative information, there are legitimate limitations and restrictions which need to be addressed when interpreting media filled data. These limitations have, in some cases, been used by firms as excuses or reasons for not conducting media fills, or as the basis for justifying excessive contamination rates. Since these problems have led to problems during FDA inspections, the following is a brief review of some of the more common areas of concern to the FDA investigator when evaluating the use of media fills in aseptic process validation. It is no coincidence that these same concerns were expressed in the FDA proposed aseptic processing guideline, because FDA inspections continued to find problems in these areas.

Contamination Rates:

The FDA recognizes that aseptic processes cannot with certainty exclude all microorganisms from the aseptic environment. Thus, there is always the possibility that personnel, equipment, and the manufacturing environment may contribute viable microorganisms that are capable of entering the exposed products during manufacturing. However, the likelihood that a product may become contaminated during aseptic exposure can, with available technology, be kept at very low probability levels. But since this probability exists, it is important that validation testing employ valid statistical methods that are able to predict (i.e., confidence intervals) the likelihood that the observed contamination rates reflect the true contamination rates.

While there may be legitimate practical and statistical limitations with the methods used to predict contamination rates, these should not be considered as unsurmountable or as reasons for not employing such testing. Properly applied testing methods can provide an increased degree of confidence that such probability of contamination is at levels which are generally adequate to assure the safety for the ultimate user. This is especially true if the statistical limitations are taken into account.

In the absence of an official published FDA standard or regulation that defines acceptable aseptic validation criteria, there have been during recent years controversies about what constituted acceptable media fill contamination rates. These differing positions by individual firms have led to a multiplicity of criteria being established, some of which satisfy FDA requirements and others which do not. The following is a brief review of the background and problems that are commonly found during FDA inspections of media fill test methods.

In 1973, the World Health Organization (WHO, 1973) published a document which cited media fill contamination rates of 0.3%. While this value has received attention and has become the subject of controversy, the FDA did not consider this to be an official requirement. In 1980, the Parenteral Drug Association (PDA, 1980) published Technical Monograph No. 2 which referenced the existence of the WHO 0.3% figure, but suggested that a manufacturer should strive for a contamination level of less than 0.1%. Neither the WHO document nor the PDA tecnical monograph include provisions for applying statistical treatments to media fill contamination rate data.

In recent times, the FDA has found firms that were using the 0.3% observed contamination rate criteria as the basis for validation acceptance. The FDA does not consider this position to be reasonable for a number of reasons. First, as pointed out by Tetzlaff (1984), an observed contamination rate on the order of 0.3% is generally indicative of poorly controlled environmental and manufacturing conditions that are usually apparent during FDA inspections. Secondly, the use of observed contamination rates, without determining statistical confidence limits, does not take into account random variation that may occur. The basis for determining statistical confidence limits for media fill data was discussed in detail by Tetzlaff (1984).

The FDA aseptic guideline (1987) does not provide specific values for observed contamination rates for media fills. Instead, the FDA considers as an acceptable process as being one in which validation test results show with a high degree of confidence that the probability of a unit becoming contaminated during aseptic processing is held at a very low level; i.e., one in which the probability of contamination is no greater than one unit in 1,000. In providing this guidance, the FDA points out that it would not consider acceptable batches in which one in 1000 containers were, in fact, nonsterile. Fry (1985) provides further insight into the current FDA philosophies regarding media fills and aseptic process validation criteria.

Number of Units Tested:

FDA expects that aseptically filled drugs should provide SAL's of at least 10^{-3}. Media fill test data can be used to provide such assurances but the probability of detecting low incidences of contamination is a function of the number of units tested. Unless sufficient number of units are tested, there may not be a valid statistical basis to establish contamination rates on the order of 10^{-3}. The following equation can be used for determining the probability (P) that at least one unit in a random sample of (n) units will be nonsterile if the proportion of non sterile units is X, (Parzen, 1960; Tetzlaff, 1983)

$$P = 1 - (1-X)^n$$

Tetzlaff (1983) has provided the rational for the FDA expectation that at least 3,000 units need be tested in order to provide a sound statistical basis for media fill validation. If at least 3000 units are tested is is possible at the 0.95 probability level to detect contamination rates on the order of 10^{-3} (ie. 1 in 1000), but if less than 3000 units are tested then the probability of detecting contamination may be significantly reduced. For example, the probability (P) of detecting a contamination rate of 1/1000 (0.001) is 0.63 if 1000 units were tested [$P = 1-(1-.001)^{1000} = 0.63$], and the probability would be further reduced to 0.1 if only 100 units were tested [$P = 1-(1-.001)^{100} = 0.1$].

Duration:

In addition to a minimum number of units tested, the FDA expects that media fill test runs should be of sufficient duration to include all of the processing and manipulations that are normally performed during actual production operations. Included in "worst case' simulations would be filling rates that are equivalent to or slower than actual production conditions (to simulate maximum exposure times), simulation of in-process adjustments and duplication of personnel change practices (including breaks), or any other condition or practice that may expose the product to increased potential of contamination.

Frequency/Reproducibility:

While three validation runs would generally be considered acceptable for a new filling line, there are no recognized official guidelines which specify absolute requirements for revalidation. This would depend largely upon numerous environmental factors such as changes in personnel, equipment and process modifications, environmental test data results, sterility test results, or any other data which may reflect the degree of control of an aseptic process. If there have been no major changes in any manufacturing or environmental systems and production data reflects a continued state of control, then it would not be necessary to repeat validation testing with three runs. In such cases, single runs conducted at intervals of at least twice per year for each personnel shift and each processing line have generally been considered as acceptable. However, if the interim data reflected problems or a lack of control, then it would be appropriate to conduct multiple runs to establish reproducibility.

Media Selection:

The media chosen for validation runs must be capable of supporting microbial growth. It is customary to utilize a growth medium that has been demonstrated as being able to support microbial growth for a broad spectrum of aerobic microorganisms. For example, soybean casein digest medium is commonly used. However, it is the responsibility of each manufacturer to establish that whatever medium is utilized does, in fact, support microbial growth for the mircroorganisms that are encountered in the firm's own particular environments. In addition, it would be appropriate for manufacturers to determine the growth promoting qualities of the media on a regular on-going basis since there is ample evidence showing variations in the ability of different media to support microbial growth (Pflug, et. al., 1981; and Cook and Gilbert, 1968). The FDA proposed aseptic guideline also suggests that consideration be given to selecting media based upon its ability to grow the specific microorganisms that have been identified or isolated from environmental monitoring and from any positive sterility tests.

Special Concerns:

FDA inspections have revealed a number of unique or unusual situations which have special bearing upon media fills and aseptic pro cess validation. These deserve attention because some firms have not adequately validated their processes based upon erroneous arguments that media fills are not amenable to their processes or that validation is not possible. The FDA expects that all aseptic processes must be validated to provide suitable sterility assurance levels. If the conventional methods are not amenable to a particular firm's process, then it would be considered appropriate to devise special techniques that are. For example, lyophilization is a unique process involved in many aseptic processes. Some firms have failed to adequately validate the lyophilization process with respect to sterility assurances, and sterility problems have been associated with the manufacture and control of lyophilized products (FDA, 1986). Frequently, this is based upon the claim that liquid medium cannot be processed through the conventional lyophilization process. Since lyophilizers may leak or may have non-sterile surfaces on the interior, it would be appropriate to at least introduce media to the lyophilization chamber and to subject the open vials to the vacuum process even if the product were not frozen and/or lyophilized per se. In this case, the product would at least have been exposed to simulated "normal" conditions to the extent practical (FDA, 1986; Avallone and Wolk, 1986; Gold Sheet, 1986; Flamberg, 1986; Couriel, 1980; Moore, 1983; Williams and Polli, 1984).

Another common problem area encountered during FDA inspections involves aseptic powder filling. Again, some firms have not properly validated the aseptic powder filling based upon the contention that media fills cannot be performed for conventional powder filling. While not all powder filling operations would be amenable to liquid media fills per se, there are a number of recognized acceptable alternatives which can provide a high degree of sterility assurance. For example, sterile powders such as lactose, PEG, or even dry microbiological medium may be employed to simulate dry powder filling (Prout, 1982).

Some firms have been successful in validating dry aseptic powder filling by utilizing conventional media filling techniques inside the powder filling room. In such cases, the powder filling equipment is bypassed (the sterilization of which is validated separately) and the containers are subjected to "normal" handling with liquid medium being substituted for dry powder. Opponents of this method argue that this does not simulate normal conditions which is true. However, proponents point out that employees are normally the major source of product contamination and, therefore, this method can at least detect microbial contamination from the aseptic environment. Admittedly, there are limitations with this method, but these should not be used as excuses for not validating the process. Opponents of the use of dry powder to validate aseptic powder filling argue that the reconstitution necessary to permit microbial growth introduces potential for adventitious contamination (i.e. false positives).

Additional problems found during FDA inspections include the failure to validate all processing lines. This is usually based on the argument that filling lines are identical, and therefore, it is not necessary to validate each individual processing line. The FDA does not consider this to be a reasonable argument. Each filling line would be considered a separate entity, and therefore, should be validated separately. Firms with slow-speed filling lines or unusual product sizes sometimes argue that it is not practical to simulate normal production conditions for media fill runs. In such cases, it may be appropriate to extend production times to provide for a sufficient number of containers to be filled or container sizes should be chosen in a manner that simulated "worst case". The Parenteral Drug Association Technical Report No. 6, Validation of Aseptic Drug Powder Filling Processes (PDA, 1984) provides guidance in some of the philosophies, materials, equipment, etc. that can be used for validating dry powder filling processes.

C. GMP documentation systems

Even before the promulgation of the drug GMP regulations in 1963, the FDA recognized that the maintenance of adequate written documentation was an essential good manufacturing practice. During the past two decades there have been dramatic improvements in the documentation systems used to insure that the intended manufacturing and control procedures have been employed. While the importance and value of effective documentation systems have long been recognized by the aseptic industry and the FDA alike, the following describes some of the documentation problems found during FDA inspections of aseptic processes. These are being emphasized not only because inadequate documentation can seriously compromise sterility assurances, but especially because finished product microbial quality attributes (sterility) cannot quantitatively be measured by testing the product. The USP XXI (1985) recognizes the statistical limitations of the sterility test and points out the benefits of maintaining proper documentation and validation systems.

Documentation systems are being emphasized here because of their important bearing upon aseptic process validation which is unlike any of the other sterilization validation methods. Terminal sterilization processes may employ overkill cycles and the sterilization parameters such as time, temperature, pressure (steam), gas concentrations (ETO), and dose (radiation) can usually be physically measured and SAL's can be derived quantitatively by direct means with relatively high SAL's (e.g., 10^{-6} or better). In contrast, current aseptic process validation methods must rely upon indirect means to determine the contamination rate probabilities such as the use of process simulation tests (media fills), and SAL's are normally in the much lower range (i.e. on the order of 10^{-3}).

Finally, documentation systems for aseptic validation methods become especially important when it is realized that available methods cannot precisely or reproducibly measure or detect all possible sources of product microbial contamination. These limitations, if fully recognized, can be largely overcome by the utilization of effective documentation systems. FDA inspections of aseptic processes usually concentrate upon the documentation systems that are in place to demonstrate a state of control. The diversity of manufacturing and quality control systems for aseptic processing have led to numerous different styles and types of documentation systems, many of which satisfy the FDA GMP requirements.

One of the most serious aseptic process documentation problems is the failure to have fail-safe systems to detect out-of-limit conditions in a timely manner. There should be formal systems in place to summarize, organize, and tabulate the large amount of environmental data that is normally collected on a regular ongoing basis. These systems will vary with each user, but all have the objective of presenting the data in a fashion such that trends become apparent and problems can be readily seen. The firms that have been the most sucessful in properly validating aseptic processes have without exception developed such documentation systems. They have been able to immediately recognize problems as they develop and react before the problems adversely impact upon products being produced.

The drug GMP Regulations, Part 211.180(e) apply to all drug products, but particular emphasis should be given to application of this requirement to those produced by aseptic processing. This section requires that firms maintain documentation in a manner such that the data can be used for evaluating periodically (at least annually) the quality standards of each drug product to determine the need for changes in drug product specifications or manufacturing or control procedures. This section is especially pertinent to aseptically produced drugs, since the environment used to produce the drug products is a dynamic one and is subject to change at any time. There is a very real chance that the microbiological or physical environmental conditions may change with time, which places special importance on the system used to periodically evaluate that the quality contol procedures and environmental conditions are being maintained in an adequate state of control.

FDA inspections continue to find firms that are having difficulty satisfying this GMP requirement: especially significant is the failure to establish systems that are adequate to permit detection of trends or problems quickly enough to allow timely corrective action. The documentation problems found during FDA inspections usually can be classified into one of the following three categories:

i. Failure to detect out-of-limit conditions

Many firms have been found to lack systems that are sufficiently organized or formalized to detect out-of-limit conditions. While these firms almost always have systems in place to record the original data and to file it, it is not uncommon during FDA inspections to find that the data are not maintained such that out-of-limit data becomes highlighted so responsible management can react in an appropriate and timely fashion. If these problems go undetected by responsible management, it is possible for out-of-control conditions to develop which may seriously jeopardize product sterility assurances. The most effective systems are those that tabulate or organize the physical and microbiological environmental data on a regular or continuing basis (such as daily, weekly or monthly) using graphs or charts showing the cumulative data such that any out-of-limit results are visibly highlighted.

ii. Failure to correct out-of-limit conditions

Once out-of-limit conditions have been detected from analysis of samples or physical testing, it is essential that there be formal written documentation systems for the follow-up actions taken. Too frequently the follow-up notification may be verbal at the time of occurrence rather than being reduced to writing. If the corrective action follow-up is not written, serious problems may develop during FDA inspections because the absence of supportive documentation may prevent the FDA from reaching the same conclusions. This may lead to possible regulatory actions if sterility assurances cannot be adequately demonstrated. The most effective systems are those which require the personnel who detect an out-of-limit condition to prepare a formal written notification record (using standardized forms) to alert the affected department. This permits the responsible department to react to this data such as to resample as necessary, to review/evaluate any related data or documents, and to decide course of action. Finally, recording on these forms the substance of this followup, corrective action, and investigation enables responsible management to conveniently review, evaluate, and intelligently decide the necessary action. Once the investigation is completed and corrective action is taken, it is desirable that responsible management review the overall documentation, and prepare a formal written approval record or have sign-off documentation showing the justification for continuing (or resuming) the use of the affected system.

Particular attention is given during FDA inspections to evaluating the basis used to justify any decision to continue use of any systems that have been found by testing to possibly be operating out of control. Unless documentation exists showing the specific basis or justification for each such decision, the FDA evaluation of the same circumstances may reach different conclusions. Some firms do not prepare corrective action reports at the time of occurrence, but instead prepare summaries afterwards (frequently days or weeks later).

Summaries can be a valuable (if not an essential) tool during an evaluation process, but should not be considered as a substitute for adequate documentation prepared at the time of occurrence.

Examples of documentation problems found during FDA inspections include insufficient documentation for microbiological samples found to exhibit growth (such as media fills or sterility samples) or for those exceeding alert or action limits (such as environmental samples of air, surfaces, equipment, personnel, etc.). Too frequently these test results are considered as being likely false positives or artifacts of testing and are not afforded the appropriate degree of documentation. In such cases, retesting may be an appropriate action, but careful consideration should be given to the possibility that the results obtained may be indicative of actual contamination rather than a testing artifact. In this instance, appropriate followup would be to issue a written notification that an out-of-limit condition (or positive test) was found, including a complete description of the sample, date and location(s) tested (specific sampling site), and laboratory test results. There should be written instructions to immediately resample the affected system (as well as any appropriate related systems), and the retest results need to be properly recorded. Microbiological test documentation systems need to allow for the necessary delays in obtaining test results, but can be designed to facilitate data retrieval.

Although many microbiological tests require several days (or even weeks) to enable detection of slow growing organisms, daily examination of incubating samples can permit early detection and immediate reaction to samples found to exhibit growth. Some firms do not examine the incubating samples until the completion of the requisite incubation period:, once positive growth is found, several days or weeks have elapsed. This prevents timely resampling of the affected system which may have changed appreciably since the previous sampling. It is prudent to monitor incubating samples frequently enough to allow timely reaction in order to maintain suitable control of the system. Processing normally continues during this incubation period and the products made during the intervening period may become at risk and sterility assurances may be jeopardized while samples are incubating. The disposition of microbiological samples having growth may affect the ability to properly follow-up or investigate the potential origin of contamination. Firms that routinely discard microbiological samples exhibiting growth before initiating/completing follow-up investigations may be prevented from reaching valid conclusions if such testing becomes indicated at a later date. This is especially significant for environmental and sterility test samples because conclusive determinations of causes or origin of contamination is difficult at best. If samples have been discarded it may be virtually impossible to reach valid conclusions.

The decision to continue the use of a system (or the affected portion) after finding microbiological test data that exceeds limits requires careful consideration and proper documentation. Since the microbiological test results may actually reflect that the system is contaminated, it is appropriate to have a formal written evaluation which provides the justification for continuing the use of the system. FDA inspections have revealed instances where firms continued to use systems when their own data showed out-of-limit conditions in the absence of conclusive data to demonstrate that the positive findings were false positives or testing artifacts.

iii. Failure to document justification that data were testing artifacts
Microbiological monitoring of aseptic environments involves the collection and

testing of a large number of samples and the FDA recognizes that there is a possibility of adventitious contamination during the sampling/testing (i.e. false positives). However, the failure of firms to properly justify or document the basis for concluding that observed growth was a false positive or testing artifact continues to be observed during FDA inspections. If the finding of growth is suspected as being a false positive, it is essential that there be formal written documentation prepared at the time occurence which shows the specific basis for reaching this conclusion. After completing the test, responsible personnel should carefully evaluate all applicable circumstances surrounding this data and should reference the specific data that was used as justification to conclude the observed growth was a testing artifact. It is not uncommon during FDA inspections of firm's environmental monitoring or sterility test systems to find positive microbiological test results that were attributed to being an artifact of the test without any written documentation or incomplete written justification to support this conclusion.

Media fill validation testing poses special documentation problems and deserves special consideration if testing exhibits growth in excess of allowable limits. FDA inspections have revealed instances where firms have found media fill contamination rates in excess of their specifications and the firms failed to demonstrate (document) that these results were invalid. In such cases, the firms continued to produce product for commercial distribution using the same equipment, facilities, and personnel that were involved in the media fill failure, without supportive evidence to invalidate the failure.

The practice of continuing production (at risk) after validation media fills have failed should be discouraged or not allowed since the product made under nonvalidated conditions during this intervening period may fail to have adequate assurances of sterility. For example, a major pharmaceutical manufacturer was found to continue production for three months while five of seven successive media fills failed, with virtually no written documentation showing any followup investigation, evaluation, or justification to invalidate the positive findings. The FDA evaluation of the same test results reached a different conclusion, and serious issues were raised concerning the placing product at risk of excessive contamination.

Any decision to invalidate data of this importance should only be done after careful consideration of a well documented set of data, and only if there is a formal review process. This documentation must necessarily include the complete written details showing which specific data was reviewed, the specific scientific basis for concluding the data was invalid, and formal written authorization/approval by responsible management. The failure to have any one of these important documentation elements may result in the FDA reaching different conclusions. If the FDA deems the products made under such conditions lack adequate sterility assurances, regulatory proceedings may be initiated as discussed above.

D. Microbiological environmental monitoring systems

Microbiological monitoring of the equipment, personnel and environment represents one of the most important features of any control program for aseptic processes. Despite this importance, FDA inspections continue to find firms that do not have adequate environmental monitoring programs. The literature is replete with information about microbiological monitoring methods (Lieberman, 1977; Abdou, 1980; Newman and Schimpff, 1982; Carlberg, 1984; Dell, 1979), sampling methods (Placencia et. al., 1982; Delmore and Thompson, 1981), and routes of microbial contamination (Whyte, 1981; Whyte et. al., 1982). Therefore, these issues will not be addressed in this presentation, but their overall importance cannot be overstressed. The failure to establish written specifications or limits or the establishment of inappropriate limits is a relatively common FDA inspectional observation. This ranges from the absence of written microbiological quality specifications for important processing areas including the nonaseptic controlled areas (such as raw material and component preparation areas, mixing and formulation rooms and component washing areas) to those areas which would be considered critical such as aseptic filling rooms, and other processing areas where exposed sterile components or products are exposed. Firms which lack such specifications normally do have microbiological monitoring programs, but they are not complete and important areas that should be tested on a regular basis sometimes are not. During an FDA investigation, it is customary to perform a systematic evaluation of the microbiological data for each of the controlled and critical aseptic processing areas. This would include determining whether specifications existed for the following important areas.

The controlled but non-aseptic areas should be maintained at a reasonable microbiological level to prevent presence of excessive microorganisms that may reflect inadequate cleaning, sanitization, and disinfection practices as well as contributing to the possibility of pyrogen formation. Since these areas are not considered to be aseptic, the microbiological levels would be expected to be of a lesser quality than the aseptic areas, but some firms erroneously consider it to be unnecessary to routinely monitor these areas and therefore have not established written specifications for room air quality, surfaces and other areas. The FDA does not expect that these areas be tested with the same frequency as for aseptic areas, but a routine monitoring program would be considered as appropriate to demonstrate adequacy of environmental conditions.

The aseptic processing areas should be monitored on a daily basis, or more frequently as necessary, to assure that microbiological environmental conditions are maintained under a suitable state of control. Since personnel and equipment conditions may change without notice at any time, it is essential that the monitoring programs be capable of detecting excursions from the firm's quality specifications in a timely manner. Sometimes FDA inspections reveal that firms have not established written specifications for aseptic room air quality or do not test air quality on a daily basis. Such firms usually rely instead upon settling plates as an indicator of room environmental quality. The FDA does not consider settling plates alone to be an adequate monitoring measure for aseptic room air quality. Quantitative sampling methods such as volumetric air samplers (slit-to-agar, centrifugal, impingers, etc.) which draw known volumes of air across a microbiological medium are considered to be essential for adequate monitoring. Settling plates have value as a qualitative test but should not be considered as an alternative to regular volumetric air sampling.

The issue of aseptic room air quality specifications is frequently raised during FDA inspections. Prior to the FDA publication of the Guideline on Sterile Drug Products Produced by Aseptic Processing (FDA, 1985), there were no published official FDA standards or regulations which specified air quality requirements. This guideline suggests that clean room air quality microbiological levels of 0.1 organism per cubic foot would be considered reasonable by the FDA. It is interesting to note that this same quality specification of 0.1 viable microorganism per cubic foot in class 100 processing areas had been established as early as 1967 by the NASA for its standards for clean rooms and work stations used for spacecraft (NASA, 1967). In 1980 the Parenteral Drug Association, Technical Monograph No. 2, references the NASA standard of 0.1 organisms per cubic foot as being obtainable and desirable.

FDA inspections continue to find firms that do not routinely collect enough representitive samples to adequately demonstrate a state of control. For example, some firms do not routinely collect microbiological samples from the nonsterile controlled environments such as mixing rooms, formulation rooms, container/closure preparation areas, or container washing areas, or fail to monitor critical areas within the aseptic areas which represents a more serious problem. For example, some, albeit the minority, still do not routinely collect microbiological samples of the room air in the aseptic filling rooms. Instead, such firms rely on settling plates.

E. Sterility testing

Sterility testing of aseptic products continues to generate controversy and misunderstandings. It is beyond the scope of this presentation to discuss the limitations of the sterility test (Brown and Gilbert, 1977; Pflug, 1973; Bowman, 1973; Bryce, 1956). Instead, special emphasis is given to the unique nature of aseptic processing and its relationship to sterility test results. Aseptic processing represents an unusual situation in that the product does not receive a terminal process to assure sterility. The possibility that contamination may occur during the aseptic assembly places special significance upon the sterility test results once growth is observed in samples. The FDA recognizes that the manipulations involved in conducting the sterility test do, in fact, create the possibility of adventitous contamination occurring (i.e., false positives), but this incidence should be at a very low level.

Once a sterility test indicates the presence of growth in a sample, it is incumbent upon the firm to exercise sound scientific practices when interpreting these results. Too frequently, FDA investigations reveal that there is a failure to characterize or identify the isolates found in the initial sterility test results and the failure to conduct documented investigations to determine the origin of the contamination. The FDA Guideline on Sterile Drug Products Produced by Aseptic Processing (1985) provides considerable insight into the FDA concerns about sterility retesting and interpretation of results. Tetzlaff (1983 and 1984) and Avallone (1983 and 1984) provide specific examples of sterility retesting problems encountered during FDA inspections.

ACKNOWLEDGEMENT: This work was supported under the FDA SARAP Fellowship program.

6. References

Abdou, M.A.F., "Determination of airborne microorganisms in a pharmaceutical plant using standard, elective, and selective culture media," Pharm. Tech., pp. 93-100, November, 1980.

Anon., "Committee to revise 209b," MD & DI, 4, 26-28, 1982.

Anon., "Federal Standard 209B revision: an update," MD & DI, 6, 41-93, 1984.

Association for the Advancement of Medical Instrumentation (AAMI), "Process Control Guidelines for Gamma Radiation Sterilization of Medical Devices," AAMI, Arlington, VA 22209, 1984.

Association for the Advancement of Medical Instrumentation (AAMI), "Guideline for Industrial Ethylene Oxide Sterilization of Medical Devices," AAMI, Arlington, VA 22209, 1981.

Avallone, H.L., and Wolk, A.E., "Regulatory aspects of lyophilization," J. Parenter. Sci. Tech., 40, 81-82, 1986.

Avallone, H.L., "Control aspects of aseptically produced products," J. Parenter. Sci. Tech., 39, 77-79, 1985.

Avallone, H.L., "Regulatory issues arising from recent FDA inspections," Pharm. Manuf., 16-22, Oct. 1984.

Avallone, H.L. "GMP inspections: a field investigator's view," Pharm. Tech., pp. 48-53, Mar. 1983.

Avallone, H.L., "Clean room design, control and characterization," Pharm. Eng., 33-46, Sept-Oct, 1982.

Avallone, H.L., "Inspectional guidelines for sterile bulk antibiotics," J. Parenter. Drug Assn., 34, 447-451, 1980.

Ballentine, C., "Taste of raspberries, taste of death: The 1937 elixir sulfanilamide incident," FDA Consumer, 18-21, June, 1981.

Betts, W.A., "A new approach to quality training," J. Parenter. Sci. Technol., 35, 248-250, 1981.

Block, S.S.(Editor), Part 2, Antiseptics and Disinfectants, Chapters 7-19, In Disinfection, Sterilization and Preservation, Lea & Febiger, Philadelphia, pp. 157-400, 1983.

Bowman, F.W., "Sterility testing," In Industrial Sterilization, Phillips, G.B. and Miller, W.S. (Eds.), Duke University Press, Durham, N.C., pp. 35-47, 1973.

British Pharmacopoeia, Vol. II, Her Majesty's Stationery Office, London, Appendix XVIII, Methods of Sterilization, pp. A196-A197, 1980.

British Pharmacopoeia, Her Majesty's Stationery Office, London, Appendix XVI, pp. 630-632, 1932.

Brown, M.R.W., and Gilbert, P., "Increasing the probability of sterility of medicinal products," J. Pharm. Pharmacol., 29, 517-523, 1977.

Bryce, D.M., "Tests for the sterility of pharmaceutical preparations," J. Pharm. Pharmacol., 8, 561-572, 1956.

Byers, T.E., "GMP's and design for quality," J. Parenter. Drug Assn.,32, 22-25, 1978.

Carlberg, D.M., "The microbiological assessment of biocleanroom quality," Pharm. Mfg., 1, 14-17, 1984.

Code of Federal Regulations, Title 21, Part 211, "Current Good Manufacturing Practice for Finished Pharmaceuticals," U.S. Government Printing Office, Washington DC.

Code of Federal Regulations, Title 21, Part 820, "Good Manufacturing Practice for Medical Devices: General," U.S. Government Printing Office, Washington DC.

Code of Federal Regulations, Title 21, Part 10.90, "Food and Drug Administration regulations, guidelines, recommendations, and agreements," U.S. Government Printing Office, Washington DC.

Cook, A.M., and Gilbert, R.J., "Factors affecting the heat resistance of Bacillus stearothermophilus spores I. The effect of recovery conditions on colony count of unheated and heated spores," J. Food Tech., 3, 285-293, 1968.

Couriel, B., "Freeze-drying: Past, present and future," J Parenter Drug Assoc, 34, 352-357, 1980.

Dell, L.A., "Aspects of microbiological monitoring for nonsterile and sterile manufacturing environments," Pharm. Tech., 47-51, August, 1979.

Delmore, R.P., and Thompson, W.N., "A comparison of air-sampler effeciencies," M D & D I, 45-53, February, 1981.

DeLuca, P.P., "Microcontamination control: A summary of an approach to training," J. Parenter. Sci. Technol., 37, 218-224, 1983.

DeVecchi, F.A., "Training personnel to work in sterile environments," Pharm. Tech., 41-44, August, 1978.

Dirksen, J.W., and Larsen, R.V., "Filling vials aseptically while monitoring for bacterial contamination," Am. J. Hosp. Pharm., 32, 1031-1032, 1975.

The Dispensatory of the United States of America, J.B. Lippincott & Co., Philadelphia, PA., pp. 1075, 1883.

Federal Register, Vol. 50, Feb. 1, 1985, 4799-4800, 1985.

Federal Register, Vol. 48, March 29, 1983, 13096, 1983.

Federal Register, Vol. 43, No. 190, Sept. 29, 1978, 45014-45087, 1978.

Federal Register, Vol. 41, No. 31, Feb.13, 1976, 6878-6894, 1976.

Federal Register, Vol. 41, No. 106, June 1, 1976, 22202-22219, 1976.

Federal Register, Vol. 36, No. 10, Jan. 15, 1971, 601-605, 1971.

Federal Register, Vol. 28, June 20, 1963, 6385, 1963.

Federal Food Drug and Cosmetic Act, As Amended, United States Code, Title 21, U.S. Government Printing Office, Washington DC 20402.

Federal Standard 209b, "Clean room and Work Station Requirements, Controlled Environment", 1973.

Flamberg, D.W., "Manufacturing considerations in the lyophilization of parenteral products," Pharm Manuf, 3, 28-48, 1986.

Flosdorf, E.W., Freeze Drying, Reinhold Publishing Corp., New York, 1949.

Flosdorf, E.W., Stokes, F.J., and Mudd, S., J. Am Med Assoc., 115, 1095-1097, 1940.

Food and Drug Administration, Inspection Technical Guide, Number 43, "Lyophilization of Parenterals," Food and Drug Administration, 5600 Fishers Lane, Rockville, MD 20857, April 18, 1986.

Food & Drug Administration, "Guideline on sterile drug products produced by aseptic processing," FDA, 5600 Fishers Lane, Rockville, MD 20857, 1985.

Food & Drug Administration, "Guideline on general principles of process validation," FDA, 5600 Fishers Lane, Rockville, Md, 20857, 1984.

Food and Drug Administration, FDA Consumer Memo, "Thalidomide," March, 1984.

Food Drug and Law Reporter, 38-068, Commerce Clearing House, Inc., 1976.

Fry, E.M., "An FDA update on GMP's for aseptic processing," J. Parenter. Sci. Technol., 39, 154-157, 1985.

Fry, E.M., "The parenteral drug industry: Recent findings," J. Parenter. Sci. Technol., 36, 55-58, 1982.

The Gold Sheet, Vol 20, No. 6, June, 1986.

The Gold Sheet, Vol 19, No. 2, February, 1985.

Groves, M.J., Parenteral Products, William Heinemann Medical Books Ltd, London, 1973.

Health Industry Manufacturers Association (HIMA), "Medical Device Sterilization Monographs Validation Of Sterilization Systems," Report No. 78-4.1, HIMA, Washington DC, 1978.

Health Industry Manufacturers Association (HIMA), "Microbial Control in the Manufacturing Environment," Report No. 78-4.3, HIMA, Washington DC, 1978.

Janssen, W.F., "The story of the laws behind the labels," FDA Consumer, 32-45, June, 1981.

Kitt, M.T., "An approach to GMP training," J. Parenter. Drug Assoc., 33, 341-345, 1979.

Krzyzyk, V., "The history of drug regulations," J. Parenter. Drug Assoc., 31, 156-160, 1977.

Lawless, E.W., "The thalidomide tragedy," In Technology and Social Shock, Rutgers Univ. Press, New Brunswick, N.J., 140-148, 1977.

Leahy, T.J., and Sullivan, M.J., "Validation of bacterial retention capabilities of membrane filters," Pharm. Tech., Nov. 1978.

Lieberman, A., "Verifying the efficiency of air-cleanliness control systems," Pharm. Tech. 33-41, September, 1977.

Loftus, B.T., "Human injectable drugs: an FDA perspective," Pharm. Tech., 45-49, Nov, 1977.

Loughhead, H., "Training of clean room personnel," Bull. Paren. Drug Assoc., 23, 228-232, 1969.

Luna, C.J., "Training the cleanroom employee," MD & DI, 6, 59-61, 1984.

Michels, D.L., "Compliance issues in 1985", J. Paren. Sci. Technol., 39, 158-160, 1985.

Moore, D.W., "The state of the science of pharmaceutical freeze-drying," Pharm Tech, 84-88, March 1983.

National Aeronautics and Space Administration (NASA), "NASA standard procedures for the microbiological examination of space hardware," NASA, Washington DC, 1980.

National Aeronautics and Space Administration (NASA), "NASA standards for clean rooms and work stations for the microbially controlled environment," Publication No. NHB 5340.2, NASA, Washington DC, August, 1967.

National Formulary, First Issue, American Pharmaceutical Assoc., pp. 76-77, 1888.

National Formulary, Fifth Edition, American Pharmaceutical Assoc., pp. 2-7, 1932.

Newman, K.A., and Schimpff, S.C., "Microbiological evaluation of laminar airflow rooms," P & MC Hospitals, 77-82, Sept/Oct, 1982.

Pall, D.B., Kirnbauer, E.A., and Allen, B.T., Colloids and Surfaces, Elsevier Scientific Publishing Company, Amsterdam, 235-256, 1980.

Parenteral Drug Association (PDA), "Technical Monograph No. 1, Validation of Steam Sterilization Cycles," PDA, Philadelphia, PA, 1978.

Parenteral Drug Association (PDA), "Technical Monograph No. 2, Validation of Aseptic Filling for Solution Drug Products," PDA, Philadelphia, PA, 1980.

Parenteral Drug Association (PDA), "Technical Report No. 3, Validation of Dry Heat Processes Used for Sterilization and Depyrogenation," PDA, Philadelphia, PA, 1981.

Parenteral Drug Association (PDA), "Technical Report No. 6, Validation of Aseptic Drug Powder Filling Processes, " PDA, Philadelphia, PA, 1984.

Parzen, E., Modern Probability Theory and its Applications, John Wiley & Sons, Inc., New York, pp. 102-103, 1960.

Pelczar, M.J., Reid, R.D., and Chan, E.C.S., Microbiology, McGraw-Hill Book Company, New York, 1977.

Pflug, I.J., Smith, G.M., and Christensen, R., "Effect of soybean casein digest agar lot on number of Bacillus stearothermophilus spores recovered," Appl. and Envir. Micro., 42, 226-230, 1981.

Pflug, I.J., "Heat sterilization," In Industrial Sterilization, Phillips, G.B., and Miller, W.S.,(Eds.), Duke University Press, Durham, N.C., pp. 239-282, 1973.

Placencia, A.M., Peeler, J.T., Oxborrow, G.S., and Danielson, J.W., "Comparison of bacterial recovery by Reuter Centrifugal air sampler and slit-to-agar sampler," Appl. and Envir. Micro., 44, 512-513, 1982.

Prout, G., "Validation and Routine Opertion of a Sterile Dry Powder Filling Facility," J. Paren. Sci. Tech. 36, 199-204, 1982.

Reti, A.R., "An assessment of test criteria for evaluating the performance and integrity of sterilizing filters," Bull. Paren. Drug Assoc., 31, 1977.

Schmitt, R.F., "Does personnel training reduce device bioburden ?", P & M C, 36-40, March/April, 1983.

Sorenson, R.L., "Federal Standard 209B and the need for a bioclean classification, Pharm. Mfg., 14-17, July, 1984.

Sorenson, R.L., "FS 209B: A part of total environmental Control," Pharm. Eng., 18-40, Nov-Dec, 1984.

Strumia, M.M., In Biological Applications of Freezing and Drying, Harris, R.J. (Ed.), Academic Press, New York, pp. 129-149, 1954.

Tetzlaff, R.F., "The advisory role of FDA district offices in the planning of a new parenteral facility," J. Paren. Sci. Technol., 38, 94-97, 1984.

Tetzlaff, R.F., "Regulatory aspects of aseptic processing," Pharm. Tech., 38-44, Nov., 1984.

Tetzlaff, R.F., "Aseptic process validation," Particulate & Micro. Control Indust., 24-38, 1983.

Tetzlaff, R.F., "Systems validation for parenteral clinical drugs–Application to R & D and QC Laboratories, J. Paren. Sci. Technol., 37, 45-50, 1983.

Tetzlaff, R.F., "Developing a systematic approach to GMP training," Pharm. Tech., 42-51, Nov., 1982.

Tyndall, J., Essays on the Floating Matter of the Air, reprinted from the New York Edition of 1882, Johnson Reprint Corp., New York, The Sources of Science, No. 16, 1966.

United States Pharmacopia, 9th revision, P. Blakiston's Son & Co., Philadelphia, pp. 616-617, 1916.

United States Pharmacopia, XVI, Mack Publishing Co., Eaton, PA, pp 817-819, 1960.

United States Pharmacopia, XIX, U.S. Pharmacopeial Convention Inc., Rockville, MD, 1975.

United States Pharmacopia, XX, U.S. Pharmacopeial Convention Inc., Rockville, MD, 1980.

United States Pharmacopia, XXI, U.S. Pharmacopeial Convention Inc., Rockville, MD, 1985.

U.S. Air Force Technical Order No. 00-25-203, U.S. Government Printing Office, Washington DC, 1963.

U.S. Air Force Manual No. AFM 88-4, Chapter 5, "Criteria for Air Force Clean Facility Design and Construction," U.S. Air Force, Washington DC, 9 September 1968.

U.S. DHEW, FDA Consumer Memo, "Thalidomide," DHEW Publication No. (FDA)74-3017, March 1974.

U.S. Government Printing Office, "Elixir Sulfanilamide-Letter from the Secretary of Agriculture transmitting in response to Senate Resolution No. 194 A report on elixir sulfanilamide-Massengill," Document No. 24, 1937.

U.S. Government Printing Office, "A Brief Legislative History of the Food, Drug, and Cosmetic Act," Committee Print No. 14, Jan. 1974.

Whyte, W., "Settling and impaction of particles into containers in manufacturing pharmacies," J. Paren. Sci. Tech., 35, 255-261, 1981.

Whyte, W., Bailey, P.V., and Tinkler, J., "An evaluation of the routes of bacterial contamination occurring during aseptic pharnaceutical manufacturing," J. Paren. Sci. Tech., 36, 102-107, 1982.

Williams, N.A., and Polli, G.P., "The Lyophilization of pharmaceuticals," J Paren Sci Tech, 38, 48-59, 1984.

World Health Organization (WHO), "General Requirements for the Sterility of Biological Substances (Requirements for Biological Substances No. 6), WHO, Geneva, 1973.

Appendix A

Sources of Equipment and Services Available to Aseptic Pharmaceutical Manufacturers

Many vendors are mentioned throughout the various chapters of this text. In most instances, the vendors are not sole sources. The following lists, while not comprehensive, are intended to mitigate any impression of sole-sourcing. To those vendors to the healthcare and pharmaceutical industries that have been omitted, we extend our sincere apologies; the omission is unintentional. The listing of a company, or the absence of a company from the lists, does not indicate a bias. The editors would be grateful for information concerning vendors not listed, so that correction can be made in subsequent editions.

1. Autoclaves

AMSCO (American Sterilizer Co.)
2425 West 23rd Street
Erie, PA 16514, USA
Ph: (814) 452–3100
Telex: 914532

Castle Co.
1777 E. Henrietta Road
Rochester, NY 14623, USA
Ph: (716) 475–1400
Telex: 2835 CASTLE UF

Getinge International Inc.
1100 Towbin Avenue
Lakewood, NJ 08701, USA
Ph: (201) 370–8800

Gruenberg Inc.
2121 Reach Road
Williamsport, PA 17701, USA
Ph: (717) 326–1755

Santasolo-Sohlberg Corp.
Hankasuontie 4
SF-00390 Helsinki, FINLAND

2. Aseptic Manufacturing (Contract)

Connaught Laboratories
Route 411
Swiftwater, PA 18370, USA
Ph: (717) 839–7187

Steris Laboratories, Inc.
620 N. 51st Avenue
Pheonix, AZ 85043, USA
Ph: (602) 939-7565

Elkins-Sinn
2 Esterbrook Lane
Cherry Hill, NJ 08003–4099, USA
Ph: (800) 257–8349
TWX: 710–896–0804

Summa Manufacturing Sciences
4272 Balloon Park Road, NE
Alburquerque, NM 87109, USA
Ph: (800) 843–4339
Telex: 910 380 9912

Pharma-Hameln
Langes Feld 30–38
D-3250 Hameln 1, WEST GERMANY
Ph: (05151) 581–255

Survival Technology
8101 Glenbrook Road
Bethesda, MD 20814, USA
Ph: (301) 656-5600

Schering-Plough
US Pharmaceutical Products Div.
Kenilworth, NJ 07033, USA
Ph: (201) 558–4811/4809
Telex: 138316/138280

Taylor Pharmacal
P.O. Box 1230
Decatur, IL 62525, USA
Ph: (217) 428-1100

Vitamed
P.O. Box 16085
IL-61160 Tel Aviv, ISRAEL
Ph: (03) 551-8042
Telex: 35770 ATTN: MRZ

Smith-Kline and French
Call Box SKF
Cidra, PR 00639, USA
Ph: (809) 766–4000

3. Centrifuges

Alfa Laval
Box 1008
S-221 03 Lund, SWEDEN
Ph: (046) 105000
Telex: 32145 ALLUND S

Pennwalt (Sharples Div.)
955 Mearns Road
Warminster, PA 18974, USA
Ph: (215) 443–4000
Telex: 4761193

Electro-Nucleonics Inc.
368 Passaic Ave.
Fairfield, NJ 08520, USA
Ph: (800) 346–4364
Telex: 138302

Spinco Inc.
1050 Page Mill Road
Palo Alto, CA 94304
Ph: (415) 857–1150
Fax: (415) 859–1550

Rousselet & Cie
17 Rue Montalivet
F-07100 Annonay, FRANCE
Ph: (75) 334221
Telex: 345670 F

Sulzer-Escher Wyss, Ltd.
Process Engineering Division
Escher Wyss Platz
CH-8023 Zurich, SWITZERLAND
Ph: (01) 2462211
Telex: 82290011

Westphalia Separator AG
1 Werner Habig Strasse
Oelde, WEST GERMANY
Ph: (049) 2522770
Telex: 84189474

4. Chromatographic Media and Systems

Amicon Corp.
25 Hartwell Ave.
Lexington, MA 02173, USA
Ph: (617) 861–9600
Telex: 923541

BioRad Laboratories
2200 Wright Ave.
Richmond, CA 94804, USA
Ph: (415) 234–4130
Telex: 335358

Cuno Inc.
400 Research Parkway
Meriden, CT 06450, USA
Ph: (800) 243–6894
Telex: 962457

LKB Producter
Box 305
S-161 26 Bromma, SWEDEN
Ph: (08) 98–0040
Telex: 85410492

Millipore Corp.
Ashby Road
Bedford, MA 01730, USA
TWX: 710–326–1938
Ph: (800) 225-1380
Telex: 923457

Pharmacia AB
Box 175
S–75104 Upsalla 1, SWEDEN
Ph: (018) 155660
Telex: 85476070

Whatman Ltd
Sprinfield Mill, Maidstone
Kent ME14 2LE, UNITED KINGDOM
Ph: (0622) 61681
Telex: 96113

5. Clean Room Design, Construction, etc.

Cambridge Filter Corp.
P. O. Box 4906
Syracuse, NY 13221–4906, USA
Ph: (315) 457–1000

Clean Room Technology, Inc.
4003 Eastbourne Drive
Syracuse, NY 13206, USA
Ph: (315) 437–2152

Comp-Aire Systems, Inc.
4185 44th SE
Grand Rapids, MI 49508, USA
Ph: (616) 698–9660

Flanders
P. O. Box 1708
Washington, NC 27889, USA
Ph: (919) 946–8081
TWX: 510-924-1898

Liberty Industries, Inc.
133 Commerce Street
East Berlin, CT 06023, USA
Ph: (203) 828-6361
TWX: 710–430–9011

6. Clean-in-Place/Steam-in-Place (CIP/SIP)

BLH Electronics
42 Fourth Avenue
Waltham, MA 02254, USA

Clenesco
P. O. Box 2918
Cincinnati, OH 45201, USA

Degussa Corporation
P. O. Box 2004
Teterborough, NJ 07608, USA

Diversey Wyandotte Corporation
1532 Biddle Avenue
Wyandotte, MI 48192, USA

Electrol Specialties Company
441 Clark Street
South Beloit, IL 61080, USA

Endress & Hauser, Inc.
2350 Endress Place
Greenwood, IN 46142, USA

Foxboro Company
38 Neponsett Avenue
Foxboro, MA 02035, USA

Klenzade
Osborn Building
St. Paul, MN 55102, USA

Ladish-Triclover
9201 Wilmot Road
Kenosha, WI 53141, USA

National Sonics
250 Marcus Boulevard
Hauppage, NY 11787, USA

Pyromation
5211 Industrial Road
Fort Wayne, IN 46895, USA

Viatran Corporation
300 Industrial Drive
Grand Island, NY 14072, USA

Sarco Company
1951 26th S. W.
Allentown, PA 18105, USA

7. Closure Washing and Sterilization

Huber Machinenfabrik
Angerstrasse 16, P. O. B. 1544
D-8050 Freising, WEST GERMANY
081 6113063
Telex: 526533

Huber
Seidenader Equipment, Inc.
35 Airport Park
Morristown, NJ 07960, USA
Ph: (201) 267–8730
TWX: 710–986–7401

Paxall Schubert Division
P. O. Box 836
Pine Brook, NJ 07058, USA
Ph: (201) 227–4677

Pharma-Technik-Smeja
Postfach 2029
D-4172 Straelen-Herongen
  WEST GERMANY
Ph: (609) 921–1220
Telex: 466 750 (WU)

8. Consultants

Bio-Separation Consultants
3935 Falcon Ave.
Long Beach, CA 90807, USA
Attn: Fred Rothstein
Ph: (213) 427–2844

Filtration Specialists Ltd
Pump Green House, Evenlode
Moreton-in-Marsh,
Gloustershire GL56 0NN, ENGLAND
Attn: Derek B. Purchase
Ph: (0608) 51217
Telex: 477719

International Consultants Assoc.
199 N. El Camino Real #F–318
Encinitas, CA 92024, USA
Attn: Hans G. Schroeder
Ph: (619) 753–0790

Interpharm International Ltd.
P. O. Box 530
Prairie View, IL 60069, USA
Attn: Michel H. Anisfeld
Ph: (312) 459–8480
Fax: (312) 459–4536
Telex: 499 5880 [INTPHRM]
[Associate offices in England,
  Israel, Italy and Japan]

Lachman Consultant Services
591 Stewart Avenue
Garden City, NY 11530, USA
Attn: Leon Lachman
Ph: (516) 222-6222

Magid-Haffner Associates
4400 Kerrybrooke Drive
Alexandria, VA 22310, USA
Attn: Ira Peine
Ph: (703) 971–3988

Pharmaceutical Education Group
P. O. Box 216
Saugus, CA 91350-0216, USA

Planning Masters
3343 William Drive
Newbury Park, CA 91320, USA
Attn: Chase Lichtenstein
Ph: (805) 499–7526

R&D Engineering Associates
22 Foxwood Drive
Somerset, NJ 08873, USA
Attn: Julius Z. Knapp
Ph: (201) 545–2002

Skyland Scientific Services
Gallatin Field, Box 34
Belgrade, MT 59714, USA
Ph: (406) 388–4051

Swift Technical Services Ltd.
7 Manor Close, Oadby
Leicester LE 2 4FE, ENGLAND
Ph: (0533) 712500

9. Disinfectants and Preservatives

Alcide, Inc.
One Willard Road
Norwalk, CT 06851, USA
Ph: (203) 847–2555
Telex: 510 1003 219

Alfa Products
152 Andover Street
Danvers, MA 01923, USA
Ph: (617) 777–1970

Lonza Inc.
22–10 Route 208
Fairlawn, NJ 07410, USA
Ph: (201) 794–2400

Mallinckrodt, Inc.
Box 5439
St. Louis, MO 63147, USA
Ph: (314) 895–2000

Spectrum Chemical Mfg Co.
14422 South San Pedro Street
Gardena, CA 90248, USA
Ph: (800) 543–0652

Sporicidin International
4000 Massachusetts Avenue NW
Washington, DC 20016, USA
Ph: (800) 424–3733
Telex: 904059

Vestal Laboratories, Inc.
5035 Manchester Ave.
St. Louis, MO 63110, USA
Ph: (800) 325–8690

10. Distillation Equipment

Aqua-Chem, Inc.
P. O. Box 421
Milwaukee, WI 53201, USA
Ph: (414) 961–2829
Telex: 26679 AQM MIL

Consolidated Stills/Sterilizers
76 Ashford Street, P. O. Box 297
Boston, MA 02134, USA
Ph: (617) 782–6072
Telex 951521

Finn-Aqua America, Inc.
11105 Main Street
Bellevue, WA 98004, USA
Ph: (206) 451–1900
Telex: 152218 Vaponics, Inc.

MECO
861 Carondelet St.
New Orleans, LA 70130, USA
Ph: (504) 523–7271
Telex: 58377

Pennwalt Corp.
Stokes Vacuum Components Dept.
5500 Tabor Road
Philadelphia, PA 19120, USA

Santasalo-Sohlberg Oy
Hankasuontie 4-6
SF-00390 Helsinki 39, FINLAND
Ph: (0) 25851
Telex: 125724

Stilmas S.p.a.
Viale delle Industrie
I-20090 Settala
Milano, ITALY

Vaponics, Inc.
Cordage Park
Plymouth, MA 02360, USA
Ph: (617) 746–7555
Telex: 921755 VAPONICS PLTH

11. Engineering and Construction

CRS Sirrine, Inc.
P. O. Box 5456
Greenville, SC 29606
Ph: (803) 281–8518

Daniel Engineering Services
Daniel Building
Greenville, SC 29602, USA
Ph: (803) 298–3262

Davy McKee Engineers
300 S. Riverside Plaza
Chicago, IL 60606, USA
Ph: (312) 902–1218
Telex: 254562

Kling Lindquist, Inc.
2301 Chestnut Street
Philadelphia, PA 19103, USA
Ph: (215) 665–9930
Telex: 244423 KLIN UR

12. Fermentation Equipment

Chemap AG
CH–8604 Volketswil,
SWITZERLAND
Ph: (01) 9472222
Telex: 58861 CHN CH

New Brunswick Scientific
44 Talmadge Road
P. O. Box 4005
Edison, NJ 08818–4005
Ph: (201) 287–1200

Chemap Inc.
230 Crossways Park Drive
Woodbury, NY 11787, USA
Ph: (201) 757–7000
Telex: 271308

13. Filling Machines

Adtech, Inc.
1170 Church Road
Lansdale, PA 19446, USA
Ph: (215) 368–7040
Telex: 988441

Perry Industries
1163 Glory Road
P. O. Box 19043
Green Bay, WI 54307–9043, USA
Ph: (414) 336–4343
            Telex: 6974420 Perryind

Bausch und Strobel
P. O. Box 20
D-7174 Ilshoven, WEST GERMANY
Ph: (07904) 701 256
Telex: 74894 BASMA D

TL Systems
5617 Corvallis Avenue North
Minneapolis, MN 35429, USA
Ph: (612) 535–51232

Cozzoli Machine Co.
401 East 3rd Street
Plainfield, NJ 07060, USA
Ph: (201) 757–2040
Telex: 178007

Vetter Pharma Fertigung
P. O. Box 2380
D-7980 Ravensburg, W GERMANY
Ph: (0751) 3700-0
Telex: 732964

14. Filter Aids

Cuno Inc.
400 Research Parkway
Meriden, CT 06450, USA
Ph: (800) 243–6894
Telex: 962457

Eagle-Picher Industries
580 A Walnut St.
Cincinnati, OH 45202, USA
Ph: (513) 721–7010

Filter Media Co.
3603 Westcenter Drive
Houston, TX 77042, USA
Ph: (713) 780–9000
Telex: 775144 FEMCO

Manville Corp.
Ken-Caryl Ranch
Denver, CO 80217, USA
Ph: (303) 979–1000
Telex: 454404

15. Flowmeters (Sanitary)

Foxboro Co.
120 Norfolk Street
Foxboro, MA 02035, USA
Ph: (617) 543–8750

Micro Motion Inc.
7070 Winchester Circle
Boulder, CO 80301, USA
Ph: (800) 522-6277

Leeds & Northrup
Sumneytown Park
North Wales, PA 19454, USA
Ph: (215) 643–2000

16. Freeze-Dryers (Sterilizable)

Edwards High Vacuum
Manor Royal, Crawley
West Sussex BH10 2LW, ENGLAND
Ph: (0293) 28844
Telex: 87123 EDIVAC G

Pennwalt (Stokes Division)
5500 Tabor Road
Philadelphia, PA 19120, USA
Ph: (215) 831–5400
Telex: 834 470

Hull Corp.
Davisville Road
Hatboro, PA 19040, USA
Ph: (215) 672–7800
TWX: 510–665–6822

Usifroid
Rue Claude Bernard
Z. A. de Coignieres-Maurepas
78310 Maurepas, FRANCE
Ph: (33–3) 051.21.27
Telex: USIF 696322 F

Leybold-Heraeus GmbH
Postfach 1555
D-6450 Hanau 1, WEST GERMANY
Ph: (06181) 34–0
Telex: 06181/34–1690

VirTis
Route 208
Gardiner, NY 12525, USA
Ph: (800) 431–8232
Telex: 926474

17. Microfiltration Equipment and Filters

Alsop Engineering Co.
Route 10
Milldale, CT 06467, USA
Ph: (203) 628–9661
Cable: Speedhy

Ametek, Plymouth Products Div
502 Indiana Avenue
Sheboygan, WI 53081, USA
Ph: (414) 457–9435
Telex: 910–264–3878

Ballston, Inc.
P. O. Box C
Lexington, MA 02173, USA
Ph: (617) 861–7240
Telex: 923481

Brunswick GmbH
Mergenthalerallee 45–47
D-6236 Eschborn,
WEST GERMANY
Ph: (06196) 427–0
Telex: 418334

Cox Instrument
see Ametek

Cumo Inc.
400 Research Parkway
Meriden, CT 06450, USA
Ph: (800 243–6894
Telex: 962457

Domnick Hunter Filters, Ltd
Durham Road D-3400
Birtley, County Durham DH3 2SF
    UNITED KINGDOM
Ph: (091) 4105121
Telex: 537282

Ertel Engineering
20 Front Street
Kingston, NY 12401, USA
Ph: (914) 331–4552

Filterite Corp.
4116 Sorrento Valley Blvd.
San Diego, CA 92121, USA
Ph: (800) 854–1571
TWX: (910) 335–1706

Filtrox Werk AG
CH-9001 St. Gallen
SWITZERLAND

FPI (Filter Products Inc.)
8314 Tiogawoods Drive
Sacramento, CA 95828, USA
Ph: (916) 689–2328

Fuji Filter Mfg Co. Ltd
Shiu-Muromachi Bldg. 4
Nihombahi-Huroshi 2-Chome
Cuo-Ku, Tokyo 103, JAPAN
Ph: (03) 241–4201
Telex: 02 22 60 93

Gelman Sciences
600 S. Wagner Road
Ann Arbor, MI 48106, USA
Ph: (800) 521–1520
TWX: (810) 223–6037

Ghia Corp.
see Gelman Sciences

Gusmer-Cellulo Co.
27 North Ave. East
Cranford, NJ 07016, USA
Telex: 96113
Telex: 13 91 06

Kurita Machinery, Mfg Co.
1-44 2-Chome, Sakaigawa,
Nishi-ku, Osaka 550, JAPAN
Ph: (06) 582–3001

Membrana (USA)
see Gelman Sciences

Millipore Corp.
Ashby Road
Bedford, MA 01730, USA
Ph: (800) 225–1380
Telex: 92 34 57

Nuclepore Corp.
2036 Commerce Circle
Pleasanton, CA 94566, USA
Ph: (415) 462-2230
Telex: 337751

Pall Corp.
30 Sea Cliff Ave.
Glen Cove, NY 11542, USA
Ph: (800) 645–6262

PTI (Purolator Technologies)
2323 Teller Road
Newbury Park, CA 91320, USA
Ph: (800) 235–3518
TWX 510–601–3161

Sartorius GmbH
Postfach 19
Gottingen, WEST GERMANY
Ph: (0551) 30 82 19
Telex: 96830

Sartorius Filters, Inc.
30940 San Clemente Street
Hayward, CA 94544
Ph: (800) 227–2842
Telex: 338534

Schenk Filterbau GmbH
Postfach 95
D-7070 Schwabisch Gmund
WEST GERMANY
Ph: (07171) 82091
Telex: 7248818

Schleicher u. Schull GmbH
Postfach
D-3354 Dassel, WEST GERMANY
Ph: (05564) 8995
Telex: 0965632

Seitz-Filter-Werke GmbH
Planiger Str. 137
D-6550 Bad Kreuznach,
WEST GERMANY
Ph: (0671) 66026

Sperry Filter Presses
112 North Grant Street
North Aurora, IL 60542, USA
Ph: (312) 892–4361
Telex: 720436

Star Systems
P. O. Box 518
Timmonsville, SC 29161, USA
Ph: (803) 346–3101
Cable: Starfilter

Toyo Roshi Kaisha
7, Nihonbacki Honcho 3-Chome
Chuo-Ku, Tokyo, JAPAN
Ph: (03) 270–7441

Whatman Ltd
Springfield Mill, Maidstone
Kent ME14 2LE, UNITED KINGDOM
Ph: (0622) 62692
Telex: 96113

18. Pumps (Sanitary)

Abex Corp.
Waukesha Foundry
5510 Lincoln Avenue
Waukesha, WI 53186, USA
Ph: (414) 542–0741
Telex: 269552

Alfa-Laval
Box 1008
S–221 03 Lund, SWEDEN
Ph: (046) 105000
Telex: 32145 ALLUND S

American Lewa
132 Hopping Brook Road
Holliston, MA 01746, USA
Ph: (617) 429–7403
Telex: 948420

The Ladish Co.
9201 Wilmot Road
Kenosha, WI 53141, USA
Ph: (414) 694–5511
Fax: 414–694–7104

Randolph Corp.
1112 Rosine Street
Houston, TX 77019, USA
Ph: (713) 461–3400
Telex: 762034

Warren Rupp-Houdaille Co.
P. O. Box 1568 TR
Mansfield, OH 44901, USA
Ph: (419) 524–8388
Telex: 987458

Wilden Pump & Engineering
22069 Van Buren Street
Colton, CA 92324, USA
Ph: (714) 783–0621

19. Sterile Tanks and Related Stainless Equipment

Bioengineering AG
Tannerstrasse 1
CH-8630 Rueti, SWITZERLAND
Ph: (055) 95 35 81
Telex: 875977

Cherry-Burrell
P. O. Box 1028
Little Falls, NY 13365
Ph: (315) 823-2000
FAX: 315-823-2666

Paul Mueller Co.
P. O. Box 828
Springfield, MO 65801, USA
Ph: (800) 641-2830

Pfaudler Co.
P. O. Box 1600
Rochester, NY 14692
Ph: (716) 235-1000

Stainless Metals, Inc.
43-49 10th Street
Long Island City, NY 11101
Ph: (718) 784-1454

Valex
6080 Leland Street
Ventura, CA 93003
Ph: (805) 658-0944
FAX: 805-658-1376

Walker Stainless Equipment
New Lisbon, WI 53950, USA
Ph: (608) 562-3151

20. Sterility Test Equipment

Gelman Sciences
600 Wagner Road
Ann Arbor, MI 48106, USA
Ph: (800) 521-1520
TWX: (810) 223-6037

MFS Division-Toyo Roshi
6800 Sierra Court
Dublin, CA 94566, USA
Ph: (415) 828-6010
Telex: 171348

Millipore Corp.
Ashby Road
Bedford, MA 01730, USA
Telex: 923457
Ph: (800) 225-1380

Sartorius GmbH
Postfach 19
D-3400 Gottingen, WEST GERMANY
Ph: (0551) 308219
Telex: 96830

Toyo Roshi Kaisha
7, Nihonbacki Honcho 3-Chome
Chuo-Ku, Tokyo, JAPAN
Ph: (03) 270-7441

21. Sterilizing and Drying Tunnels (Hot Air)

Calumatic BV
3 Steenstraat
NE-5107 Dongen, NETHERLANDS
Ph: (031) 1623 13454

H. Strunck Machinenfabrik
7 Postfach 301269
D-5000 Koln 30, WEST GERMANY

Hans Gilowy Maschinefabrik
"Meteorwerk" GmbH & Co.
Schmalenbachstrasse 12-16
D-1000 Berlin 44
Ph: (030) 6 84 60 71
Telex: 184910

22. Stoppering Machines

Adtech Inc.
1170 Church Road
Lansdale, PA 19446, USA
Ph: (215) 368–7040
Telex: 988441

Perry Industries
1163 Glory Road
P. O. Box 19043
Green Bay, WI 54307–9043, USA
Ph: (414) 336–4343

Calumatic BV
3 Steenstraat 7
NE-5107 Dongen, NETHERLANDS
Ph: (031) 1623 13454
TWX: 844 54316

TL Systems
5617 Corvallis Ave. North
Minneapolis, MN 55429–3594
Ph: (612) 535-5123

22. Vial and Bottle Washers

Bausch und Strobel
P. O. Box 20
D-7174 Ilshofen, WEST GERMANY
Ph: (07904) 701 256

Hans Gilowy Maschinefabrik
"Meteorwek" GmbH & Co.
Schmalenbachstrasse 12–16
D-1000 Berlin 44, WEST GERMANY
Ph: (030) 6846071
Telex: 184910

Calumatic BV
3 Steenstraat 7
NE-5107 Dongen, NETHERLANDS
Ph: (031) 1623 13454

Cozzoli Machine Co.
401 East 3rd Street
Plainfield, NJ 07060, USA
Ph: (201) 757–2040
Telex: 178007

Dawson Bros. MMP Ltd.
406 Roding Lane South
Woodford Green, Essex
UNITED KINGDOM

Schubert & Co.
Vallenbaksvej 24
DK-2600 Glostrup, DENMARK

H. Strunck Maschinenfabrik
Postfach 301269
D-5000 Koln 30, WEST GERMANY

☐ Appendix B

Figure B-1 — HP5898R Automated Gas Chromatograph for Microbial Identification

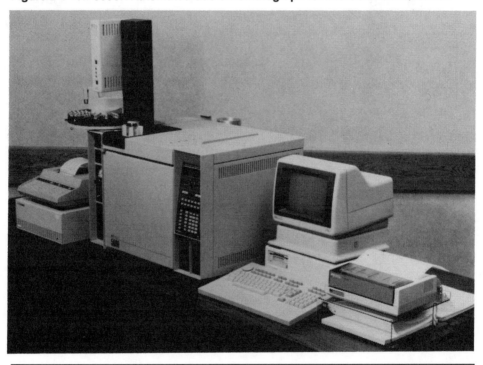

Figure B-2—Separation by GC of Fatty Acids

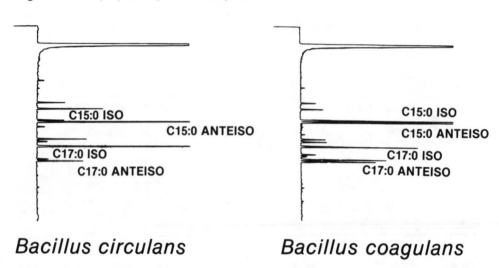

Bacillus circulans   *Bacillus coagulans*

Figure B-3—HP5898R Sample Print-out

HEWLETT-PACKARD HP 5898A Microbial Identification System

*** SAMPLE ***

File: FLOPPY:F85923372   Date of report: 19-OCT-85 03:51:13
Bottle: 23   Date of run: 23-SEP-85 15:57:21
ID: 74
Name: P. AERUGINOSA

RT	Area	Ar/Ht	Respon	ECL	Name	Area %	Comment 1	Comment 2
1.499	41771000	0.083	. . .	7.010	SOLVENT PEAK	. . .	< min rt	
1.784	541	0.015	. . .	7.572	. . . .	. . .	< min rt	
4.107	7809	0.035	0.991	11.420	10:0 30H	2.84	ECL deviates -0.003	
4.646	8499	0.036	0.982	12.001	12:0	3.07	ECL deviates 0.001	Reference 0.000
6.049	11194	0.038	0.971	13.174	12:0 20H	3.99	ECL deviates -0.004	
6.434	8476	0.039	0.969	13.453	12:0 30H	3.02	ECL deviates -0.002	
7.188	2871	0.039	0.967	13.999	14:0	1.02	ECL deviates -0.001	Reference -0.001
10.106	39325	0.045	0.971	15.817	16:1 CIS 9	14.03	ECL deviates 0.000	
10.168	14075	0.041	0.971	15.854	16:1 TRANS 9	5.02	ECL deviates -0.002	Sum In Feature 4
10.413	71812	0.044	0.973	16.001	16:0	25.66	ECL deviates 0.001	Reference 0.000
13.596	111420	0.052	0.999	17.823	18:1 CIS 11	40.89	ECL deviates 0.001	Sum In Feature 7
13.906	1216	0.046	1.003	17.999	18:0	0.45	ECL deviates -0.001	Reference -0.002
*******	14075	. .	. . .	. . .	SUMMED FEATURE 4 . .	5.02		
*******	111420	. .	. . .	. . .	SUMMED FEATURE 7 . .	40.89		

Solvent Ar	Total Area	Named Area	% Named	Total Amnt	Nbr Ref	Ref ECL Shift	ECL Deviation
41771000	276697	276697	100.00	272135	4	0.001	0.002

MOST LIKELY MATCHES   SIMILARITY

Pseudomonas 0.874
  P. aeruginosa 0.874

☐ Index

HTLV-I, 355
HTLV-III, 355
Human chorionic gonadotropin, 126
Human immunodeficiency virus, 355
Human serum albumin, 326
Hydrophobic attraction, 85
Hydrogen peroxide, 31, 187, 321
Hydrophobic interactions, 64
Hypochlorite, 329

Immersion test, 187.
Immune serum globulins, 357
Impendance, 340
Inactivation, thermal, 3
Incompatibilities, physical/chemical, 381
Influenza, 358
Injunctions, 376
Inorganic oxides, 17
Inspections, 375
Insulin zinc, 328
Integrity testing, 382
Interactions, chemical, 9
Intermittent positive pressure, 326
Intramuscular injection, 1
Iodophor sanitizers, 262
Iodophores, 7
Ion exchange, 19, 20, 88
Ionic interactions, 63
Ionizing radiation, 43, 93, 101
Irradiation sterilization, 40, 68
Irradiation, gamma, 41, 101
Isoelectric point, 116
Isolation technology, 219
Isopropyl myristate, 324
IV Pumps, 10

Kefauver-Harris amendments, 374
Kinetics, 4
Klebsiella-Enterobacter, 9

LAL, 207-209
LAL Sepharose, 88
Laminar flow, 7, 35, 44-46
Large volume parenterals, 7, 8, 14
Latent heat of vaporization, 38, 39
Leaching and dissolution of glass, 22
Leaching, 14, 19, 20, 25, 26
Limulus amebocyte lysate (LAL) test, 75, 137
Limulus challenge, 209

Linear accelerators, 41
Lipid A, biological activity, 79
Lipid emulsions, 9
Lipids, 120
Lipopolysaccharide (LPS), 76
Lipoproteins, 120
Liposomes, 115
Liquid impinger, 343
Luciferase, 336, 337, 340
Luciferin, 336, 337
Lyophilization, 235, 239

Mandrel, 205
Mandrel, blow/fill, 213
Manhole openings, 256
Mannitol, 6
Matrix solubilization, 137
Measles, 358
Media fills, 152, 154, 383
Media migration, 140
Media selection, 386
Membrane filter, analytical, 333
Membrane method, 320
Mesothelioma, 109
Microbial aerobiology test, 188
Microbial analysis monitor, 335
Microbial bioburden, 330
Microbial death rate, 4
Microbial growth inhibitors, 321
Microbial immersion test, 186
Microbial retention test, 131
Microbiological assessment of air, 341
Microfiberglass filters, 108
Microfiltration equipment and filters, 412
Microfiltration, 101
Microorganism sterilization, 41
Microorganisms, 38
Microorganisms, identification, 345
Microwave heating, 52
Minibag, 6
Mitomycin, 6
Moist heat, 90
Monomers, 23
Morphine, 1
Motile organisms, 335
Multi-tank, 250, 252
Mumps viruses, 358
Mycoplasmas, 130

NASA, 372, 394
NDA, 367